Early Diagnosis and Treatment of Cancer: Ovarian Cancer

Early Diagnosis and Treatment of Cancer

Series Editor: Stephen C. Yang, MD

Breast Cancer
Edited by Lisa Jacobs and Christina A. Finlayson

Colorectal Cancer
Edited by Susan Lyn Gearhart and Nita Ahuja

Head and Neck Cancer
Edited by Wayne M. Koch

Ovarian Cancer
Edited by Robert E. Bristow and
Deborah K. Armstrong

Prostate Cancer
Edited by Li-Ming Su

EARLY DIAGNOSIS AND TREATMENT OF CANCER

Series Editor: Stephen C. Yang, MD

Ovarian Cancer

Edited by

Robert E. Bristow, MD

Professor and Director
The Kelly Gynecologic Oncology Service and Ovarian Cancer Center of Excellence
Department of Gynecology and Obstetrics
The Johns Hopkins Medical Institutions
Baltimore, Maryland

Deborah K. Armstrong, MD

Associate Professor of Oncology, Gynecology, and Obstetrics
The Sidney Kimmel Comprehensive Cancer Center
The Johns Hopkins Medical Institutions
Baltimore, Maryland

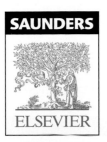

SAUNDERS

ELSEVIER

SAUNDERS
ELSEVIER

1600 John F. Kennedy Blvd.
Ste 1800
Philadelphia, PA 19103-2899

EARLY DIAGNOSIS AND TREATMENT OF CANCER: ISBN-13: 978-1-4160-4685-1
OVARIAN CANCER

Notices

Knowledge and best practice in this field are constantly changing. As new research and experience
broaden our understanding, changes in research methods, professional practices, or medical
treatment may become necessary.

  Practitioners and researchers must always rely on their own experience and knowledge in
evaluating and using any information, methods, compounds, or experiments described herein.
In using such information or methods they should be mindful of their own safety and the safety
of others, including parties for whom they have a professional responsibility.

  With respect to any drug or pharmaceutical products identified, readers are advised to check
the most current information provided (i) on procedures featured or (ii) by the manufacturer of
each product to be administered, to verify the recommended dose or formula, the method and
duration of administration, and contraindications. It is the responsibility of practitioners, relying on
their own experience and knowledge of their patients, to make diagnoses, to determine dosages and
the best treatment for each individual patient, and to take all appropriate safety precautions.

  To the fullest extent of the law, neither the Publisher nor the authors, contributors, or editors,
assume any liability for any injury and/or damage to persons or property as a matter of products
liability, negligence or otherwise, or from any use or operation of any methods, products,
instructions, or ideas contained in the material herein.

Library of Congress Cataloging-in-Publication Data

Ovarian cancer / edited by Robert E. Bristow, Deborah K. Armstrong.
    p. ; cm.—(Early diagnosis and treatment of cancer)
    Includes bibliographical references.
    ISBN 978-1-4160-4685-1
    1. Ovaries—Cancer. I. Bristow, Robert E. II. Armstrong, Deborah K. III. Series: Early diagnosis
and treatment of cancer series.
    [DNLM: 1. Ovarian Neoplasms—diagnosis. 2. Early Diagnosis. 3. Ovarian Neoplasms—therapy.
WP 322 O9633 2010]
    RC280.O8O8833   2010
    616.99'465—dc22

                                                           2009032162

Acquisitions Editor: Dolores Meloni
Design Direction: Steven Stave

Printed in China.

Last digit is the print number: 9 8 7 6 5 4 3 2 1

Contents

Series Preface

Seen on a graph, the survival rate for many cancers resembles a precipice. Discovered at an early stage, most cancers are quickly treatable, and the prognosis is excellent. In late stages, however, the typical treatment protocol becomes longer, more intense, and more harrowing for the patient, and the survival rate declines steeply. No wonder, then, that one of the most important means in fighting cancer is to prevent or screen for earlier stage tumors.

Within each oncologic specialty, there is a strong push to identify new, more useful tools for early diagnosis and treatment, with an emphasis on methods amenable to an office-based or clinical setting. These efforts have brought impressive results. Advances in imaging technology, as well as the development of sophisticated molecular and biochemical tools, have led to effective, minimally invasive approaches to cancer in its early stages.

This series, *Early Diagnosis and Treatment of Cancer*, gathers state-of-the-art research and recommendations into compact, easy-to-use volumes. For each particular type of cancer, the books cover the full range of diagnostic and treatment procedures, including pathologic, radiologic, chemotherapeutic, and surgical methods, focusing on questions like these:

- What do practitioners need to know about the epidemiology of the disease and its risk factors?
- How do patients and their families wade through and interpret the many tests they face?
- What is the safest, quickest, least invasive way to reach an accurate diagnosis?
- How can the stage of the disease be determined?
- What are the best initial treatments for early-stage disease, and how should the practitioner and the patient choose among them?
- What lifestyle factors might affect the outcome of treatment?

Each volume in the series is edited by an authority within the subfield, and the contributors have been chosen for their practical skills as well as their research credentials. Key Points at the beginning of each chapter help the reader grasp the main ideas at once. Frequent illustrations make the techniques vivid and easy to visualize. Boxes and tables summarize recommended strategies, protocols, indications and contraindications, important statistics, and other essential information. Overall, the attempt is to make expert advice as accessible as possible to a wide variety of health care professionals.

For the first time since the inception of the National Cancer Institute's annual status reports, the 2008 "Annual Report to the Nation on the Status of Cancer," published in the December 3 issue of the *Journal of the National Cancer Institute*, noted a statistically significant decline in "both incidence and death rates from all cancers combined." This mark of progress encourages all of us to press forward with our efforts. I hope that the volumes in *Early Diagnosis and Treatment of Cancer* will make health care professionals and patients more familiar with the latest developments in the field, as well as more confident in applying them, so that early detection and swift, effective treatment become a reality for all our patients.

Stephen C. Yang, MD
The Arthur B. and Patricia B. Modell
Professor of Thoracic Surgery
Chief of Thoracic Surgery
The Johns Hopkins Medical Institutions
Baltimore, Maryland

Preface

Worldwide, 204,449 new cases of ovarian cancer are diagnosed each year, with an estimated 124,860 disease-related deaths.[1] In the United States, ovarian cancer is the leading cause of gynecologic cancer–related morbidity and mortality in large part due to the difficulty in detecting early-stage disease. One of the primary reasons that ovarian cancer is associated with such a significant burden of disease for the individual and for society is that it is a difficult disease to prevent, or at the very least diagnose in the early stages, when cure is still an attainable goal for the majority of patients. This volume discusses the full range of diagnostic and therapeutic considerations, including epidemiologic, pathologic, radiologic, surgical, and chemotherapeutic aspects. The volume is intended as a practical guide and overview to the diagnosis, staging, and management of patients with both early-stage and advanced-stage ovarian cancer.

Despite recent advances, the pathogenesis of ovarian cancer is still unclear, and one of the difficulties in studying ovarian cancer is the lack of a comprehensive tumor progression model. Ovarian cancer is a heterogeneous collection of tumors, which are primarily classified by cell type into serous, mucinous, endometrioid, clear cell, and Brenner (transitional) tumors corresponding to different types of epithelia in the organs of the female reproductive tract.[2-4] The tumors in each of the categories are further subdivided into three groups—benign, malignant, and intermediate (border-line tumor, or low-malignant-potential)—based on their clinical behavior. On the basis of a review of recent clinical, histopathologic, and molecular genetic findings, a research team has proposed a new carcinogenesis model that reconciles the relationship of borderline tumors to invasive carcinoma, discussed in Chapter 2.

The epidemiology of ovarian cancer has been extensively studied, and the most clinically relevant observations are presented in this volume. It is known that the incidence of ovarian cancer increases with age. Epithelial ovarian cancer is predominantly a disease of perimenopausal and postmenopausal women, with 80% of ovarian cancers occurring after the age of 40. There are a number of demographic characteristics and factors related to reproductive history and health, including the so-called "incessant ovulation" theory and the associated effect of oral contraceptive use on reduction in risk, parity as a risk factor, and the interaction with infertility. Several environmental risk factors for ovarian cancer have also been targeted as potential contributors to pathogenesis. Perhaps the most significant known risk factor for ovarian cancer is a family history of the disease (or breast cancer) and the likelihood of a genetic predisposition. Approximately 10% of all ovarian cancers can be associated with a familial genetic predisposition. At present, the majority of hereditary ovarian cancers can be linked to two currently known syndromes, hereditary breast and ovarian cancer (HBOC) and hereditary nonpolyposis colorectal cancer (HNPCC).[5,6] HBOC syndrome is associated primarily with an increased risk for breast cancer, while HNPCC is associated with an increased risk for colorectal cancer. The most up-to-date information on ovarian cancer family syndromes is presented in Chapter 3. In addition, the indications and options for genetic testing of women at risk for ovarian cancer are also covered in detail.

At the current time, there have been no studies that demonstrate sufficient efficacy for ovarian cancer screening in the general population. Therefore, ovarian cancer screening is not recommended for women at general population risk. However, the urgency of ovarian cancer screening is greater for women with *BRCA1* and *BRCA2* mutations, given the significantly increased risk of ovarian cancer among these women. In Chapter 6, the basic principles of cancer screening, the challenges associated with ovarian cancer screening, and studies of screening strategies in high- and low-risk populations are reviewed. Because of the challenges of early detection of disease and the fact that genetic testing and screening will identify only a minority of patients who will ultimately develop ovarian cancer, chemical or surgical ovarian cancer prophylaxis may be considered for selected women. The various options for ovarian cancer prevention are reviewed in Chapter 4.

Radiographic imaging is an integral part of ovarian cancer detection, diagnosis, management, and treatment follow-up. A number of imaging modalities are available, and a variety of new techniques, especially molecular imaging approaches, are being developed. Each imaging modality has its unique advantages and limitations; therefore, evidence-based use of imaging is essential for achieving the greatest possible benefit without over- or underuse of specific modalities. New developments in radiographic imaging of ovarian cancer and the associated clinical applications are covered in Chapter 5.

Surgery is a cornerstone of the diagnosis and treatment of ovarian carcinoma. The surgical goals differ based on the nature and stage of disease. For patients with apparent early-stage disease, the primary surgical objective is to obtain sufficient pathologic documentation of the true extent of disease through a rigorous staging procedure. Accurate staging information allows low-risk patients to safely defer adjuvant chemotherapy and identifies patients at high risk of recurrence as those who will benefit from systemic treatment following surgery. Unfortunately, approximately 65% of patients will be diagnosed with International Federation of Gynecology and Obstetrics (FIGO) Stage III (T3N0/1M0) or IV (any T, any N, M1) disease.[7] For this group, the most important clinician-driven prognostic factors are the extent of residual disease following primary cytoreductive surgery and the administration of adjuvant platinum-based chemotherapy.[8,9] The most critical considerations for surgical intervention and selection of a chemotherapy treatment regimen for patients with both early-stage and advanced-stage ovarian cancer are reviewed in Chapters 7 and 8.

This volume is intended for all clinicians caring for women with ovarian cancer, including attending surgeons and physicians, fellows, and residents in the disciplines of gynecologic oncology, medical oncology, and primary care. Ultimately, the optimal management of ovarian cancer is dependent on multiple factors, including demographic prognostic factors, the age and general medical condition of the patient, the extent of disease at the time of detection, the biologic aggressiveness of disease, and available access to an appropriately skilled multidisciplinary care team. We hope that you enjoy this volume and benefit from the extensive experience of the elite team of contributors who have authored its contents.

References

1. IARC. GLOBOCAN 2002. Cancer incidence, mortality and prevalence worldwide (2002 estimates). 2006 accessed (http://www-dep.iarc.fr/).
2. Seidman JD, Russell P, Kurman RJ: Surface epithelial tumors of the ovary. In Kurman RJ (ed): Blaustein's Pathology of the Female Genital Tract, 5th ed. New York: Springer Verlag, 2002, p 791.
3. Scully RE: International Histological Classification of Tumuors: Histological Typing of Ovarian Tumuors. Geneva: World Health Organization, 1999.

4. Scully RE: World Health Organization International Histological Classification of Tumours. New York: Springer, 1999.
5. Reedy M, Gallion H, Fowler JM, et al: Contribution of BRCA1 and BRCA2 to familial ovarian cancer: a gynecologic oncology group study. Gynecol Oncol 85:255–259, 2002.
6. Pal T, Permuth-Wey J, Betts JA, et al: BRCA1 and BRCA2 mutations account for a large proportion of ovarian carcinoma cases. Cancer 104:2807–2816, 2005.
7. Pecorelli S, Creasman WT, Petterson F, et al: FIGO annual report on the results of treatment in gynaecological cancer. J Epid Biostat 3:75–102, 1998.
8. Hunter RW, Alexander ND, Soutter WP: Meta-analysis of surgery in advanced ovarian carcinoma: is maximum cytoreductive surgery an independent determinant of prognosis? Am J Obstet Gynecol 166:504–511, 1992.
9. Bristow RE, Tomacruz RS, Armstrong DK, et al: Survival effect of maximal cytoreductive surgery for advanced ovarian carcinoma during the platinum era: a meta-analysis. J Clin Oncol 20:1248–1259, 2002.

Robert E. Bristow, MD
Deborah K. Armstrong, MD

Contributors

Deborah K. Armstrong, M.D.
Associate Professor of Oncology, Gynecology, and
Obstetrics, The Sidney Kimmel Comprehensive Cancer
Center, The Johns Hopkins Medical Institutions,
Baltimore, Maryland

Jennifer E. Axilbund, M.S.
Research Associate, The Johns Hopkins University;
Genetic Counselor, The Johns Hopkins Hospital,
Baltimore, Maryland

Jeffrey G. Bell, M.D.
Clinical Professor, Ohio State University; Medical
Director, Cancer Services, Riverside Methodist Hospital,
Columbus, Ohio

Robert E. Bristow, M.D.
Professor and Director, The Kelly Gynecologic Oncology
Service and Ovarian Cancer Center of Excellence,
Department of Gynecology and Obstetrics, The Johns
Hopkins Medical Institutions, Baltimore, Maryland

Dennis S. Chi, M.D.
Associate Professor, Weill Medical College of Cornell
University; Associate Attending Surgeon, Memorial
Sloan-Kettering Cancer Center, New York, New York

Teresa Diaz-Montes, M.D.
Assistant Professor, Department of Gynecology and
Obstetrics, The Johns Hopkins Medical Institutions,
Baltimore, Maryland

Ram Eitan, M.D.
Attending Physician, Gynecologic Oncology Division,
The Helen Schneider Hospital for Women,
Rabin Medical Center, Petah Tikva; Sackler School of
Medicine, Tel Aviv University, Tel Aviv, Israel

J. Stuart Ferriss, M.D.
Fellow in Gynecologic Oncology, Obstetrics and
Gynecology, University of Virginia; Fellow Physician,
Obstetrics and Gynecology, University of Virginia Health
System, Charlottesville, Virginia

Robert L. Giuntoli II, M.D.
Assistant Professor, Department of Gynecology and
Obstetrics, The Johns Hopkins Medical Institutions,
Baltimore, Maryland

Amy L. Gross, M.H.S.
Johns Hopkins Bloomberg School of Public Health,
Baltimore, Maryland

Hedvig Hricak, M.D., Ph.D., Dr. HC
Professor of Radiology, Weill Medical College of
Cornell University; Chair, Department of Radiology,
Memorial Sloan-Kettering Cancer Center, New York,
New York

Namita Jhamb, M.D.
Clinical Fellow, Sylvester Comprehensive Cancer Center,
Miami, Florida

N. Jinawath, M.D., Ph.D.
Lecturer, Research Center, Faculty of Medicine,
Ramathibodi Hospital, Mahidol University, Bangkok,
Thailand; Clinical Cytogenetics Fellow, McKusick-Nathan
Institute of Genetic Medicine, The Johns Hopkins
Medical Institutions, Baltimore, Maryland

Amer K. Karam, M.D.
Fellow, Gynecologic Oncology, UCLA/Cedars-Sinai
Medical Center, Los Angeles, California

Beth Y. Karlan, M.D.
Professor and Director, Division of Gynecologic Oncology,
Department of Obstetrics and Gynecology, Cedars-Sinai
Medical Center; Professor of Obstetrics and Gynecology,
Geffen School of Medicine at UCLA, Los Angeles,
California

Elizabeth R. Keeler, M.D.
Assistant Professor, Department of Gynecologic Oncology,
University of Texas M.D. Anderson Cancer Center,
Houston, Texas

Erin R. King, M.D., M.P.H.
Department of Obstetrics and Gynecology, University of
Virginia, Charlottesville, Virginia

Nicholas C. Lambrou, M.D.
Former Associate Professor, Division of Gynecologic
Oncology, University of Miami; Gynecologic Oncologist,
Baptist Health South Florida, Miami, Florida

Karen H. Lu, M.D.
Associate Professor, Department of Gynecologic
Oncology, The University of Texas M.D. Anderson Cancer
Center, Houston, Texas

Christopher V. Lutman, M.D.
Riverside Methodist Hospital, Columbus, Ohio

Maurie Markman, M.D.
The University of Texas M.D. Anderson Cancer Center,
Houston, Texas

Susan C. Modesitt, M.D.
Associate Professor and Director, Gynecologic Oncology
Division, University of Virginia Health System,
Charlottesville, Virginia

Le-Ming Shih, M.D., Ph.D.
Professor of Pathology, Oncology, and Gynecology, The
Johns Hopkins University School of Medicine; Attending
Physician, Department of Pathology, The Johns Hopkins
Hospital, Baltimore, Maryland

Kala Visvanathan, M.B.B.S., M.H.S.
Assistant Professor of Epidemiology and Oncology, The
Johns Hopkins Medical Institutions, Baltimore, Maryland

Christine Walsh, M.D.
Attending Physician, Division of Gynecologic Oncology,
Department of Obstetrics and Gynecology, Cedars-Sinai
Medical Center, Los Angeles, California

Jingbo Zhang, M.D.
Assistant Professor of Radiology, Weill Cornell Medical
College; Memorial Sloan-Kettering Cancer Center,
New York, New York

1

Epidemiology and Clinical Presentation of Ovarian Cancer

Namita Jhamb and Nicholas C. Lambrou

KEY POINTS

- Ovarian cancer is the leading cause of death from all gynecologic cancers in the United States.
- Median age of diagnosis is 63 years. Survival is related to race, age, and stage at diagnosis.
- Risk factors for ovarian cancer can be categorized as genetic, environmental, and reproductive.
- Nulliparity and infertility have been associated with an increased risk of ovarian cancer, whereas oral contraceptive use has a strong protective association.
- Family history is the most significant known risk factor. Hereditary breast-ovarian cancer syndrome and hereditary nonpolyposis colorectal cancer syndrome are the two clinically distinct syndromes associated with ovarian cancer.
- Environmental factors such as diet, obesity, and endometriosis have been associated with increased risk of ovarian cancer.
- The most common presenting symptoms include abdominal distention and bloating. Palpable pelvic mass is a common presenting sign.
- Serous papillary histology is the most common subtype of ovarian cancer, whereas mucinous and endometrioid histologies have been associated with improved prognosis in comparison.
- Optimal cytoreduction defined by residual disease less than 1 cm is associated with improved survival.
- CA-125 is well established for assessment of tumor response and detection of recurrent disease.

Introduction

Ovarian cancer is the leading cause of mortality from gynecologic cancers in the United States. In 2009, an estimated 21,550 women will be diagnosed with ovarian cancer and 14,600 will die of the disease.[1] It is the fifth most common cancer in women in the United States, and the fourth most common cause of death from malignancy[2] (Fig. 1-1). In the United States, an estimated 1 in 72 women will develop ovarian cancer in their lifetime (Table 1-1), and 1 in 100 will die from the disease.

Epidemiology

The incidence of ovarian cancer increases with age. Epithelial ovarian cancer is predominantly a disease of perimenopausal and postmenopausal women, with 80% of ovarian cancers occurring after age 40. Based on the cancer registry data collected by the Surveillance, Epidemiology and End Results (SEER) program of the National Cancer Institute, the median age at diagnosis for cancer of the ovary is 63 years. Age-specific incidence analysis reveals the following percentages of age at diagnosis of ovarian cancer:

1.2%—20 years
3.5%—20 to 34 years
8.1%—35 to 44 years
18.6%—45 to 54 years

21.4%—55 to 64 years
20.8%—65 to 74 years
19.4%—75 to 84 years
7.0%—≥85 years

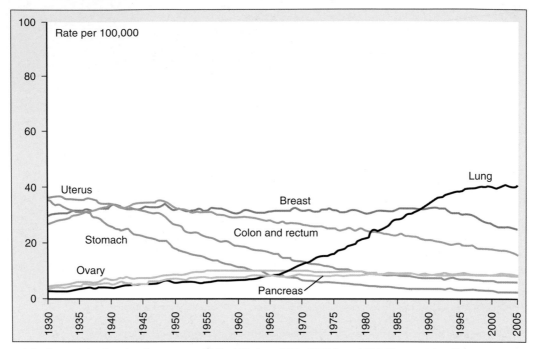

Figure 1-1. Cancer death rates for women, United States, 1930–2005 (per 100,000 women). Rates are age-adjusted to the 2000 U.S. standard population. (From US Mortality Public Use Data Tapes, 1960–2005, US Mortality Volumes, 1930–1959, National Center for Health Statistics, Centers for Disease Control and Prevention, 2008. American Cancer Society, *Cancer Facts & Figures 2009*. Atlanta: American Cancer Society, Inc., 2009.)

Table 1-1. Lifetime Probability of Developing Cancer by Site in Women, United States, 2002–2004*	
Site	**Risk**
All sites[†]	1 in 3
Breast	1 in 8
Lung and bronchus	1 in 16
Colon and rectum	1 in 20
Uterine corpus	1 in 40
Non-Hodgkin lymphoma	1 in 53
Melanoma[§]	1 in 58
Ovary	1 in 72
Pancreas	1 in 75
Urinary bladder[‡]	1 in 84
Uterine cervix	1 in 145

*For those free of cancer at beginning of age interval.
[†]All sites exclude basal and squamous cell skin cancers and in situ cancers except urinary bladder.
[‡]Includes invasive and in situ cancer cases.
[§]Statistic for white women.
From DevCan: Probability of Developing or Dying of Cancer Software, Version 6.2 Statistical Research and Applications Branch, NCI, 2007, http://srab.cancer.gov/devcan. Copyright 2009 American Cancer Society, Inc. Reprinted with permission. All rights reserved.

Table 1-2. Incidence Rates by Race	
Race/Ethnicity	Incidence
All races	13.3 per 100,000 women
White	14.1 per 100,000 women
Black	10.1 per 100,000 women
Asian/Pacific Islander	9.8 per 100,000 women
American Indian/Alaska native	11.3 por 100,000 women
Hispanic	11.7 per 100,000 women

Data from Ries LAG, Harkins D, Krapcho M, et al: (eds): SEER Cancer Statistics Review, 1975–2005, National Cancer Institute. Bethesda, MD. http://seer.cancer.gov/csr/1975_2005/, based on November 2007 SEER data submission, posted to the SEER web site 2008. http://www.seer.cancer.gov/

Women with ovarian cancer and age younger than 50 have a 5-year survival rate of 70.5% compared with 40.6% in those 50 or older.[3] Survival is related to stage at diagnosis. In recent studies of the Gynecologic Oncology Group (GOG), the progression-free survival after platinum-paclitaxel chemotherapy following optimal cytoreduction was 21 to 22 months, and the median overall survival was 52 to 57 months.[4,5]

The average incidence of ovarian cancer in African-American women is 10.1 per 100,000 women compared with 14.5 per 100, 000 white women.[1] However African-American women have poorer survival rates compared with whites regardless of socioeconomic status.[6] A review of cases of epithelial ovarian cancer submitted to the National Cancer Database between 1985 and 1988 and between 1990 and 1993 revealed that African-American women were two times more likely than white women not to receive appropriate treatment. They had poorer survival rates than white women from the same or different hospitals, regardless of income. Among staged cases, African-American women were more often diagnosed with stage IV disease than were white women. The incidence rates by race are shown in Table 1-2. The majority of ovarian cancers are sporadic. The overall risk of developing ovarian cancer for women in the United States is 1.0% to 1.8%. For women with family history of ovarian cancer, the risk increases to 9.4%.[7]

Risk Factors

The epidemiology of ovarian cancer is multifactorial, with genetic, environmental, and reproductive factors directly or indirectly related to carcinogenesis.

Reproductive Factors

Incessant ovulation has been proposed as one of the primary causes of epithelial ovarian cancer. The ovarian epithelial cells proliferate after ovulation, which may propagate mutations or promote carcinogenesis.[8] Ovulation itself has been implicated in malignant transformation of the epithelium. Various epidemiologic studies have attempted to estimate women's total duration of ovulatory life based on reproductive and contraceptive histories. Purdie and associates[9] considered the effects of age-specific ovulation on ovarian cancer risk and found the highest risk for ovulations in the 20- to 29-year age group (odds ratio [OR] = 1.20 for each ovulatory year in this age group). For age groups 30 to 39 and 40 to 49 years, the odds ratios were 1.06

and 1.04, respectively. Therefore, suppression of ovulation in the 20- to 29-year age group would provide maximal reduction in risk of developing ovarian cancer.

Nulliparity is a known risk factor for ovarian cancer. Women who have ever been pregnant have a 30% to 60% reduction in ovarian cancer risk compared with nulliparous women.[10] Ovarian cancer risk is inversely related to parity (OR = 0.59 for four or more pregnancies compared with nulliparous women).[11] No significant association between ovarian cancer risk and young age at menarche has been seen in recent studies. However late menopause may be associated with a trend toward higher risk for ovarian cancer risk.[11,12]

There is a strong protective association between oral contraceptives and ovarian cancer. The decline in incidence and mortality rates in ovarian cancer among younger women in the United States has been associated with increased oral contraceptive use. The overall estimated protection from cohort and case-control studies is approximately 40% in women who have ever used oral contraceptives and increases with duration of use to more than 50% for users of 5 years or longer. The favorable effect of oral contraceptives against ovarian cancer risk persists for at least 10 to 15 years after use has ceased, and it is not confined to any particular type of oral contraceptive formulation.[13] The risks in ever-users is appreciably lower in women who reported their first oral contraceptive use before 25 years of age (relative risk [RR] = 0.3 for first use before age 25, 0.8 for first use at age 25 to 34, and 0.7 at 35 years or after).[14] The Cancer and Steroid Hormone Study suggested that 10 years of oral contraceptive use by women with a family history of ovarian cancer appeared to reduce their risk to levels lower than those of women with no family history of ovarian cancer who never used oral contraceptives. Similarly, 5 years of oral contraceptives by nulliparous women was projected to reduce their risk to the levels seen for parous women who never use oral contraceptives.[15] Lactation has been associated with a slight additional reduction in risk of ovarian cancer.[16] Women who breastfeed only 1 to 2 months have a relative risk of ovarian cancer of 0.6 compared with that of women who never breastfed, with this effect being most prominent with the first exposure.[17]

Infertility alone is an independent risk factor for ovarian cancer. The possible link between fertility drugs and ovarian cancer remains controversial. Various studies have focused on the risk of ovarian cancer after use of fertility agents. A meta-analysis of eight case-control studies showed that neither longer duration of fertility drug use nor unsuccessful fertility drug use was independently associated with significant elevations in adjusted cancer risk. Women who did not achieve a pregnancy after prolonged use of infertility drugs had a higher risk of developing borderline serous tumors, but not invasive tumors.[18] No association between fertility drugs, ovulation-inducing agents, and clomiphene citrate and ovarian cancer has been observed when comparing parous with nulliparous women.[19]

Few studies have examined the association of ovarian cancer after in vitro fertilization (IVF). During in vitro fertilization, multiple folliculogenesis is achieved by intensive ovulation induction. Both ovulation induction and ovarian puncture have been associated in the past with ovarian cancer.[20] However, more recent studies show no excessive risk of ovarian cancer in patients after completion of IVF when compared with the general population.[21,22]

Data from earlier epidemiologic studies did not show a clear association between hormone replacement therapy and ovarian cancer.[23] However, more recent studies suggest an association between long duration of use of unopposed estrogen and ovarian cancer.[24-26] The Women's Health Initiative Randomized Trial provided additional support regarding the effects of estrogen and progesterone on risks of ovarian cancer. The hazard ratio (HR) for invasive ovarian cancer in women assigned to estrogen plus progestin compared with placebo was 1.58 (95% confidence interval [CI] =

0.77 to 3.24).[27] The National Institutes of Health–AARP Diet and Health Study Cohort included 97,638 women age 50 to 71 years. Use of unopposed estrogen for fewer than 10 years was not associated with ovarian cancer. Compared with no hormone therapy, use of unopposed estrogen for 10 or more years was statistically significantly associated with ovarian cancer among all women (RR = 1.89, 95% CI = 1.22 to 2.95; P = .004; 56 versus 72 ovarian cancers per 100,000 person-years, respectively) and, though not statistically significant, among women with hysterectomy (N = 19,359, RR = 1.70, 95% CI = 0.87 to 3.31; P = .06). Compared with women with intact uteri who never used hormone therapy, women who used estrogen and progestin had a statistically significant increased risk of ovarian cancer. (RR = 1.50, 95% CI = 1.03 to 2.19; P = .04). Risks of ovarian cancer were higher for women taking sequential (RR = 1.94, 95% CI = 1.17 to 3.22; P = .01) than continuous (RR = 1.41, 95% CI = .90 to 2.22; P = .14) regimens[28] (Table 1-3). Given the data, women who take hormone replacement therapy for more than 10 years should consider the potential increased risk for ovarian cancer when deciding to discontinue.

Genetic Factors

A family history of ovarian cancer is the most significant known risk factor. Approximately 10% of all ovarian cancers can be associated with a familial genetic predisposition. The risk depends on the number of first- and second-degree relatives with ovarian cancer and their age at diagnosis. A woman with a single family member affected by ovarian cancer has a 4% to 5% lifetime risk of developing the disease. This risk increases to about 7% if two family members are affected[3] (Table 1-4).

Approximately 7% of ovarian cancer patients have a positive family history of ovarian cancer, of whom 3% to 9% may eventually manifest certain hereditary cancer syndromes. Two clinically distinct syndromes are associated with hereditary ovarian cancer for which pedigree analysis suggests an autosomal dominant transmission with variable penetrance. Therefore, inheritance of these genetic mutations may occur from the maternal or paternal side. The hereditary breast-ovarian cancer syndrome (HBOC) is the more common of the two and is associated with germline mutations in *BRCA1* and *BRCA2* tumor suppressor genes. A lesser proportion is associated with the inherited form of endometrial and colorectal cancer known as hereditary non-polyposis colorectal cancer (HNPCC).

The *BRCA1* gene is located on the long (q) arm of chromosome 17 at position 21 (17q21), and the *BRCA2* gene is localized to the long arm of chromosome 13 (13q12). Both *BRCA1* and *BRCA2* gene mutations are associated with a predisposition to breast and ovarian cancer. These mutations are mainly of the frameshift or nonsense variety. *BRCA1* is a tumor suppressor gene that acts as a negative regulator of tumor growth. Following the recognition of DNA damage, *BRCA1* is activated, which then may be involved in the transcription-coupled repair of oxidative DNA damage. Activated *BRCA1* is also likely to function as a transcription factor in regulation of complex genetic program that responds to DNA damage. Without a functional *BRCA1* or *BRCA2* gene, repair fails, leading to activation of p53-dependent DNA damage. A clinically significant mutation in *BRCA1* confers a lifetime risk of ovarian cancer of 40% to 50% compared with 20% to 30% risk associated with a *BRCA2* mutation.[29] In women with a *BRCA1* or *BRCA2* mutation, the risk of ovarian and breast cancer may be as high as 54% and 82%, respectively.[30] Most ovarian cancers associated with germline *BRCA* mutations are diagnosed at a younger age and are high-grade, advanced-stage serous carcinomas. Mutation rates for these genes have been reported to be as high as 8% to 10% in the general population.[31,32]

Women of Ashkenazi Jewish descent have been found to have an increased risk of inheriting *BRCA* mutations. About 40% of ovarian cancers in this population are

Table 1-3. Associations between Unopposed Estrogen Therapy-Only Use and Ovarian Cancer among Women Enrolled in the National Institutes of Health–AARP Diet and Health Study Cohort*

Exposure	All Women (N = 97,638)				Women with Hysterectomy (N = 19,359)			
	No. of Cancers	Person-years	RR† (95% CI)	P Value‡	No. of Cancers	Person-years	RR§ (95% CI)	P Value‡
No HT use	87	176,376	1.00 (referent)		14	25,030	1.00 (referent)	
Only ET	49	71,815	1.33 (0.89–2.00)	.17	37	51,455	1.23 (0.67–2.27)	.43
Recency of use								
Former	14	23,539	1.15 (0.65–2.05)		6	10,355	1.03 (0.40–2.70)	
Current	34	47,284	1.46 (0.89–2.38)	.13	31	40,638	1.37 (0.72–2.62)	.32
Duration of use (yr)								
<10	23	43,458	1.15 (0.72–1.82)		11	25,971	0.84 (0.38–1.88)	
≥10	26	27,501	1.89 (1.22–2.95)	.004	26	24,990	1.70 (0.87–3.31)	.06
Recency and duration								
Former	14	23,539	1.16 (0.65–2.07)		6	10,355	1.07 (0.41–2.78)	
Current (yr)								
<10	10	22,497	1.00 (0.49–2.03)		7	17,481	0.83 (0.33–2.09)	
≥10	24	24,603	1.88 (1.08–3.27)	.06	24	22,994	1.71 (0.87–3.35)	.14

CI, confidence interval; ET, unopposed estrogen therapy; HT, hormone therapy; RR, relative risk.

*Among all women, recency of use was unknown for one woman who developed ovarian cancer and 992 person-years, duration of use was unknown for 857 person-years, and recency and duration were unknown for 1177 person-years. Among women with hysterectomy, recency of use was unknown for 462 person-years, duration of use was unknown for 494 person-years, and recency and duration were unknown for 625 person-years.

†Relative risks adjusted for continuous age (years), race (white, other/unknown), duration of oral contraceptive use (none, <10 years, ≥10 years, or unknown), body mass index (BMI) (<25, 25–29, ≥30 kg/m² or unknown), and menopause and hysterectomy (natural menopause, surgical menopause, premenopause, or unknown); models include terms for ever use of other HT formulations (ET followed by estrogen plus progestin, estrogen plus progestin only, progestin followed by estrogen plus progestin, ET and estrogen plus progestin but order unknown, other formulations, or unknown).

‡P values (two-sided) were calculated using Wald chi-square tests of categorical (ever-use) or ordinal (recency of use and recency and duration) variables based on the categories and referent group shown. The P value (two-sided) for duration of use was based on an ordinal variable for total years of use at baseline (none, 1, 2, 3,..., 9, 10, or >10).

§Relative risks adjusted for continuous age (years), race (white, other/unknown), duration of oral contraceptive use (none, <10 years, ≥10 years, or unknown), and BMI (<25, 25–29, ≥30 kg/m² or unknown).

From Lacey JV, Brinton LA, Leitzmann MF, et al: Menopausal hormone therapy and ovarian cancer risk in the National Institutes of Health-AARP Diet and Health Study Cohort. NCI J Natl Cancer Inst 98:1397–1405, 2006.

Table 1-4. Ovarian Cancer: Family History and Relative Risk (RR)

Relation	RR	Lifetime
One second degree	2.8	3.5%
One first degree	3.6	5%
Two relatives	5	7%
Two first degree		40%

From NIH Consensus Conference: Ovarian Cancer. Screening, treatment, and follow-up. NIH Consensus Development Panel on Ovarian Cancer. JAMA 273:491–497, 1995.

of hereditary nature. For these women, the risk of carrying a *BRCA* mutation is approximately 1 in 40. Three specific mutations have been carried by the Ashkenazi Jewish population: 185delAG and 5382insC on *BRCA1* and 6174delT on *BRCA2*. The increased risk is a result of what has been defined as "founder effect" (higher rate of mutations have occurred within a defined geographic area).[33] Hereditary nonpolyposis colorectal cancer (Lynch II syndrome) combines familial colon cancer with increased risk of ovarian and endometrial cancer, as well as other malignancies of the gastrointestinal and genitourinary system. It is caused by inherited mutations in DNA mismatch repair genes (MMR), *hMLI1* and *hMSH2* and to a lesser extent *hPMS1* and *hPMS2*. The risk of developing ovarian cancer has been reported to be 12%. With *MSH2* mutation, the risk is reported to be higher (10%) compared with *MLH1*, where the risk is about 3%.[34]

Environmental Factors

Additional variables have been associated with an increased risk of ovarian cancer. An example is saturated fat consumption (OR = 1.20 for each 10 g/day of intake; 95% CI = 1.03 to 1.40; $P = .008$).[35] Clinical and epidemiologic studies have conflicting views on an association between ovarian carcinoma and talcum powder use.[36,37] Coffee and tobacco consumption has not been found to be associated with an increased risk.[38] Obesity is a risk factor for several hormone-related cancers, but evidence of an effect on risk of epithelial ovarian cancer remains inconclusive. Some studies have shown a positive correlation between early adulthood obesity and ovarian cancer.[39] Alcohol consumption has not been associated with increased risk.[40,41] A history of pelvic inflammatory disease and endometriosis (endometrioid and clear cell histologies) has been associated with ovarian cancer.[42,43]

Clinical Presentation

Symptoms

The symptoms of ovarian cancer are vague and commonly occur in benign conditions. Patients with ovarian cancer often present late and are diagnosed at an advanced stage. In early-stage disease, patients may present with common gynecologic symptoms such as vaginal bleeding or discharge. Urinary frequency or constipation may be the result of compression of the bladder or rectum. Patients at all stages may present with abdominal pain and distention. Gastrointestinal symptoms such as nausea, anorexia, early satiety, and abdominal bloating are usually associated with advanced-stage disease and are related to ascites and peritoneal carcinomatosis[44] (Table 1-5). In a study by Olson and colleagues,[45] nearly all patients (93%) reported

Table 1-5. Symptoms Most Commonly Associated with Ovarian Cancer

	All Symptoms Reported (%)				First Symptom Reported (%)			
	Borderline (n = 146)	Invasive Stage I–II (n = 218)	Invasive Stage III–V (n = 447)	χ^2 test	Borderline (n = 146)	Invasive Stage I–II (n = 218)	Invasive Stage III–IV (n = 447)	χ^2 test
Gynecologic symptoms	15.5	15.4	9.5	P = .03	9.8	10.4	6.5	P = .1
Abdominal symptoms	80.5	78.2	78.1	P = .6	72.4	64.4	66.1	P = .3
Pain or pressure	43.9	46.0	42.6	P = .7	39.0	34.2	34.0	P = .6
Swelling or tightening	42.3	31.2	40.9	P = .04	23.6	18.3	25.4	P = .1
Mass	13.0	19.3	8.8	P = .0009	9.8	11.9	6.5	P = .07
Gastrointestinal symptoms	11.4	11.9	17.9	P = .03	6.5	7.9	10.7	P = .1
Urinary/bladder symptoms	4.9	11.4	5.6	P = .02	3.3	6.9	3.7	P = .1
General malaise	4.9	9.4	13.0	P = .008	4.1	5.9	6.3	P = .1
Other symptoms	5.7	7.4	9.8	P = .1	4.1	4.5	6.5	P = .1

From Webb PM, Purdie DM, Grover S, et al: Symptoms and diagnosis of borderline, early and advanced epithelial ovarian cancer. Gynecol Oncol 92(1):232–239, 2004.

at least one symptom. The most common symptoms are abdominal bloating, fullness, and pressure (71%). Other symptoms included abdominal or lower back pain (52%), lack of energy (43%), frequent urination, urgency or burning (33%), constipation (21%), decreased appetite (20%), and nausea (13%). If the disease has progressed to involve the lungs, as exemplified by the presence of pulmonary metastasis or malignant pleural effusions, the patient may present with complaints of shortness of breath.

Signs

The diagnosis of early-stage ovarian cancer usually occurs by palpation of an asymptomatic adnexal mass during routine pelvic examination.[2] In premenopausal women, the majority of these palpable pelvic masses are benign. Therefore, management of adnexal masses less than 8 cm in premenopausal women is generally to repeat the pelvic examination and imaging studies in 1 to 2 months. However, in postmenopausal women, a complex adnexal mass is more likely to be malignant, and surgical exploration is indicated.[3] A fixed, solid, irregular pelvic mass is suggestive of ovarian cancer, especially in the presence of ascites.

Prognostic Factors

Stage

The 5-year survival rate of patients with epithelial ovarian cancer correlates directly with the International Federation of Gynecology and Obstetrics (FIGO) surgical stage of disease. The stage can be determined only after exploratory laparotomy and thorough evaluation of all areas except in stage IV disease, which can be diagnosed by cytologically positive pleural fluid or CT-guided biopsy of parenchymal liver lesion. The technique of surgical staging involves making a vertical midline incision, obtaining peritoneal lavage or aspiration of ascites, intact tumor removal, complete abdominal exploration with biopsy of suspicious lesions, random peritoneal biopsies, and pelvic and para-aortic lymph node dissection. The FIGO staging system, revised in 1985, is presented in Box 1-1. Five-year survival rates for early-stage (presumptive stage I and II) disease have been reported as 50% to 90% and for late-stage disease (stages III and IV), 21%.[46] A review of 5156 patients in a study based on National Survey of Ovarian Cancer showed a 5-year survival rate of 89%, 58%, 24%, and 12% for stages I, II, III, and IV, respectively. When survival data for ovarian cancer were substratified further to substage division, the 5-year survival rates were 92% for stage IA, 85% for stage IB, 83% for stage IC, 67% for stage IIA, 56% for stage IIB, 51% for stage IIC, 39% for stage IIIA, 26% for stage IIIB, 17% for stage IIIC, and 12% for stage IV.[47] The 5-year survival rates based on the SEER cancer statistics review by the National Cancer Institute are 93.1% for localized disease, 69.0% for regional disease, 29.6% for distant disease, and 23.3% for unstaged disease[1] (Fig. 1-2).

Patient Characteristics

In a population-based analysis of patients with ovarian cancer between 1988 and 2001, age was identified as an independent prognostic factor with a survival advantage in younger women compared with older patients. Of 28,165 patients, 400 were under 30 years of age (very young), 11,601 were 30 to 60 (young), and 16,164 were over 60 (older). Of the very young, young, and older patients, 261 (65.3%), 4664 (40.2%), and 3643 (22.5%) had stage I-II disease, respectively ($P < .001$). Across all stages, very young women had a significant survival advantage over the young and

Box 1-1. Carcinoma of the Ovary (FIGO Staging)

Stage I   Growth limited to the ovaries
    IA Growth limited to one ovary; no ascites present containing malignant cells. No tumor on the external surface; capsule intact.
    IB Growth limited to both ovaries; no ascites present containing malignant cells. No tumor on the external surface; capsule intact.
    IC Tumor classified as either Stage IA or IB but with tumor on the surface of one or both ovaries; or with ruptured capsule(s); or with ascites containing malignant cells or with positive peritoneal washings.

Stage II   Growth involving one or both ovaries, with pelvic extension
    IIA Extension and/or metastases to the uterus and/or tubes.
    IIB Extension to other pelvic tissue.
    IIC Tumor classified as either Stage IIA or IIB but with tumor on the surface of one or both ovaries; or with capsule(s) ruptured; or with ascites containing malignant cells or with positive peritoneal washings.

Stage III   Tumor involving one or both ovaries with peritoneal implants outside the pelvis and/or positive retroperitoneal or inguinal nodes. Superficial liver metastasis equals Stage III. Tumor is limited to the true pelvis but with histologically proven malignant extension to small bowel or omentum.
    IIIA Tumor grossly limited to the true pelvis with negative nodes but with histologically confirmed microscopic seeding of abdominal peritoneal surfaces.
    IIIB Tumor of one or both ovaries with histologically confirmed implants of abdominal peritoneal surfaces, none exceeding 2 cm in diameter; nodes are negative.
    IIIC Abdominal implants greater than 2 cm in diameter and/or positive retroperitoneal or inguinal nodes.

Stage IV   Growth involving one or both ovaries, with distant metastases. If pleural effusion is present, there must be positive cytological findings to allot a case to Stage IV. Parenchymal liver metastasis equals Stage IV.

older groups, with 5-year disease-specific survival rate estimates at 78.8% versus 58.8% and 35.3%, respectively ($P < .001$). This survival difference among age groups persists even after adjusting for race, stage, grade, and surgical treatment. Reproductive-age (16 to 40 years) women with stage I-II epithelial ovarian cancer who received uterine-sparing procedures had similar survival rates compared with those who underwent standard surgery (93.3% versus 91.5%; $P = .26$).[48] In another national survey of ovarian carcinoma in patients less than 25 years of age, younger patients appeared to have favorable stage and histologic grade. These factors, combined with good performance status and optimal cytoreduction, resulted in improved survival from cancer.[49] Thigpen and associates[50] reviewed 2123 patients enrolled in six GOG trials and identified age, volume of residual disease, and performance status as the three major prognostic factors affecting outcome in patients with ovarian cancer. Age over 69 years exhibited poorer survival even after correcting for stage, residual disease, and performance status.

Histology and Grade

Patients with mucinous, endometrioid, and mesonephric ovarian cancers have the best prognosis, all with 5-year survival rates higher than 50%. On the other hand, the serous papillary and anaplastic variant cancers are associated with much worse prognoses, with 5-year survival rates of 34% and 29%, respectively.[51] Serous and mucinous tumors of low malignant potential have excellent survival rates. When comparing survival in patients with low malignant potential tumors of serous and mucinous variety with survival in women with invasive carcinoma, the overall relative

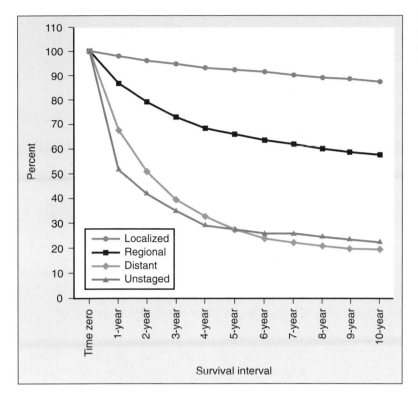

Figure 1-2. Survival rates for ovarian cancer by stage at diagnosis, all races, all ages. (From SEER 9 Registries for 1988–2002.)

survival rates at 10 years for low malignant potential-serous tumors are 98% compared with 31% for women with invasive serous cancers. For women with low malignant potential-mucinous tumors, the 10-year survival rate was 95% compared with 65% for women with mucinous carcinoma. For distant-stage disease, survival rates were between 86% and 90%.[52] Histologic grade of tumor is an important prognostic factor in early-stage disease. Patients with stage I disease with poorly differentiated tumors have worse survival and need adjuvant therapy compared with patients with well-differentiated tumors. The 5-year survival rates for women with early-stage ovarian cancer (I and II) are 90%, 80%, and 75% for grades 1, 2, and 3, respectively. For advanced ovarian cancer (stage III and IV), the reported 5-year survival rates are 57%, 31%, and 28%, respectively.[53]

Residual Disease after Cytoreductive Surgery

The volume of residual disease after cytoreductive surgery has been strongly associated with survival. Optimal cytoreduction is defined as residual disease of less than 1 cm. The GOG reported 37- and 31-month median survival times for patients with residual disease less than 1 cm and 1 to 2 cm, respectively. In an analysis of patients presenting with stage IV disease median survival of optimally cytoreduced patients was 38.4 months compared with 10.3 months for patients with suboptimal residual disease.[54] In a prospective study of 465 patients with stage IIIC ovarian cancer, Chi and colleagues[55] examined the significance of residual disease diameter on survival. Their analysis revealed that median overall survival in relation to the five residual disease categories was no gross residual—106 months; gross 0.5 cm or less—66 months; 0.6 to 1.0 cm—48 months; 1 to 2 cm—33 months; and more than 2 cm—34 months. Although the difference in survival did not reach statistical significance,

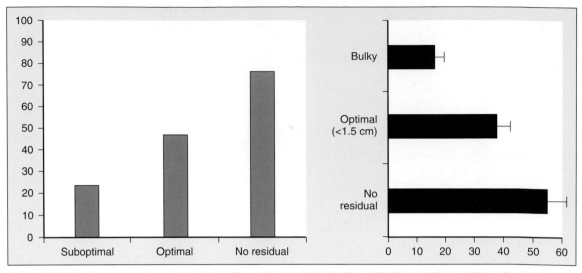

Figure 1-3. Ovarian cancer: tumor debulking. (From Hoskins WJ, McGuire WP, Brady MF, et al: The effect of diameter of largest residual disease on survival after primary cytoreductive surgery in patients with suboptimal residual epithelial ovarian carcinoma. Am J Obstet Gynecol 170(4):974–979, 1994; discussion 979–980.)

within the gross 1 cm or less residual group, there was a trend toward improved survival in patients with smaller-volume residual, that is, less than 0.5 cm compared with 0.6 to 1.0 cm ($P = .06$). In patients with suboptimal debulking, the difference in survival between those with less than 2 cm residual disease and those with more than 2 cm residual disease has been reported to be significant, although no difference in the risk of dying between groups was observed[56] (Fig. 1-3). A meta-analysis of 6885 patients with stage III or IV ovarian cancer showed a statistically significant positive correlation between percent maximal cytoreduction and median survival time after controlling for all other variables ($P < .001$). Each 10% increase in maximal cytoreduction was associated with a 5.5% increase in median survival time. Cohorts with less than 25% maximal cytoreduction had a median survival time of 22.7 months compared with 33.9 months for cohorts with more than 75% cytoreduction[57] (Table 1-6; see also Fig. 7-1).

CA-125

Serum levels of CA-125 loosely correlate with the volume of disease. Although there is controversy regarding the value of CA-125 before surgery as a predictor of survival, its role in assessment of treatment response is well established. Looking at the usefulness of the preoperative value of CA-125 in predicting optimal cytoreduction, it has been shown that preoperative CA-125 values of less than 500 U/mL had a positive predictive value for optimal cytoreduction of 82%, but a poor negative predictive value of 48%.[58] In another study, the sensitivity of this test in predicting optimal cytoreduction was 58%, and the specificity was 54%.[59] CA-125 levels have been shown to correlate with survival in patients receiving platinum-based chemotherapy. In a study of patients with suboptimally debulked stage III and IV ovarian cancer, the levels of this tumor marker 8 weeks after therapy was of significant prognostic value. The median survivals for patients with a CA-125 level of less than 35 U/mL compared with patients with a CA-125 level of more than 35 U/mL were 26 months and 15 months, respectively. Furthermore, women with serum CA-125 values less than 50% of their pretreatment concentration at 8 weeks experienced a median survival of 21 months compared with only 10 months for individuals with tumor marker levels above 50% of their baseline value.[60]

Table 1-6. Multiple Linear Regression Analysis				
	Change in Median Survival Time			
Variable	%	Increase	95% CI or CL	P
Percent maximal cytoreduction	5.5	10%	3.3–7.8	<.001
Year of publication	2.8	1 year	0.9–4.6	.004
Platinum dose-intensity	0.8	10%	–0.7, 2.3	.911
Cumulative platinum dose	1.4	1 U	–1.9, 4.7	.377
Percent stage IV disease	–2.2	10%	–8.5, 4.1	.495
Median age	–0.9	1 year	–3.1, 1.2	.371

CI, confidence interval; CL, confidence limits.
From Bristow RE, Tomacruz RS, Armstrong DK, et al: Survival effect of maximal cytoreductive surgery for advanced ovarian carcinoma during the platinum era: a meta-analysis. J Clin Oncol 20(5):1248–1259, 2002, Table 2.

The rate of decline in CA-125 during primary chemotherapy has been an important independent prognostic factor in several multivariate analyses. Data suggest that rapid normalization within 1 month of initiation of treatment is of major prognostic significance. Persistent elevation of CA-125 at the time of a second-look surgical surveillance procedure predicts residual disease with more than 95% specificity. Rising CA-125 values have preceded clinical detection of recurrent disease by at least 3 months, but not in all studies. Rising CA-125 during subsequent chemotherapy has been associated with progressive disease in more than 90% of cases.[61]

Tumor Biology

Various biologic factors have been associated with prognostic significance in ovarian cancer. The role of ploidy in predicting outcome in ovarian cancer remains controversial. In many studies, diploid tumors have been associated with better survival rates. Recurrence-free survival of patients with DNA-diploid primary ovarian cancer was significantly better compared with that of patients with DNA-aneuploid tumors in univariate analysis (47% versus 18%; P = .01). The tumor-dependent overall survival rate of patients with DNA-diploid tumors was 57% compared with 30% with DNA-aneuploid tumors.[62] Mutations of the p53 tumor suppressor genes have been found in epithelial ovarian cancer, but the clinical significance of p53 overexpression in ovarian carcinoma is uncertain. In univariate analysis, p53 overexpression was a significant prognostic factor. However, in multivariate analysis, after adjustment for stage and size of residual tumor following cytoreductive surgery, p53 overexpression did not retain statistical significance. Survival curves for patients with different stages and grades of tumor differentiation did not demonstrate a difference in survival among patients with no p53 overexpression compared with those who demonstrated any degree of p53 overexpression.[63] Overexpression of the HER2/neu proto-oncogene occurs in 20% to 30% of ovarian epithelial cancers, in which it may be of prognostic significance. The incidence of HER2/neu amplification in late-stage (III–IV, 77%) is significantly higher than that in early-stage (I-II, 21%) invasive epithelial carcinoma and is associated with a worse prognosis.[64] However, use of trastuzumab targeting the HER2/neu amplification has failed to show a benefit.[65]

References

1. Jemal A, Siegel R, Ward E, et al: Cancer Statistics, 2009. CA Cancer J Clin 59:225–249, 2009.
2. Berek J: Epithelial ovarian cancer. In Berek JS, Hacker NF (eds): Practical Gynecologic Oncology, 4th ed. Philadelphia: Lippincott Williams & Wilkins, 2005, pp 443–509.
3. Ozols R, Rubin S, Thomas G, Robboy S: In Hoskins W et al (eds): Principles and Practice of Gynecologic Oncology, 4th ed. Philadelphia: Lippincott Williams & Wilkins, 2005, pp 895–987.
4. Ozols RF, Bundy BN, Greer BE, et al: Gynecologic Oncology Group. Phase III trial of carboplatin and paclitaxel compared with cisplatin and paclitaxel in patients with optimally resected stage III ovarian cancer: a Gynecologic Oncology Group study. J Clin Oncol 21(17):3194–3200, 2003.
5. Markman M, Bundy BN, Alberts DS, et al: Phase III trial of standard-dose intravenous cisplatin plus paclitaxel versus moderately high-dose carboplatin followed by intravenous paclitaxel and intraperitoneal cisplatin in small-volume stage III ovarian carcinoma: an intergroup study of the Gynecologic Oncology Group, Southwestern Oncology Group, and Eastern Cooperative Oncology Group. J Clin Oncol 19(4):1001–1007, 2001.
6. Parham G, Phillips JL, Hicks ML, et al: The National Cancer Data Base report on malignant epithelial ovarian carcinoma in African-American women. Cancer 80(4):816–826, 1997.
7. Hartge P, Whittemore AS, Itnyre J, et al: Rates and risks of ovarian cancer in subgroups of white women in the United States. Obstet Gynecol 84:760–764, 1994.
8. Fathalla MF: Incessant ovulation-a factor in ovarian neoplasia? Lancet 2(7716):163, 1971.
9. Purdie DM, Bain CJ, Siskind V, et al: Ovulation and risk of epithelial ovarian cancer. Int J Cancer 104:228–232, 2003.
10. Greene MH, Clark JW, Blayney DW: The epidemiology of ovarian cancer. [Review]. Semin Oncol 11(3):209–226, 1984.
11. Pelucchi C, Galeone C, Talamini R, et al: Lifetime ovulatory cycles and ovarian cancer risk in 2 Italian case-control studies. Am J Obstet Gynecol 196(1):83.e1–83.e7, 2007.
12. Franceschi S, La Vecchia C, Booth M, et al: Pooled analysis of 3 European case-control studies of ovarian cancer: II. Age at menarche and at menopause. Int J Cancer 49(1):57–60, 1991.
13. La Vecchia C: Oral contraceptives and ovarian cancer: an update, 1998–2004. [Review]. Eur J Cancer Prev 15(2):117–124, 2006.
14. Franceschi S, Parazzini F, Negri E, et al: Pooled analysis of 3 European case-control studies of epithelial ovarian cancer: III. Oral contraceptive use. Int J Cancer 49(1):61–65, 1991.
15. Gross TP, Schesseleman JJ: The estimated effect of oral contraceptive use on the cumulative risk of epithelial ovarian cancer. Obstet Gynecol 83(3):419–424, 1994.
16. Rosenblatt KA, Thomas DB: Lactation and the risk of epithelial ovarian cancer. The WHO Collaborative Study of Neoplasia and Steroid Contraceptives. Int J Epidemiol 22(2):192–197, 1993.
17. Gwinn ML, Lee NC, Rhodes PH, et al: Pregnancy, breast feeding, and oral contraceptives and the risk of epithelial ovarian cancer. J Clin Epidemiol 43(6):559–568, 1990.
18. Ness B, Cramer DW, Goodman MT, et al: Infertility, fertility drugs, and ovarian cancer: a pooled analysis of case-control studies. Am J Epidemiol 155(3):217–224, 2002.
19. Rossing MA, Tang MT, Flagg EW, et al: A case-control study of ovarian cancer in relation to infertility and the use of ovulation-inducing drugs. Am J Epidemiol 160(11):1070–1078, 2004.
20. Shoham Z: Epidemiology, etiology and fertility drugs in ovarian epithelial carcinoma: Where are we today? Fertil Steril 62:433–448, 1994.
21. Dor J, Lerner-Geva L, Rabinovici J, et al: Cancer incidence in a cohort of infertile women who underwent in vitro fertilization. Fertil Steril 77(2):324–327, 2002.
22. Venn A, Jones P, Quinn M, Healy D: Characteristics of ovarian and uterine cancers in a cohort of in vitro fertilization patients. Gynecol Oncol 82(1):64–68, 2001.
23. Kaufman DW, Kelly JP, Welch WR, et al: Noncontraceptive estrogen use and epithelial ovarian cancer. Am J Epidemiol 130(6):1142–1451, 1989.
24. Lacey JV, Jr, Mink PJ, Lubin JH, et al: Menopausal hormone replacement therapy and risk of ovarian cancer. JAMA 288(3):334–341, 2002. Erratum in: JAMA 288(20):2544, 2002.
25. Moorman PG, Schildkraut JM, Calingaert B, et al: Menopausal hormones and risk of ovarian cancer. Am J Obstet Gynecol 193(1):76–82, 2005.
26. Glud E, Kjaer SK, Thomsen BL, et al: Hormone therapy and the impact of estrogen intake on the risk of ovarian cancer. Arch Intern Med 164(20):2253–2259, 2004.
27. Anderson GL, Judd HL, Kaunitz AM, et al: Women's Health Initiative Investigators. Effects of estrogen plus progestin on gynecologic cancers and associated diagnostic procedures: the Women's Health Initiative Randomized Trial. JAMA 290(13): 1739–1748, 2003.
28. Lacey JV, Jr, Brinton LA, Leitzmann MF, et al: Menopausal hormone therapy and ovarian cancer risk in the National Institutes of Health-AARP Diet and Health Study Cohort. J Natl Cancer Inst 98(19):1397–1405, 2006.
29. Boyd J: Specific keynote: hereditary ovarian cancer: what we know. [Review]. Gynecol Oncol 88(1 Pt 2):S8–S10, 2003; discussion S11–S13.
30. King MC, Marks JH, Mandell JB: New York Breast Cancer Study Group. Breast and ovarian cancer risks due to inherited mutations in BRCA1 and BRCA2. Science 302 (5645):643–646, 2003.
31. Szabo CI, King MC: Population genetics of BRCA1 and BRCA2. Am J Hum Genet 60(5):1013–1020, 1997.
32. Rubin SC, Blackwood MA, Bandera C, et al: BRCA1, BRCA2, and hereditary nonpolyposis colorectal cancer gene mutations in an unselected ovarian cancer population: relationship to family history and implications for genetic testing. Am J Obstet Gynecol 178(4):670–677, 1998.
33. Robles-Diaz L, Goldfrank DJ, Kauff ND, et al: Hereditary ovarian cancer in Ashkenazi Jews. Fam Cancer 3(3–4):259–264, 2004.
34. Lynch HT, Casey MJ, Lynch J, et al:: Genetics and ovarian carcinoma. [Review]. Semin Oncol 25(3):265–280, 1998.
35. Risch HA, Jain M, Marrett LD, Howe GR: Dietary fat intake and risk of epithelial ovarian cancer. J Natl Cancer Inst 86(18):1409–1415, 1994.
36. Cramer DW, Liberman RF, Titus-Ernstoff L, et al: Genital talc exposure and risk of ovarian cancer. Int J Cancer 81(3):351–356, 1999.
37. Wong C, Hempling RE, Piver MS, et al: Perineal talc exposure and subsequent epithelial ovarian cancer: a case-control study. Obstet Gynecol 93(3):372–376, 1999.
38. Whittemore AS, Wu ML, Paffenbarger RS, Jr, et al: Personal and environmental characteristics related to epithelial ovarian cancer. II. Exposures to talcum powder, tobacco, alcohol, and coffee. Am J Epidemiol 128(6):1228–1240, 1988.
39. Olsen CM, Green AC, Whiteman DC, et al: Obesity and the risk of epithelial ovarian cancer: a systematic review and meta-analysis. Eur J Cancer 43:690–709, 2007.
40. Chang ET, Canchola AJ, Lee VS, et al: Wine and other alcohol consumption and risk of ovarian cancer in the California Teachers Study cohort. Cancer Causes Control 18(1):91–103, 2007.
41. Peterson NB, Trentham-Dietz A, Newcomb PA, et al: Alcohol consumption and ovarian cancer risk in a population-based case-control study. Int J Cancer 119(10):2423–2437, 2006.
42. Risch HA, Howe GR: Pelvic inflammatory disease and risk of epithelial ovarian cancer. Cancer Epidemiol Biomarkers Prev 4(5):447–451, 1995.
43. Yoshikawa H, Jimbo H, Okada S, et al: Prevalence of endometriosis in ovarian cancer. Gynecol Obstet Invest 50(Suppl 1):11–17, 2005.
44. Webb PM, Purdie DM, Grover S, et al: Symptoms and diagnosis of borderline, early and advanced epithelial ovarian cancer. Gynecol Oncol 92(1):232–239, 2004.
45. Olson SH, Mignone L, Nakraseive C, et al: Symptoms of ovarian cancer. Obstet Gynecol 98(2):212–217, 2001.
46. Munoz KA, Harlan LC, Trimble EL: Patterns of care for women with ovarian cancer in the United States. J Clin Oncol 15(11): 3408–3415, 1997.
47. Nguyen HN, Averette HE, Hoskins W, et al: National survey of ovarian carcinoma. VI. Critical assessment of current International Federation of Gynecology and Obstetrics staging system. Cancer 72(10):3007–3011, 1993.
48. Chan JK, Urban R, Cheung MK, et al: Ovarian cancer in younger vs older women: a population-based analysis. Br J Cancer 95(10): 1314–1320, 2006.

49. Rodriguez M, Nguyen HN, Averette HE, et al: National survey of ovarian carcinoma XII. Epithelial ovarian malignancies in women less than or equal to 25 years of age. Cancer 73(4):1245–1250, 1994.

50. Thigpen T, Brady MF, Omura GA, et al: Age as a prognostic factor in ovarian carcinoma. The Gynecologic Oncology Group experience. Cancer 71(2 Suppl):606–614, 1993.

51. Sorbe B, Frankendal B, Veress B: Importance of histologic grading in the prognosis of epithelial ovarian carcinoma. Obstet Gynecol 59(5):576–582, 1982.

52. Sherman ME, Mink PJ, Curtis R, et al: Survival among women with borderline ovarian tumors and ovarian carcinoma: a population-based analysis. Cancer 100(5):1045–1052, 2004.

53. Heintz A, Odicino F, Maisonneuve P, et al: Carcinoma of the ovary. Int J Gynecol Obstet 95(Suppl 1):S161–S192.

54. Bristow RE, Montz FJ, Lagasse LD, et al: Survival impact of surgical cytoreduction in stage IV epithelial ovarian cancer. Gynecol Oncol 72(3):278–287, 1999.

55. Chi DS, Eisenhauer EL, Lang J, et al: What is the optimal goal of primary cytoreductive surgery for bulky stage IIIC epithelial ovarian carcinoma (EOC)? Gynecol Oncol 103(2):559–564, 2006.

56. Hoskins WJ, McGuire WP, Brady MF, et al: The effect of diameter of largest residual disease on survival after primary cytoreductive surgery in patients with suboptimal residual epithelial ovarian carcinoma. Am J Obstet Gynecol 170(4):974–979, 1994; discussion 979–980.

57. Bristow RE, Tomacruz RS, Armstrong DK, et al: Survival effect of maximal cytoreductive surgery for advanced ovarian carcinoma during the platinum era: a meta-analysis. J Clin Oncol 20(5):1248–1259, 2002.

58. Cooper BC, Sood AK, Davis CS, et al: Preoperative CA125 as a prognostic factor in stage I epithelial ovarian cancer. APMIS 114(5):359–363, 2006.

59. Memarzadeh S, Lee SB, Berek JS, Farias-Eisner R: .CA125 levels are a weak predictor of optimal cytoreductive surgery in patients with advanced epithelial ovarian cancer. Int J Gynecol Cancer 13(2):120–124, 2003.

60. Markman M, Federico M, Liu PY, et al: Significance of early changes in the serum CA-125 antigen level on overall survival in advanced ovarian cancer. Gynecol Oncol 103(1):195–198, 2006.

61. Bast RC, Jr, Xu FJ, Yu YH, et al: CA 125: the past and the future. [Revised]. [Int J Biol Markers 13(4):179–187, 1998.

62. Kimmig R, Wimberger P, Hillemanns P, et al: Multivariate analysis of the prognostic significance of DNA-ploidy and S-phase fraction in ovarian cancer determined by flow cytometry following detection of cytokeratin-labeled tumor cells. Gynecol Oncol 84(1):21–31, 2002.

63. Eltabbakh GH, Belinson JL, Kennedy AW, et al: p53 overexpression is not an independent prognostic factor for patients with primary ovarian epithelial cancer. Cancer 80(5):892–898, 1997.

64. Wong YF, Cheung TH, Lam SK, et al: Prevalence and significance of HER-2/neu amplification in epithelial ovarian cancer. Gynecol Obstet Invest 40(3):209–212, 1995.

65. Bookman MA, Darcy KM, Clarke-Pearson D, et al: Evaluation of monoclonal humanized anti-HER2 antibody, trastuzumab, in patients with recurrent or refractory ovarian or primary peritoneal carcinoma with overexpression of HER2: a phase II trial of the Gynecologic Oncology Group. J Clin Oncol 21(2):283–290, 2003.

2

Biology and Pathology of Ovarian Cancer

Natini Jinawath and Ie-Ming Shih

KEY POINTS

- Ovarian carcinomas are heterogeneous and are primarily classified by cell type into serous, mucinous, endometrioid, clear cell, and Brenner (transitional) tumors corresponding to different types of epithelia. The tumors in each category are further subdivided into three groups—benign, malignant, and intermediate—based on their clinical behavior.
- Recent molecular genetic studies provide the basis for a more comprehensive model of ovarian carcinogenesis, which proposes two main pathways of tumorigenesis, corresponding to the development of type I and type II tumors.
- Type I tumors (low-grade serous carcinoma) develop in a stepwise manner from well-accepted precursors. They are slow-growing and often confined to the ovary at the time of diagnosis.
- Type II tumors are clinically high-grade at presentation (high-grade serous carcinoma). They evolve rapidly, metastasize early in their course, and are highly aggressive.
- Type I tumors frequently exhibit *BRAF/KRAS* gene mutations and low cellular proliferation. They usually have a gradual increase in cervical intraepithelial neoplasia (CIN) and are associated with a relatively long 5-year survival rate (~55%).
- Type II tumors have frequent *p53* mutations, HLA-G expression, and high cellular proliferation. They also show high cervical intraepithelial neoplasia and have a relatively short 5-year survival rate (~30%).
- Protein kinase inhibitors are a promising novel therapy for ovarian cancers especially in type II tumors. It is interesting to see whether *BRAF* inhibitors and other MEK inhibitors can prolong disease-free interval and overall survival in patients with advanced-stage of SBTs.

Introduction

Ovarian cancer is the most lethal gynecologic malignancy, and carcinoma is the most common type of ovarian cancer. The pathogenesis of ovarian carcinoma is still unclear, and one of the difficulties in studying ovarian cancer is the lack of a comprehensive tumor progression model. Ovarian carcinomas are heterogeneous and are primarily classified by cell type into serous, mucinous, endometrioid, clear cell, and Brenner (transitional) tumors corresponding to different types of epithelia in the organs of the female reproductive tract.[1-3] The tumors in each of the categories are further subdivided into three groups, benign, malignant, and intermediate (borderline tumor or low-malignant-potential) based on their clinical behavior. It has been well known that mucinous and endometrioid borderline tumors are often associated with invasive carcinomas, but serous borderline tumors (SBTs) are rarely associated with serous carcinomas.[1] The latter observation, as well as recent molecular genetic studies showing a very different mutation frequency of *p53* and *KRAS/BRAF/ERBB2* in serous carcinoma compared with serous borderline tumors, has led most investigators to conclude that serous borderline tumors and serous carcinomas are biologically unrelated.[4-8] The uncertainty about the nature of the borderline tumor groups, reflected by the ambiguous term "borderline," is a major shortcoming of the current classification. Based on a review of recent clinical, histopathologic, and molecular genetic findings, a research team has proposed a new carcinogenesis model that reconciles the relation of borderline tumors to invasive carcinoma.

Clinical and Pathologic Observations Supporting the Dualistic Ovarian Carcinogenesis Model

Comprehensive efforts have been made in analyzing histopathologic and clinical features of a large number of noninvasive and invasive epithelial ovarian tumors to delineate their pathogenesis and behavior.[1,9-11] One of the main conclusions from these studies is the recognition of a subset of low-grade serous tumors designated *micropapillary serous carcinoma* (MPSC), which displays characteristic histopathologic features, low proliferative activity, and an indolent behavior that contrasts dramatically with the conventional type of serous carcinoma.[1,9-11] The term MPSC was originally proposed by Dr. Kurman and colleagues to distinguish this tumor from the more common noninvasive tumor, termed an atypical proliferative serous tumor, both of which have been classified as borderline or low malignant potential tumor.[9,11] Histologic transitions from adenofibromas and atypical proliferative serous tumors to noninvasive MPSCs are observed and areas of infiltrative growth (stromal invasion) immediately adjacent to the noninvasive component are found in a significant proportion of cases.[12] Subsequent studies have suggested that these invasive MPSCs are synonymous with invasive low-grade serous carcinoma. The histopathologic findings suggest a morphologic and biologic spectrum of tumor progression beginning from a benign serous cystadenoma/adenofibroma through a proliferative tumor (atypical proliferative serous tumor) to a noninvasive low-grade carcinoma (noninvasive MPSC), and ending with an invasive low-grade serous carcinoma (invasive MPSC).

In contrast to conventional high-grade serous carcinoma that is a clinically aggressive neoplasm, invasive low-grade serous carcinomas typically pursue a relatively indolent course that may go on for years.[11,12] Approximately 50% to 60% of patients with invasive low-grade carcinomas ultimately succumb to their disease because of widespread intra-abdominal carcinomatosis, but the tumor maintains its low-grade appearance and low proliferative activity throughout its clinical course.[12] Analyses of mucinous, endometrioid, clear cell carcinomas, and malignant Brenner tumors reveal that they are often associated with cystadenomas, borderline tumors, and intraepithelial carcinomas.[1] Furthermore, it has been long recognized that endometrioid carcinoma and clear cell carcinoma are associated with endometriosis in the ovary or pelvis in 15% to 50% of cases,[13,14] leading researchers to propose that endometriosis is a precursor of these tumors. In contrast, a high-grade serous carcinoma is rarely associated with ovarian endometriosis.

A recent clinical study using serial transvaginal ultrasonography has demonstrated that approximately 50% of ovarian carcinomas develop from preexisting cystic lesions, whereas the remaining 50% develop in ovaries without apparent abnormality on ultrasound.[15] The former group was composed mainly of mucinous, endometrioid, and clear cell carcinomas, and borderline tumors, whereas the latter group was composed almost exclusively of high-grade serous carcinomas.

A Proposed Model of Ovarian Carcinogenesis

Recent clinicopathologic and molecular genetic studies as previously discussed provide the basis for a more comprehensive model of ovarian carcinogenesis, which proposes that there are two main pathways of tumorigenesis, corresponding to the development of type I and type II tumors (Tables 2-1 and 2-2 and Fig. 2-1). Note that

Table 2-1. Precursors and Molecular Genetic Alterations of Type I Tumors of the Ovary

Precursors*	Known Molecular Genetic Alterations
Low-Grade Serous Carcinoma (Invasive MPSC)	
Serous cystadenoma/adenofibroma	*BRAF* and *KRAS* mutations (~67%)
Intraepithelial carcinoma	
Noninvasive MPSC	
Mucinous Carcinoma	
Mucinous cystadenoma	*KRAS* mutations (>60%)
Atypical proliferative mucinous tumor	
Intraepithelial carcinoma	
Endometrioid Carcinoma	
Endometriosis	LOH or mutations in *PTEN* (20%)
Endometrioid adenofibroma	β-catenin gene mutations (16–54%)
Atypical proliferative endometrioid tumor	*KRAS* mutations (4–5%)
Intraepithelial carcinoma	Microsatellite instability (13–50%)
Clear Cell Carcinoma	
Endometriosis	*KRAS* mutations (5–16%)
Clear cell adenofibroma	Microsatellite instability (13%)
Atypical proliferative clear cell tumor	TGF-β RII mutation (66%)
Intraepithelial carcinoma	
Malignant Brenner (Transitional) Tumor	
Brenner tumor	Not yet identified
Atypical proliferative Brenner tumor	

LOH, loss of heterozygosity; MPSC, micropapillary serous carcinoma; TGF, transforming growth factor.
*Atypical proliferative serous tumors and noninvasive MPSC have been termed "borderline" tumors in the literature.
Similarly for mucinous, endometrioid, clear cell, and Brenner tumors, atypical proliferative tumor and intraepithelial carcinoma have been combined and designated "borderline tumor" in the literature.

Table 2-2. Precursors and Molecular Genetic Alterations of Type II Tumors* of the Ovary

Precursors	Known Molecular Genetic Alterations
High-Grade Serous Carcinoma	
Not yet identified	*p53* mutations (50–80%)
	Amplification and overexpression of *HER2/neu* (10–20%) and *AKT2* (12–18%)
	Inactivation of *p16* gene (10–17%)
Undifferentiated Carcinoma	
Not yet identified	Not yet identified
Malignant Mixed Mesodermal Tumor (Carcinosarcomas)	
Not yet identified	*p53* mutations (>90%)

*Type II tumors can contain neoplastic cells with clear cytoplasm and have sometimes been classified as "clear cell carcinoma."

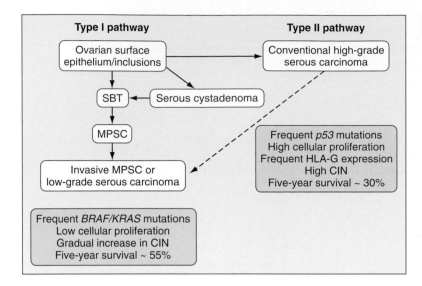

Figure 2-1. A simplified diagram of types I and II ovarian epithelial cancers. CIN, cervical intraepithelial neoplasia; MPSC, micropapillary serous carcinoma; SBT, serous borderline tumor.

type I and type II tumors describe pathways of tumorigenesis and are not specific histopathologic terms. Thus, they are not designed to replace the conventional terminology in pathology reports. Rather, the proposed model provides another view to classify ovarian epithelial tumors that may have clinical or translational implications in studying ovarian cancer.

Type I Tumors

Type I ovarian tumors (low-grade serous carcinoma, mucinous carcinoma, endometrioid carcinoma, malignant Brenner tumor, and clear cell carcinoma) develop in a stepwise manner from well-accepted precursors, namely, borderline tumors that in turn develop from cystadenomas/adenofibromas[4] (see Table 2-1 and Fig. 2-1). Serous and mucinous tumors appear to develop from the surface inclusion cysts or cystadenomas, whereas endometrioid and clear cell tumors develop from endometriosis or endometriomas. Type I tumors are slow-growing, large, and often confined to the ovary at the time of diagnosis.

Type II Tumors

Type II ovarian tumors are clinically high grade at presentation and include the morphologically defined entities such as high-grade serous carcinoma (moderately and poorly differentiated), malignant mixed mesodermal tumors (carcinosarcomas), and undifferentiated carcinomas (see Table 2-2). In addition, it is likely that some rare high-grade endometrioid and clear cell carcinoma should also be included in this group. Although malignant mixed mesodermal tumors were once thought to be mixed tumors composed of carcinoma and sarcoma, recent studies have demonstrated that they are monoclonal.[16,17] These tumors are now accordingly regarded as high-grade carcinomas with metaplastic sarcomatous elements. Type II carcinomas have been proposed to develop de novo from the surface epithelium or inclusion cysts of the ovary[6]; they are rarely associated with morphologically recognizable precursor lesions. They evolve rapidly, metastasize early in their course, and are highly aggressive (Figs. 2-2 and 2-3). It is likely that the apparent de novo conven-

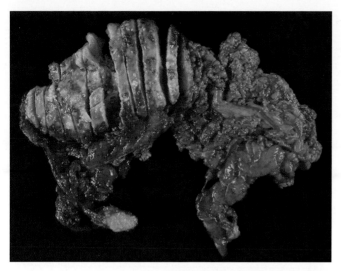

Figure 2-2. High-grade ovarian serous carcinoma involving the omentum.
High-grade serous carcinoma has a strong tendency to involve the omentum, forming a "caking" appearance. The omentum was bread-loafed to reveal the solid tumor mass.

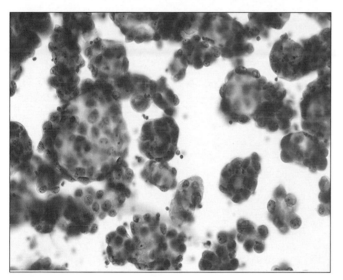

Figure 2-3. High-grade ovarian cancer cells obtained from ascites. Tumor cells in the peritoneal fluid form ball-like clusters.

tional high-grade serous carcinoma does develop in a stepwise manner, but precursor lesions have not yet been elucidated molecularly or morphologically. Presumably, this is because of rapid transit from inception as a microscopic carcinoma to a clinically diagnosed neoplasm. Thus, the window to detect the precursor lesions appears to be very small.

This dualistic model is the first step in an attempt to elucidate the molecular pathogenesis of ovarian carcinoma, but it should not be construed as implying that all ovarian carcinomas follow the proposed pathways of tumorigenesis. In fact, Dehari and colleagues[18] have demonstrated that in rare cases, a high-grade serous carcinoma is associated with either an invasive low-grade carcinoma or a serous borderline tumor. Mutational analysis of *KRAS* and *BRAF* in both low-grade/borderline component and high-grade component from the same cases shows that both areas share the same mutations in all informative cases. This finding strongly indicates that both low-grade carcinoma/borderline tumors and high-grade carcinomas are genetically related and suggests that a subset of high-grade carcinomas may likely arise from a preexisting low-grade carcinoma or a borderline tumor.[18]

Molecular Evidence Supporting the Ovarian Carcinogenesis Model

Since serous carcinoma is the most common type of ovarian carcinoma, low-grade and high-grade serous carcinomas serve as the prototypes of type I and type II carcinomas, respectively (Table 2-3). Accordingly, the molecular genetic data supporting the dualistic model are derived mainly from studies of serous carcinoma.

Mutation of *BRAF* and *KRAS*

Several unique molecular changes characterize low-grade and high-grade serous carcinomas (Table 2-4 and Fig. 2-4). Among them, the most significant molecular genetic alterations are mutations in *BRAF* and *KRAS* oncogenes. The *RAS*, *RAF*, *MEK*, *ERK*, and *MAP* cascade is important for the transmission of growth signals

Table 2-3. Summary of Clinicopathologic Features of the Prototypic Type I and Type II Tumors

Type I: Low-Grade Serous Carcinoma	Type II: High-Grade Serous Carcinoma
Frequency	
25% of serous carcinomas*	~75% of serous carcinomas*
Histologic Feature	
Micropapillary architecture	Solid nests and masses
Low-grade nuclei	High-grade nuclei
Low mitotic index	High mitotic index
Precursor Lesions	
Serous cystadenoma	Not known
Serous atypical proliferative (borderline) tumor	Probably from ovarian surface epithelium or inclusion cysts (de novo)
Clinical Behavior	
Indolent; slow progression 5-year survival 55%[†]	Aggressive; rapid progression; 5-year survival ~30%[†]
Response to Chemotherapy	
Poor	Good, although recurrence is common

*Based on a survey at the Johns Hopkins University Hospital. Most patients eventually die from the disease.
[†]Advanced-stage tumors.

Table 2-4. Summary of Molecular Features of Prototypic Type I and Type II Tumors

	Type I: Low-Grade Serous Carcinoma	Type II: High-Grade Serous Carcinoma
KRAS mutations	35%	0%
BRAF mutations	30%	0%
BRAF or *KRAS* mutations	65%	0%
TP53 mutations	0%	50–80%
HLA-G expression	0%	61%
Proliferation (Ki-67) index	10–15%	>50%

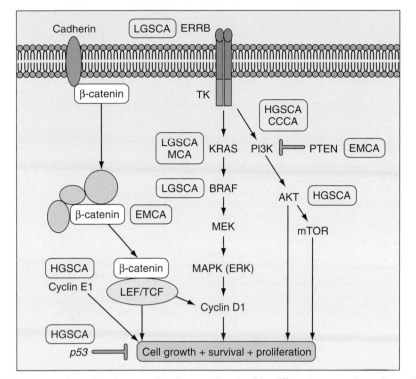

Figure 2-4. The main molecular genetic changes involved in different types of ovarian epithelial cancer. Several pathways have been known to be abnormal in ovarian cancer including p53, MAPK, cadherin/β-catenin, PI3CA/AKT, and cyclin E pathways. High-grade serous carcinoma (HGSCA) is characterized by very high frequency of mutations in *p53*, amplifications in cyclin E, AKT, and PI3CA loci. Low-grade serous carcinoma (LGSCA) harbor activating mutations in *KRAS, BRAF,* or *ERRB2*. Endometrioid carcinoma (EMCA) contains mutations in β-catenin and *PTEN*. Although the molecular genetic changes in clear cell carcinoma (CCCA) have not been extensively studied, mutations in *PI3CA* have been detected in approximately 20% of cases. Mucinous carcinoma (MCA) is characterized by mutations in *KRAS* in most cases.

into the nucleus.[19] Oncogenic (activating) mutations in *BRAF* and *KRAS* result in constitutive activation of this pathway and contribute to neoplastic transformation. Recent studies have demonstrated that *KRAS* mutations at codons 12 and 13 occur in approximately one third of low-grade serous carcinomas (invasive MPSCs) and one third of borderline tumors (atypical proliferative tumor and noninvasive MPSC) but not in high-grade serous carcinomas.[4,20] Similarly, *BRAF* mutations at codon 600 occur in 30% of low-grade serous carcinomas and 28% of borderline tumors but not in high-grade serous carcinomas.[20] Mutations in *BRAF* and *KRAS*, therefore, were found in about two thirds of low-grade invasive serous carcinomas and atypical proliferative tumors and in noninvasive MPSCs, their putative precursors, but neither of the genes was mutated in high-grade serous carcinomas. It is interesting that *BRAF* mutations were found only in tumors with wild-type *KRAS*.[20] The mutually exclusive nature of *BRAF* mutations and *KRAS* mutations in ovarian carcinoma is consistent with similar findings in melanoma and colorectal carcinoma[21,22] and lends support for the view that *BRAF* and *KRAS* mutations may have an equivalent effect on tumorigenesis. Since mutations of *BRAF* and *KRAS* can be detected in small atypical proliferative serous tumors but not in serous cystadenomas,[23] they seem to occur very early in the development of low-grade serous carcinoma. These data provide cogent evidence that the development of conventional high-grade serous carcinomas involves molecular mechanisms not related to mutations in *BRAF* and *RAS*.

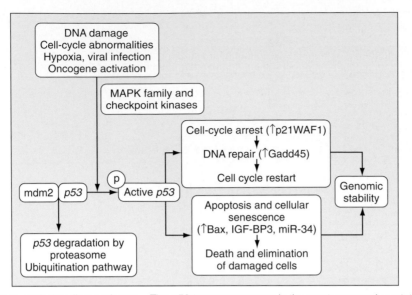

Figure 2-5. *p53* signaling pathway.   The *p53* tumor suppressor is the most commonly mutated gene in human cancer. In a normal cell, *p53* is inactivated by its negative regulator, mdm2. Upon DNA damage or other stress, various pathways lead to the dissociation of the p53 and mdm2 complex. The stable p53 protein is activated by phosphorylation, dephosphorylation, and acetylation, yielding a potent sequence-specific DNA-binding transcription factor. Once activated, p53 either induces a cell-cycle arrest to allow repair and survival of the cell or apoptosis to discard the damaged cell. The wide range of the biological effects of p53 can in part be explained by its activation of expression of a number of target genes including *p21WAFI, GADD45, 14-3-3 sigma, bax, Fas/APO1, KILLER/DR5, PIG3, Tsp1, IGF-BP3,* and others.

Mutation of *p53*

The *p53* tumor suppressor gene is the most commonly mutated gene in human cancer (Fig. 2-5). In contrast to low-grade serous carcinoma in which mutations in *p53* are rare, mutations in *p53* are common in high-grade serous carcinomas. Many studies have shown that 50% to 80% of advanced stage high-grade serous carcinomas have mutant *p53*.[24–28] It has also been reported that mutant *p53* is present in 37% of stage I and II presumably high-grade serous carcinomas.[29] Overexpression of *p53* and mutation of *p53* were found in all early invasive high-grade serous carcinomas as well as in the adjacent dysplastic surface epithelium, in a study of very early microscopic stage I serous carcinomas in ovaries removed prophylactically from women who were *BRCA* heterozygotes.[30] It is likely that inherited mutations in *BRCA* genes predispose the peritoneal surface epithelium, ovarian surface inclusion cysts, and epithelial cells of the fimbriae ends of fallopian tubes to neoplastic transformation through an increase in genetic instability. Thus, it is conceivable that conventional high-grade serous carcinoma in its very earliest stage resembles advanced-stage serous carcinoma at a molecular as well as a morphologic level. Similar to high-grade serous carcinoma, most malignant mixed mesodermal tumors (carcinosarcomas) also demonstrate *p53* mutations.[31–33] It has been reported that the same *p53* mutations occur in the epithelial and mesenchymal components.[31] Moreover, the fact that pure carcinomatous areas are often associated with sarcomatous components suggests a common derivation of both epithelial and mesenchymal components in these neoplasms.[34] The finding that metastases from these tumors nearly always are composed exclusively of carcinoma has led investigators to suggest that malignant mixed mesodermal tumors are metaplastic carcinomas.

Overexpression of Human Leukocyte Antigen G

Besides molecular genetic alterations, both low-grade and high-grade serous car-cinomas are characterized by distinct gene expression profiles. For example, transcriptome-wide gene expression profiling has demonstrated that human leuko-cyte antigen-G (HLA-G) is overexpressed in many high-grade serous carcinomas but rarely in low-grade serous carcinomas. HLA-G immunoreactivity, ranging from focal to diffuse, was detected in most high-grade ovarian serous carcinomas but not in any low-grade serous carcinomas or serous borderline tumors (atypical proliferative serous tumors) and noninvasive low-grade serous carcinomas).[35] A similar correlation of HLA-G expression with behavior has been observed in large cell carcinomas.[36] A possible mechanism that explains the association of HLA-G expression with high-grade serous carcinomas is that HLA-G seems to facilitate tumor cell evasion of the immune system by protecting malignant cells from being attacked by immune cells.[37]

Overexpression of Apolipoprotein E

Based on serial analysis of gene expression(SAGE), investigators have found apolip-rotein E (ApoE) overexpression in ovarian carcinoma. Besides the well-known role of ApoE in cholesterol transport and in the pathogenesis of atherosclerogenesis and Alzheimer's disease, ApoE may play a novel role in the development of human cancer. ApoE immunoreactivity has been detected in 66% of high-grade but only 12% of low-grade ovarian serous carcinomas, and not in normal ovarian surface epithelium, serous cystadenomas, serous borderline tumors, or other type I tumors.[38] Hence, expression of ApoE is primarily associated with the type II high-grade serous carci-nomas. Inhibition of ApoE expression in vitro induces cell-cycle arrest and apoptosis in ApoE-expressing ovarian cancer cells, suggesting that ApoE expression is important for their growth and survival.

Allelic Imbalance and Chromosomal Instability

A progressive increase in the degree of allelic imbalance (calculated as the number of SNP markers with allelic imbalance/total SNP markers examined) of chromo-somes 1p, 5q, 8p, 18q, 22q, and Xp was noted when comparing atypical proliferative tumors with noninvasive MPSCs and low-grade serous carcinomas (invasive MPSCs).[4] In particular, allelic imbalance of chromosome 5q was more frequently observed in noninvasive MPSCs compared with atypical proliferative tumors. Moreover, allelic imbalance of chromosome 1p, which harbors tumor suppressor genes, including *MYCL1* and *NOERY/ARH1*, was more frequently found in low-grade serous carci-noma (invasive MPSC) compared with noninvasive MPSCs. The allelic imbalance patterns in atypical proliferative tumors were also found in noninvasive MPSCs con-taining adjacent atypical proliferative tumor components, further supporting the view that atypical proliferative tumors are the precursors of MPSCs. On the contrary, all high-grade serous carcinomas including the very earliest tumors (less than 8 mm confined to one ovary) showed high levels of allelic imbalance. Since allelic imbalance reflects chromosomal instability (changes in DNA copy number), the previous find-ings suggest a stepwise increase in chromosomal instability in the progression to low-grade serous carcinoma in contrast to a high level of chromosomal instability in high-grade serous carcinoma, even in their earliest stage of development. Microsatel-lite instability also reflects the genetic instability in tumor cells. Microsatellite insta-bility has been studied in serous borderline tumors using 69 microsatellite markers.[39]

Similar to high-grade serous carcinoma in which frequency of microsatellite instability is rare,[40] serous borderline tumors showed no evidence of microsatellite instability. Thus, microsatellite instability is not a likely hallmark of ovarian carcinoma.

Molecular Alterations in Other Nonserous Types of Ovarian Carcinomas

The stepwise progression of borderline tumors (atypical proliferative tumor and noninvasive MPSC) to the low-grade serous carcinoma (invasive MPSC) closely approximates the adenoma-carcinoma sequence in colorectal carcinoma. This tumor progression model is also applicable to other type I carcinomas, specifically mucinous and endometrioid carcinoma. Accordingly, these mucinous and endometrioid borderline tumors have been thought to represent an intermediate stage in the stepwise progression to mucinous and endometrioid carcinoma, respectively (Table 2-5).

Mucinous Carcinoma

Morphologic transitions from mucinous cystadenoma to mucinous atypical proliferative tumor (borderline tumor), to mucinous intraepithelial carcinoma and invasive mucinous carcinoma have been recognized for some time, and an increasing frequency of *KRAS* mutations at codons 12 and 13 has been described in every stage of tumor progression.[7,41-44] In addition, the same *KRAS* mutation has been detected in mucinous carcinoma and in the adjacent mucinous cystadenoma and borderline

Table 2-5. Ovarian Borderline Tumors and Associated Molecular Genetic Changes in Tumor Progression

Summary of Major Molecular Genetic Alterations	Precursor Lesions	Progression
Serous Borderline Tumor		
BRAF and *KRAS* mutations (67%)	Serous cystadenoma/ adenofibroma	Invasive low-grade serous carcinoma
Mucinous Borderline Tumor		
KRAS mutations (>60%)	Mucinous cystadenoma	Intraepithelial carcinoma then to invasive mucinous carcinoma
Endometrioid Borderline Tumor		
LOH or mutations in *PTEN* (20%)	Endometriosis/ endometrioid	Intraepithelial carcinoma then to invasive endometrioid carcinoma
β-catenin gene mutations (50%)		
Microsatellite instability (13–50%)		
Clear Cell Borderline Tumor		
KRAS mutations (5–16%)	Endometriosis/clear cell adenofibroma	Intraepithelial carcinoma then to invasive clear cell carcinoma
Microsatellite instability (13%)		
Brenner (Transitional Type) Borderline Tumor		
Not yet identified	Brenner tumor	Malignant Brenner (transitional cell) carcinoma

LOH, loss of heterozygosity.

tumor.[41] In contrast to serous borderline tumor and serous low-grade carcinoma, *BRAF* mutations are extremely rare in ovarian mucinous tumors. Other than *KRAS* mutations, molecular genetic changes, including microsatellite instability, have rarely been reported in mucinous borderline tumors.[40]

Endometrioid Carcinoma

Mutation of β-catenin has been reported in approximately one third of cases,[45,46] and mutation of *PTEN* in 20%, rising to 46% in tumors with 10q23 loss of heterozygosity.[47] These mutations are generally detected in well-differentiated stage I tumors with a favorable prognosis, suggesting that inactivation of these genes is an early event. Moreover, similar molecular genetic alterations, including loss of heterozygosity at 10q23 and mutations in *PTEN*, have been reported in endometriosis, atypical endometriosis, and ovarian endometrioid carcinoma in the same specimen.[48–52] The molecular genetic findings together with the morphologic data showing a frequent association of endometriosis with endometrioid adenofibromas, atypical proliferative (borderline) tumors, adjacent to invasive well-differentiated endometrioid carcinoma, suggest a stepwise tumor progression toward the development of endometrioid carcinoma.

A previous study shows that mouse model expressing oncogenic *KRAS* or conditional *PTEN* deletion within the ovarian surface epithelium gave rise to preneoplastic ovarian lesions similar to endometriosis and in some mice to endometrioid carcinomas.[53] More recently, Dr. Cho's research team has further generated new transgenic mice that conditionally express mutant *PTEN* and β-catenin. Upon induction of the mutations, all mice develop endometrioid carcinomas.[54] Hence, β-catenin and *PTEN* mutations play an important role in the development of endometrioid carcinoma of the ovary.

Clear Cell Carcinoma

Clear cell carcinoma is also frequently associated with endometriosis, clear cell adenofibromas, and clear cell atypical proliferative (borderline) tumors, but molecular evidence for the stepwise progression model is still lacking. Recently, hepatocyte nuclear factor-1β and glutathione peroxidase 3 have been reported as molecular markers for ovarian clear cell carcinoma because both genes are highly expressed in ovarian clear cell carcinomas but rarely in other ovarian carcinomas.[55,56] Transforming growth factor-β receptor type II has been found to be mutated in the kinase domain in two of three clear cell carcinomas but rarely in other histologic types of ovarian carcinomas.[57] Microsatellite instability is present in endometrioid and clear cell carcinoma but is only rarely detected in serous and mucinous tumors.[58,59] These findings provide further evidence that endometrioid and clear cell carcinoma may have a common precursor lesion.

Future Study of Kinase Inhibitors in Treating Ovarian Cancer

Protein kinases are the largest superfamily of conserved genes in the genome, and many of the family members are implicated in human cancer development. The kinase genes participate in numerous and diverse signaling pathways affecting cellular growth, differentiation, adhesion, motility and survival—all key characteristics of tumorigenesis. Essentially, all structural changes in protein kinases that lead to neoplastic transformation appear to deregulate (constitutively activate) protein kinase activity, providing an attractive target for therapeutic intervention (Table 2-6). For example, therapeutic molecules or proteins have been designed to aim directly

Table 2-6. List of Kinase Genes That Are Promising as Therapeutic Targets for Cancer and Their Small Molecule Inhibitors

No.	Official Symbol	Gene Name	Inhibitor
1	AKT	v-akt murine thymoma viral oncogene homolog	Naltrindole hydrochloride
2	AURKA	Aurora Kinase A	VX-680
3	AURKB	Aurora Kinase B	VX-680
4	AMPK	AMP-activated protein kinase	Dorsomorphin dihydrochloride
5	CKI	Casein kinase I	D4476
6	CKII	Casein kinase II	DMAT
7	CHK1	Checkpoint kinase I	AZD7762
8	CHK2	Checkpoint kinase II	AZD7762
9	CDK2	Cyclin-dependent kinase 2	Seliciclib (CYC202, R-roscovitine)
10	CDK7	Cyclin-dependent kinase 7	Seliciclib (CYC202, R-roscovitine)
11	CDK9	Cyclin-dependent kinase 9	Seliciclib (CYC202, R-roscovitine)
12	DNAPK	DNA-dependent protein kinase	NU7441
13	GSK3A	Glycogen synthase kinase 3 alpha	BIO ($2'Z,3'E$)-6-Bromoindirubin-3'-oxime
14	GSK3B	Glycogen synthase kinase 3 beta	BIO ($2'Z,3'E$)-6-Bromoindirubin-3'-oxime
15	JNK1	c-Jun N-terminal kinase 1	SP600125
16	JNK2	c-Jun N-terminal kinase 2	SP600125
17	JNK3	c-Jun N-terminal kinase 3	SP600125
18	ERK1	Extracellular signal-regulated kinase 1	PD98059
19	ERK2	Extracellular signal-regulated kinase 2	PD98059
20	p38 MAPK	p38 Mitogen-activated protein kinase	SB203580
21	MEK1	Mitogen-activated protein kinase kinase 1	U0126
22	MEK2	Mitogen-activated protein kinase kinase 2	U0126
23	PI3K	Phosphatidylinositol 3-kinase	LY294002
24	PKA	Protein kinase A, cAMP-dependent protein kinase	H89 dihydrochloride
25	PKC$_\alpha$	Protein kinase C alpha-isozyme	Go6976
26	PKC$_{\beta 1}$	Protein kinase C beta 1-isozyme	LY379196
27	PKC$_{\beta 2}$	Protein kinase C beta 2-isozyme	LY379196
28	PKC$_\delta$	Protein kinase C delta-isozyme	Rottlerin

Table 2-6. List of Kinase Genes That Are Promising as Therapeutic Targets for Cancer and Their Small Molecule Inhibitors—cont'd

No.	Official Symbol	Gene Name	Inhibitor
29	PKC_ε	Protein kinase C epsilon-isozyme	GF 109203X (Bisindolylmaleimide I)
30	$PKGI_\alpha$	cGMP-dependent protein kinase type I alpha	Rp-8-pCPT-cGMPS, TEA
31	$PKGI_\beta$	cGMP-dependent protein kinase type I beta	Rp-8-pCPT-cGMPS, TEA
32	PKGII	cGMP-dependent protein kinase type II	Rp-8-pCPT-cGMPS, TEA
33	Plk1	Polo-like kinase 1	BI 2536
34	$PDGFR_\alpha$	Platelet-derived growth factor receptor alpha	Gleevec (imatinib)*
35	BCR-ABL	BCR-ABL kinase	Gleevec (imatinib)*
36	c-Kit	v-kit Hardy-Zuckerman 4 feline sarcoma viral oncogene homolog	Sutent (sunitinib)*
37	SRC	v-src sarcoma (Schmidt-Ruppin A-2) viral oncogene homolog (avian)	Sprycel (dasatinib)*
38	EPHA2	Ephrin receptor A2	Sprycel (dasatinib)*
39	EGFR	Epidermal growth factor receptor	Iressa (gefitinib)*
40	ERBB2	v-erb-b2 erythroblastic leukemia viral oncogene homolog 2	Tykerb (lapatinib)*
41	VEGFR1	Vascular endothelial growth factor receptor 1	Recentin (Cediranib)
42	VEGFR2	Vascular endothelial growth factor receptor 2	Recentin (Cediranib)
43	VEGFR3	Vascular endothelial growth factor receptor 3	Recentin (Cediranib)
44	RET	ret proto-oncogene	Zactima (vandetanib)†
45	IGF1R	Insulin-like growth factor 1 receptor	OSI-906
46	JAK2	Janus-activated kinase 2	Lestaurtinib (CEP-701)
47	JAK3	Janus-activated kinase 3	CP-690550
48	STAT3	Signal transducers and activators of transcription 3	Cucurbitacin I (JSI-124)
49	STAT5	Signal transducers and activators of transcription 5	Lestaurtinib (CEP-701)
50	FGFR1	Fibroblast growth factor receptor 1	SU5402
51	FGFR2	Fibroblast growth factor receptor 2	PD173074
52	Lck	Lymphocyte-specific protein tyrosine kinase, p56	Emodin

Table continued

Table 2-6. List of Kinase Genes That Are Promising as Therapeutic Targets for Cancer and Their Small Molecule Inhibitors—cont'd

No.	Official Symbol	Gene Name	Inhibitor
53	c-Met	Met proto-oncogene (hepatocyte growth factor receptor)	ARQ 197
54	SYK	Spleen tyrosine kinase	R406
55	TGFβR1	Transforming growth factor β type I receptor	SM16
56	TrkA	Neurotrophic tyrosine kinase, receptor, type 1	GW 441756
57	c-Raf	v-raf-1 murine leukemia viral oncogene homolog 1	Sorafenib (BAY43-9006)*
58	B-Raf	v-raf murine sarcoma viral oncogene homolog B1	Sorafenib (BAY43-9006)*
59	ROCK1	Rho-associated, coiled-coil containing protein kinase 1	Fasudil
60	ROCK2	Rho-associated, coiled-coil containing protein kinase 2	Fasudil
61	SK	Sphingosine kinase	Dimethylsphingosine (DMS)

*FDA-approved anti-cancer drugs.
†FDA fast track designation received.

at inhibiting protein kinase activity such as STI571 (Gleevec), an ATP-binding competitive inhibitor that is a potent inhibitor of the *BCR-Abl* and c-KIT tyrosine kinases. Gleevec is now used to treat chronic myelogenous leukemia and gastrointestinal stromal tumors with promising antitumor effect.[60] A number of other protein kinase inhibitors are in clinical trials for a variety of malignancies and other diseases (see Table 2-6). In most serous borderline tumors and low-grade serous carcinomas of the ovary, there is constitutive activation of the MAPK signaling pathway owing to frequent mutations in the *KRAS* and *BRAF* genes, the upstream regulators of MAPK. Accordingly, it is interesting to test whether *BRAF* inhibitors and other MEK inhibitors can prolong disease-free interval and overall survival in patients with advanced-stage serous borderline tumors. Further identification and characterization of the panoply of molecular changes associated with ovarian carcinogenesis will facilitate development of diagnostic tests for early detection of ovarian cancer and for the development of novel therapies aimed at blocking key growth-signaling pathways.

References

1. Cho K, Shih IM: Ovarian cancer. Ann Rev Pathol 4:287–313, 2009.
2. Scully RE: International Histological Classification of Tumors: Histological Typing of Ovarian Tumors. Geneva: World Health Organization, 1999, pp 3–44.
3. Tavassoli FA, Deville P: Tumours of the Breast and Female Genital Organs: World Health Organization Classification of Tumours. Lyon: IARC Press, 2003, pp 117–145.
4. Singer G, Kurman RJ, Chang H-W, et al: Diverse tumorigenic pathways in ovarian serous carcinoma. Am J Pathol 160:1223–1228, 2002.
5. Ortiz BH, Ailawadi M, Colitti C, et al: Second primary or recurrence? Comparative patterns of p53 and K-ras mutations suggest that serous borderline ovarian tumors and subsequent serous carcinomas are unrelated tumors. Cancer Res 61:7264–7267, 2001.

6. Bell DA, Scully RE: Early de novo ovarian carcinoma. A study of fourteen cases. Cancer 73:1859–1864, 1994.
7. Caduff RF, Svoboda-Newman SM, Ferguson AW, et al: Comparison of mutations of Ki-RAS and p53 immunoreactivity in borderline and malignant epithelial ovarian tumors. Am J Surg Pathol 23:323–328, 1999.
8. Dubeau L: Ovarian cancer. In Scriver CR, Beaudet AL, Sly WS (eds): The Metabolic and Molecular Bases of Inherited Disease. Toronto: McGraw-Hill, 2001, pp 1091–1096.
9. Burks RT, Sherman ME, Kurman RJ: Micropapillary serous carcinoma of the ovary. A distinctive low-grade carcinoma related to serous borderline tumors. Am J Surg Pathol 20:1319–1330, 1996.
10. Riopel MA, Ronnett BM, Kurman RJ: Evaluation of diagnostic criteria and behavior of ovarian intestinal-type mucinous tumors: atypical proliferative (borderline) tumors and intraepithelial, microinvasive, invasive, and metastatic carcinomas. Am J Surg Pathol 23:617–635, 1999.
11. Seidman JD, Kurman RJ: Subclassification of serous borderline tumors of the ovary into benign and malignant types. A clinicopathologic study of 65 advanced stage cases. Am J Surg Pathol 20:1331–1345, 1996.
12. Sehdev AES, Sehdev PS, Kurman RJ: Noninvasive and invasive micropapillary serous carcinoma of the ovary: a clinicopathologic analysis of 135 cases. Am J Surg Pathol 27:725–736, 2003.
13. Okuda T, Otsuka J, Sekizawa A, et al: p53 mutations and overexpression affect prognosis of ovarian endometrioid cancer but not clear cell cancer. Gynecol Oncol 88:318–325, 2003.
14. Modesitt SC, Tortolero-Luna G, Robinson JB, et al: Ovarian and extraovarian endometriosis-associated cancer. Obstet Gynecol 100:788–795, 2002.
15. Horiuchi A, Itoh K, Shimizu M, et al: Toward understanding the natural history of ovarian carcinoma development: a clinicopathological approach. Gynecol Oncol 88:309–317, 2003.
16. Masuda A, Takeda A, Fukami H, et al: Characteristics of cell lines established from a mixed mesodermal tumor of the human ovary. Carcinomatous cells are changeable to sarcomatous cells. Cancer 60:1697–2703, 1987.
17. Moritani S, Moriya T, Kushima R, et al: Ovarian carcinoma recurring as carcinosarcoma. Pathol Int 51:380–384, 2001.
18. Dehari R, Kurman RJ, Logani S, et al: The development of high-grade serous carcinoma from atypical proliferative (borderline) serous tumors and low-grade micropapillary serous carcinoma—a morphologic and molecular genetic analysis. Am J Surg Pathol, 31:1007–1012, 2007.
19. Peyssonnaux C, Eychene A: The Raf/MEK/ERK pathway: new concepts of activation. Biol Cell 93:53–62, 2001.
20. Singer G, Oldt R, III, Cohen Y, et al: Mutations in BRAF and KRAS characterize the development of low-grade ovarian serous carcinoma. J Natl Cancer Inst 95:484–486, 2003.
21. Davies H, Bignell GR, Cox C, et al: Mutations of the BRAF gene in human cancer. Nature 417:949–954, 2002.
22. Rajagopalan H, Bardelli A, Lengauer C, et al: RAF/RAS oncogenes and mismatch-repair status. Nature 418:934, 2002.
23. Cheng EJ, Kurman RJ, Wang M, et al: Molecular genetic analysis of ovarian serous cystadenomas. Lab Invest 84:778–784, 2004.
24. Chan W-Y, Cheung K-K, Schorge JO, et al: Bcl-2 and p53 protein expression, apoptosis, and p53 mutation in human epithelial ovarian cancers. Am J Pathol 156:409–417, 2000.
25. Kohler MF, Marks JR, Wiseman RW, et al: Spectrum of mutation and frequency of allelic deletion of the p53 gene in ovarian cancer. J Natl Cancer Inst 85:1513–1519, 1993.
26. Kupryjanczyk J, Thor AD, Beauchamp R, et al: p53 gene mutations and protein accumulation in human ovarian cancer. Proc Natl Acad Sci USA 90:4961–4965, 1993.
27. Berchuck A, Carney M: Human ovarian cancer of the surface epithelium. Biochem Pharmacol 54:541–544, 1997.
28. Wen WH, Reles A, Runnebaum IB, et al: p53 mutations and expression in ovarian cancers: correlation with overall survival. Int J Gynecol Pathol 18:29–41, 1999.
29. Shelling AN, Cooke I, Ganesan TS: The genetic analysis of ovarian cancer. Br J Cancer 72:521–527, 1995.
30. Pothuri B, Leitao M, Barakat R, et al: Genetic analysis of ovarian carcinoma histogenesis. Society of Gynecologic Oncologists 32nd Annual Meeting. Gynecol Oncol (Abstract) 80, 2001.
31. Gallardo A, Matias-Guiu X, Lagarda H, et al: Malignant mullerian mixed tumor arising from ovarian serous carcinoma: a clinicopathologic and molecular study of two cases. Int J Gynecol Pathol 21:268–272, 2002.
32. Kounelis S, Jones MW, Papadaki H, et al: Carcinosarcomas (malignant mixed mullerian tumors) of the female genital tract: comparative molecular analysis of epithelial and mesenchymal components. Hum Pathol 29:82–87, 1998.
33. Abeln EC, Smit VT, Wessels JW, et al: Molecular genetic evidence for the conversion hypothesis of the origin of malignant mixed mullerian tumours. J Pathol 183:424–431, 1997.
34. Sreenan JJ, Hart WR: Carcinosarcomas of the female genital tract. A pathologic study of 29 metastatic tumors: further evidence for the dominant role of the epithelial component and the conversion theory of histogenesis. Am J Surg Pathol 19:666–674, 1995.
35. Singer G, Rebmann V, Chen YC, et al: HLA-G is a potential tumor marker in malignant ascites. Clin Cancer Res 9:4460–4464, 2003.
36. Urosevic M, Kurrer MO, Kamarashev J, et al: Human leukocyte antigen G up-regulation in lung cancer associates with high-grade histology, human leukocyte antigen class I loss and interleukin-10 production. Am J Pathol 159:817–824, 2001.
37. Urosevic M, Willers J, Mueller B, et al: HLA-G protein up-regulation in primary cutaneous lymphomas is associated with interleukin-10 expression in large cell T-cell lymphomas and indolent B-cell lymphomas. Blood 99:609–617, 2002.
38. Chen YC, Pohl G, Wang TL, et al: Apolipoprotein E is required for cell proliferation and survival in ovarian cancer. Cancer Res 65:331–337, 2005.
39. Shih YC, Kerr J, Hurst TG, et al: No evidence for microsatellite instability from allelotype analysis of benign and low malignant potential ovarian neoplasms. Gynecol Oncol 69:210–213, 1998.
40. Allen HJ, DiCioccio RA, Hohmann P, et al: Microsatellite instability in ovarian and other pelvic carcinomas. Cancer Genet Cytogenet 117:163–166, 2000.
41. Mok SC, Bell DA, Knapp RC, et al: Mutation of K-ras protooncogene in human ovarian epithelial tumors of borderline malignancy. Cancer Res 53:1489–1492, 1993.
42. Ichikawa Y, Nishida M, Suzuki H: Mutation of KRAS protooncogene is associated with histological subtypes in human mucinous ovarian tumors. Cancer Res 54:33–35, 1994.
43. Enomoto T, Weghorst CM, Inoue M, et al: K-ras activation occurs frequently in mucinous adenocarcinomas and rarely in other common epithelial tumors of the human ovary. Am J Pathol 139:777–785, 1991.
44. Gemignani ML, Schlaerth AC, Bogomolniy F, et al: Role of KRAS and BRAF gene mutations in mucinous ovarian carcinoma. Gynecol Oncol 90:378–381, 2003.
45. Wu R, Zhai Y, Fearon ER, et al: Diverse mechanisms of beta-catenin deregulation in ovarian endometrioid adenocarcinomas. Cancer Res 61:8247–8255, 2001.
46. Moreno-Bueno G, Gamallo C, Perez-Gallego L, et al: Beta-catenin expression pattern, beta-catenin gene mutations, and microsatellite instability in endometrioid ovarian carcinomas and synchronous endometrial carcinomas. Diagn Mol Pathol 10:116–122, 2001.
47. Obata K, Morland SJ, Watson RH, et al: Frequent PTEN/MMAC mutations in endometrioid but not serous or mucinous epithelial ovarian tumors. Cancer Res 58:2095–2097, 1998.
48. Sato N, Tsunoda H, Nishida M, et al: Loss of heterozygosity on 10q23.3 and mutation of the tumor suppressor gene PTEN in benign endometrial cyst of the ovary: possible sequence progression from benign endometrial cyst to endometrioid carcinoma and clear cell carcinoma of the ovary. Cancer Res 60:7052–7056, 2000.
49. Saito M, Okamoto A, Kohno T, et al: Allelic imbalance and mutations of the PTEN gene in ovarian cancer. Int J Cancer 85:160–165, 2000.
50. Thomas EJ, Campbell IG: Molecular genetic defects in endometriosis. Gynecol Obstet Invest 50:44–50, 2000.
51. Obata K, Hoshiai H: Common genetic changes between endometriosis and ovarian cancer. Gynecol Obstet Invest 50:39–43, 2000.
52. Bischoff FZ, Simpson JL: Heritability and molecular genetic studies of endometriosis. Hum Reprod Update 6:37–44, 2000.
53. Dinulescu DM, Ince TA, Quade BJ, et al: Role of K-ras and Pten in the development of mouse models of endometriosis and endometrioid ovarian cancer. Nat Med 11:63–70, 2005.

54. Wu R, Hendrix-Lucas N, Kuick R, et al: Mouse model of human ovarian endometrioid adenocarcinoma based on somatic defects in the Wnt/beta-catenin and PI3K/Pten signaling pathways. Cancer Cell 11:321–333, 2007.

55. Tsuchiya A, Sakamoto M, Yasuda J, et al: Expression profiling in ovarian clear cell carcinoma: identification of hepatocyte nuclear factor-1beta as a molecular marker and a possible molecular target for therapy of ovarian clear cell carcinoma. Am J Pathol 163:2503–2512, 2003.

56. Hough CD, Sherman-Baust CA, Pizer ES, et al: Large-scale serial analysis of gene expression reveals genes differentially expressed in ovarian cancer. Cancer Res 60:6281–6287, 2000.

57. Francis-Thickpenny KM, Richardson DM, van Ee CC, et al: Analysis of the TGF-beta functional pathway in epithelial ovarian carcinoma. Br J Cancer 85:687–691, 2001.

58. Fujita M, Enomoto T, Yoshino K, et al: Microsatellite instability and alterations in the hMSH2 gene in human ovarian cancer. Int J Cancer 64:361–366, 1995.

59. Gras E, Catasus L, Arguelles R, et al: Microsatellite instability, MLH-1 promoter hypermethylation, and frameshift mutations at coding mononucleotide repeat microsatellites in ovarian tumors. Cancer 92:2829–2836, 2001.

60. Druker BJ: Perspectives on the development of a molecularly targeted agent. Cancer Cell 1:31–36, 2002.

3

Ovarian Cancer Family Syndromes and Genetic Testing

Jennifer E. Axilbund, Amy L. Gross, and Kala Visvanathan

KEY POINTS

- Most hereditary cancer predisposition syndromes are inherited in an autosomal dominant pattern.
- Although most families with a history suggestive of hereditary ovarian cancer do not have a currently recognizable syndrome, a significant proportion is due to one of two known syndromes, hereditary breast and ovarian cancer (HBOC) or hereditary nonpolyposis colorectal cancer (HNPCC).
- Features suggestive of HBOC include premenopausal breast cancer, ovarian cancer, and male breast cancer. Families with a significant history of young-onset colorectal or endometrial cancer are suggestive of HNPCC.
- *BRCA1* and *BRCA2* are two genes responsible for HBOC, and they appear to function as tumor suppressor genes.
- Mutations in *BRCA1* and *BRCA2* have a high penetrance, conferring a lifetime risk of ovarian cancer of between 20% and 65%. As with breast cancer, *BRCA1* mutations are associated with a higher risk of ovarian and primary peritoneal cancer and earlier age of onset compared with *BRCA2* mutations.
- The precise factors dictating which mutation carriers will develop cancer are unknown and are thought to depend on both genetic and environmental risk modifiers.
- Genetic testing for *BRCA1* and *BRCA2* is clinically available; for most families this involves full sequencing of both genes.
- Four genes have been associated with HNPCC thus far, and clinical genetic testing is available for all of these genes.
- Interventions in women who carry *BRCA1*, *BRCA2*, or HNPCC mutations include intensive cancer screening, chemoprevention, and prophylactic surgery. In *BRCA1* and *BRCA2* mutation carriers, prophylactic bilateral salpingo-oophorectomy has been shown to reduce the risk of ovarian cancer by 80% to 90% when compared with gynecologic surveillance to detect early-stage ovarian cancer. In the United States, bilateral salpingo-oophorectomy is considered the standard of care.
- Although the predominant feature of HNPCC is an increased risk of colorectal cancer—and to a lesser extent endometrial cancer—it is often forgotten that this syndrome is also associated with a 10% lifetime risk of ovarian cancer.
- Patients whose personal or family history is suggestive of HBOC or HNPCC should be referred for genetic counseling and discussion of screening and preventive strategies.
- DNA banking by women with ovarian cancer that is not explained by current genetic technology is also an option that should be discussed and undertaken by some families.

Introduction

Although most ovarian cancers are sporadic and are likely due to the combination of genetic and environmental factors, an estimated 5% to 10% of ovarian cancers are "hereditary," meaning that they are primarily attributable to mutations in a specific gene. At present, the majority of hereditary ovarian cancers can be linked to two currently known syndromes: hereditary breast and ovarian cancer (HBOC) and

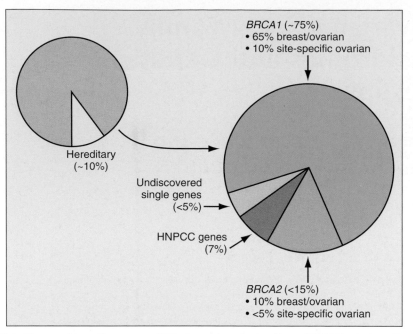

Figure 3-1. Causes of hereditary susceptibility to ovarian cancer. (From ASCO Curriculum: Cancer Genetics and Cancer Predisposition Testing, 2nd ed, 2004, Slide 6-32.)

hereditary nonpolyposis colorectal cancer (HNPCC)[1,2] (Fig. 3-1). HBOC syndrome is primarily associated with an increased risk of breast cancer, whereas HNPCC is associated with an increased risk of colorectal cancer.

Recognizing hereditary ovarian cancer not only is an academic exercise but it can be helpful to families for several reasons. For a woman with ovarian cancer, the identification of a mutation can help explain her cancer, as well as predict her risk for other related cancers. For a woman with no personal history of cancer, but with a strong family history of ovarian cancer, it can better help to define her risk of ovarian and other related cancers, enabling consideration of more specific screening and risk reduction options. In both cases, such genetic information can also be useful when assessing risk to family members, particularly children, siblings, and parents. Knowledge of a woman's cancer risk can be used to guide both screening and risk-reduction strategies. Such information may also decrease anxiety, since a woman's perceived risk of developing cancer is often much higher than her actual risk.

The overall goal of cancer risk assessment is twofold: (1) to target high-risk groups with more aggressive screening and risk-reduction strategies so as to increase their overall survival and (2) to minimize overtreatment and its associated complications in low-risk groups.

Genetics Review

Autosomal Dominant Inheritance

Most hereditary cancer predisposition syndromes are inherited in an autosomal dominant pattern (Fig. 3-2). Humans have 46 chromosomes, arranged into 23 pairs. The first 22 pairs are called autosomes and are present in both males and females. The 23rd pair comprises the sex chromosomes, with females having two X chromosomes, and males having one X and one Y chromosome. The genes for most currently recognized hereditary cancer syndromes are located on the autosomes, meaning that

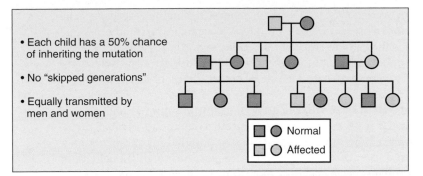

Figure 3-2. Autosomal dominant inheritance. (From ASCO Curriculum: Cancer Genetics and Cancer Predisposition Testing, 2nd ed, 2004, Slide 1-40.)

rather than being sex-linked, they can be inherited and transmitted by both males and females. For this reason, it is important to consider both maternal and paternal family history when assessing cancer risk.

When a parent has a mutation in a hereditary cancer gene, he or she has one copy of the gene with the mutation and one copy without it. Each offspring of that individual inherits one copy of the parent's gene and thus a 50% chance of inheriting the copy with the mutation and a 50% chance of inheriting the copy without the mutation. A child of a mutation carrier who inherits the mutation can pass it on to future children. However, members of a family who are shown not to have a mutation previously identified in another relative cannot pass it to their offspring.

Hereditary Ovarian Cancer Syndromes

Hereditary Breast and Ovarian Cancer

BRCA1 and *BRCA2* are two genes initially discovered by studying families strongly suggestive of hereditary breast cancer. Thus, they are named *breast ca*ncer susceptibility gene 1 (*BRCA1*) and *breast ca*ncer susceptibility gene 2 (*BRCA2*). Several hundred mutations have been reported in *BRCA1* and *BRCA2* since their identification.[3]

Functions of BRCA Genes

The *BRCA1* and *BRCA2* genes are known to be involved, both separately and coordinately, in DNA double-strand break repair. These breaks can occur in response to ionizing radiation or DNA cross-linking agents such as cisplatin, a chemotherapeutic agent. Repair occurs through homologous recombination, by which homologous, undamaged DNA strands are invaded by a damaged single-stranded DNA. Homologous sequences are then paired, resulting in an undamaged double-stranded DNA molecule. The double-stranded break repair pathway is complex and involves numerous other genes in addition to *BRCA1* and *BRCA2*.

BRCA genes are considered to act as tumor suppressor genes, because an inherited deleterious mutation in one allele represents the first "hit" in Knudsen's two-hit hypothesis of tumorigenesis.

If the second allele loses its function within a cell (through accumulation of damage), cancer can develop owing to the inability of the cell to repair acquired abnormalities. Precisely why *BRCA1* and *BRCA2* predispose specifically to breast and ovarian cancer is currently under investigation.

In light of these roles for *BRCA1* and *BRCA2*, it is interesting to note that women with *BRCA*-related ovarian cancer have a better response to cisplatin-based regimens than those with sporadic ovarian cancer.[4] Cisplatin generates a highly reactive species after intracellular aquation. This species binds to DNA, causing intrastrand crosslinks primarily between adjacent guanines in the DNA helix major groove. Among other cytotoxic effects, it is believed that the cisplatin-induced adducts may induce the mismatch repair (MMR) complex to produce single-strand DNA breaks, resulting in cytotoxicity and cell death.[5]

For genetic testing of *BRCA1* and *BRCA2* to be useful to families at high risk for a mutation in these genes, it is necessary to have accurate assessments of their prevalence (i.e., how common the mutations are in a particular population) and penetrance (i.e., the likelihood of mutation carriers developing cancer). Although thought to be responsible for most familial ovarian cancers,[6] mutations in these two genes are generally rare. Estimations of mutation prevalence in the general population range from approximately 0.1% to 0.76% (1/1000 to 1/132).[7-9] However, in women of Ashkenazi Jewish (Eastern European) descent, approximately 2.5% (1/40) are believed to be mutation carriers.[10]

BRCA1 and *BRCA2* mutations have a high penetrance. The lifetime risk of invasive breast cancer with a *BRCA1* or *BRCA2* mutation ranges from approximately 36% to 85%, depending on the study methodology.[11-14] Original data were primarily based on highly selected families, such as those used for positional cloning of the genes. In these families, the estimated lifetime risk of breast cancer was over 80%; in *BRCA1* carriers, the lifetime risk for ovarian cancer was between 40% and 65%, and for *BRCA2* carriers, 20%.[15,16] Later studies have used case-based ascertainment and, to a lesser extent, population-based data. Population-based designs to ascertain penetrance are usually performed on specific subpopulations (such as Ashkenazi Jews) known to harbor a high incidence of founder mutations to obtain an adequate number of carriers. One study of the Ashkenazim showed a 56% lifetime risk (to age 70 years) for breast cancer, and a 16% lifetime risk of ovarian cancer but did not distinguish between *BRCA1* and *BRCA2*.[10] By comparison, case-based ascertainment usually yields higher penetrance estimates, with 69% and 74% lifetime risk of breast cancer, and 54% and 23% risk of ovarian cancer in Ashkenazi Jews with mutations in *BRCA1* and *BRCA2*, respectively.[12]

A meta-analysis of case-based studies showed a 65% lifetime risk for breast cancer and 39% risk for ovarian cancer in all comers with mutations in *BRCA1*; corresponding values for *BRCA2* were 45% and 11%.[14] A recent meta-analysis (including both Ashkenazi and non-Ashkenazi populations) estimated the lifetime risk of breast cancer as 55% in *BRCA1* carriers and 47% in *BRCA2* carriers; ovarian cancer risk was estimated as 39% in *BRCA1* carriers and 17% in *BRCA2* carriers.[17]

Penetrance estimates vary, based on the populations studied and on other risk factors such as oral contraceptive use, parity, and oophorectomy[18] (Fig. 3-3). Penetrance may also vary according to the specific location of the mutation within the gene. Analysis of *BRCA1* cancer families has revealed a correlation between the mutation site and the relative risk of breast versus ovarian cancer. 3′ mutations, which cause truncation of the C-terminal region, are associated with a higher proportion of breast than ovarian cancers, whereas 5′ mutations, which delete a large segment of the BRCA1 protein, are associated with a mixture of breast and ovarian cancers.[19] Mutations in the central region of *BRCA2* (referred to as the "ovarian cancer cluster region") have been shown to be associated with a decreased risk of breast cancer relative to ovarian cancer risk[20] (Fig. 3-4).

Features and Risks of BRCA1- and BRCA2-Related Cancers

Compared with the general population, *BRCA1/2* mutation carriers have an increased risk of ovarian cancer. The lifetime risk of ovarian cancer in the general population

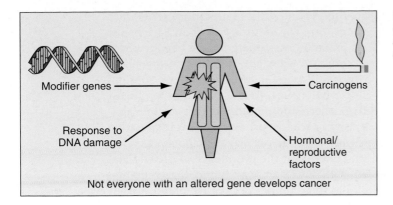

Figure 3-3. Factors affecting penetrance. (From ASCO Curriculum: Cancer Genetics and Cancer Predisposition Testing, 2nd ed, 2004, Slide 1-36.)

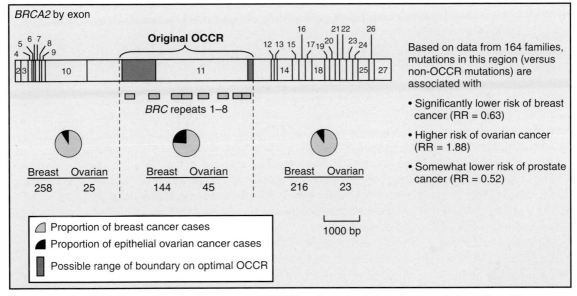

Figure 3-4. BRCA2: the ovarian cancer cluster region (OCCR) and genotype-phenotype correlations. (From Thompson D, Easton D, and the Breast Cancer Linkage Consortium: Variation in cancer risks, by mutation position, in BRCA2 mutation carriers. Am J Hum Genet 68: 410–419, 2001. Reprinted with permission from the University of Chicago Press.)

is approximately 1.3%, whereas the lifetime risk of *BRCA* mutation carriers is estimated at 10% to 65%.

BRCA1 mutations confer a higher risk of ovarian and primary peritoneal cancer compared with *BRCA2* mutations, and they are associated with earlier age of onset. Fallopian tube cancers, though much rarer than ovarian cancer, are also higher in carriers than in noncarriers[21]; again this risk is increased more in *BRCA1* carriers than in *BRCA2* carriers. *BRCA1*-associated and *BRCA2*-associated ovarian cancers are pathologically and histologically indistinguishable from one another. However, they are generally of serous histology, with endometrioid being the next most common. Mucinous tumors are unlikely to be associated with *BRCA1* or *BRCA2* mutations, whereas rarer forms such as clear cell tumors are not common enough for an association (or lack thereof) to be determined to date. In addition, borderline and low malignant potential tumors of the ovary are not believed to be associated with *BRCA1* or *BRCA2* mutations.[20]

Compared with the general population, *BRCA1* and *BRCA2* mutation carriers also have an increased risk of developing breast cancer. The lifetime risk of invasive breast cancer conferred by a *BRCA1* or *BRCA2* mutation is estimated to be between 36% and 85%. *BRCA1* and *BRCA2*-associated breast cancers are diagnosed at a younger age, often premenopausally.[22] This is particularly true for *BRCA1* carriers, approximately 20% of whom develop breast cancer before age 40 and 50% develop breast cancer by age 50.[23] A recent retrospective cohort study indicated that ductal carcinoma in situ (DCIS), with or without invasive cancer, is just as prevalent in mutation carriers (37%) as in high-risk noncarriers (34%), but that it may develop at an earlier age.[24] A population-based case-control study looked at the prevalence of *BRCA1* and *BRCA2* mutations in women diagnosed with DCIS. It was found that mutation prevalence rates in this group were similar to those found for invasive breast cancer, suggesting that the criteria used to assess eligibility for screening and risk for positive mutation-carrier status should include diagnoses of DCIS.[25] In another cohort study of mutation carriers with stage I or II breast cancer, it was found that the risk of a second primary breast cancer in the contralateral breast was approximately 30% over 10 years and was even higher in women who did not use chemoprevention or undergo oophorectomy.[26]

In addition to conferring the risk of lower age of onset of breast cancer, *BRCA1*-related breast cancers typically have features associated with a poorer prognosis, including numerous mitoses and substantial pleomorphism.[27] Compared with sporadic and *BRCA2*-related cancers, *BRCA1*-type breast cancers typically exhibit higher frequency of grade 3 tumors, lower frequency of both estrogen receptors (ER) and progesterone receptors (PR), and are rarely *HER2/neu*-positive.[28] Approximately 75% of *BRCA2*-associated breast cancers are hormone receptor–positive, whereas a similar proportion of *BRCA1*-associated breast cancers are not.[28]

The lack of estrogen receptor, progesterone receptors, and *HER2* receptor expression comprises the "triple-negative" or basal phenotype, which has been identified as having a poorer prognosis than other tumors because of the limited number of therapies that can specifically target these cells.

Men with *BRCA1* and *BRCA2* mutations are also at increased risk for cancer. Although the risk for male breast cancer is known to be increased with *BRCA1* mutations, it is higher with *BRCA2* mutations, with a lifetime risk estimate of 5% to 6% compared with 0.1% in men who are noncarriers. The lifetime risk of prostate cancer is also increased, but has not been reliably quantified. Although there is a trend toward younger-onset prostate cancer, it is not strikingly young, as is often seen with breast cancer in women.

The association of other cancers with *BRCA1* and *BRCA2* mutations has been studied in a number of cohorts. In particular, *BRCA2* mutations are associated with an increased risk of pancreatic cancer and melanoma.[10,29] Unfortunately, the lifetime risk for these malignancies has not been reliably quantified. A kin-cohort study of unselected patients newly diagnosed with ovarian cancer looked at cancer incidence in first-degree relatives of confirmed *BRCA1* and *BRCA2* mutation carriers. A higher risk ratio was associated with ovarian, female breast, and testicular cancer in *BRCA1* carriers, with higher risk for ovarian, female and male breast, and pancreatic cancers associated with *BRCA2* carriers.[30]

The precise factors that determine which mutation-positive women will and which will not develop cancer are unknown. Variation in penetrance of *BRCA1* and *BRCA2* has resulted in the identification of possible cancer risk modifiers in carriers. Both hormonal and genetic influences have been examined. The use of oral contraceptives, for example, has been reported to protect against ovarian cancer in noncarriers.[31] Studies in carriers present differential risk in regard to breast or ovarian cancer, showing a protective effect of oral contraceptive use against ovarian cancer,[32] or no reduction in risk.[33] However, a clinical dilemma is presented by data suggesting that the use of oral contraceptives in *BRCA1* carriers may also significantly increase breast cancer risk.[18] At present, oral contraceptives are not actively recommended for ovarian cancer prevention, but short-term use for contraceptive needs is not contraindicated.

The relation of endogenous hormonal factors to breast and ovarian cancer risk has also been assessed in *BRCA1* and *BRCA2* carriers. In a study of the reproductive histories of *BRCA1* carriers, the risk of breast cancer was increased in those who experienced menarche before age 12, and in those with parity of less than 3.[32] It is interesting to note that the risk of ovarian cancer in *BRCA1* carriers has been found to be lower with greater parity, in contrast to *BRCA2* carriers, in whom parity was associated with a significant increase in ovarian cancer risk.[34]

Modifier genes may also play a role in the expression and penetrance of *BRCA1* and *BRCA2* genes. For instance, in one study, *BRCA1* carriers with certain rare alleles of the *HRAS1* variable number of tandem repeats (VNTR) polymorphism had a twofold greater risk of ovarian cancer than carriers with the more common *HRAS1* alleles.[35]

Further studies to address gene-environment and gene-gene interactions are ongoing. These studies are needed to potentially make it possible to provide more personalized risk estimates to an individual woman.

Genetic Testing for Hereditary Breast and Ovarian Cancer

Family history features suggestive of a *BRCA1* or *BRCA2* mutation include premenopausal breast cancer, ovarian cancer, and male breast cancer. A referral for genetic counseling is indicated if the medical or family history is consistent with hereditary breast and ovarian cancer (Box 3-1).

Because of autosomal dominant inheritance, it is most informative to begin genetic testing in a family member who has had the cancer of concern. This is because one goal of genetic testing is to first identify the mutation in a relative with cancer in the family and to then determine which other relatives did, and did not, inherit it. Those who did inherit the mutation have an increased risk for specific malignancies, whereas the risk of cancer for those who did not inherit the mutation is much lower and based on other cancer-specific risk factors, such as age at menarche, age at menopause, body mass index (BMI), hormone replacement therapy (HRT), and other factors.

Box 3-1. Features Indicating a Need for Referral for Cancer Genetic Counseling

- Breast cancer diagnosed before menopause (typically before age 50 years)
- Member of a family with a known *BRCA1* or *BRCA2* mutation
- Two breast primaries in a single individual, particularly if one was diagnosed premenopausally
- Breast and ovarian cancer in a single individual
- Personal or family history of male breast cancer
- Two breast cancers or ovarian cancers in close relative(s) from the same side of family (maternal or paternal)
- Breast or ovarian cancer in a member of a high-risk population (i.e., Ashkenazi Jewish)
- Ovarian and colorectal cancer in the same person or in close relative(s) from the same side of the family (maternal or paternal)
- Synchronous ovarian and endometrial cancers, particularly with close relative(s) with colorectal cancer

---

Data from Daly MB, Axilbund JE, Bryant E, et al: Genetic/familial high-risk assessment: breast and ovarian. J Natl Compr Cancer Netw 4(2):156–176, 2006; and Levin B, Barthel JS, Burt RW, et al: Colorectal Cancer Screening Clinical Practice Guidelines. J Natl Compr Cancer Netw 4(4):384–420, 2006.

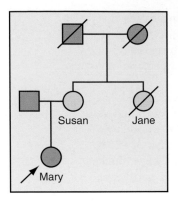

Figure 3-5. In this family, Mary is concerned about her risk for ovarian cancer because her mother, Susan, and her maternal aunt, Jane, both had ovarian cancer. Genetic testing is most informative if it begins with Susan.

Consider the following scenario, which is illustrated in Figure 3-5. A woman (Mary) is concerned about her risk for developing ovarian cancer, since her mother (Susan) was recently diagnosed with the disease. Her maternal aunt (Jane) is deceased from ovarian cancer, suggesting a hereditary component to the family history. If Mary chooses to undergo genetic testing and no mutations are detected (i.e., a negative result), there are two possible explanations for this result. One, Susan's and Jane's ovarian cancers may be due to a mutation in the gene for which Mary was tested. However, owing to autosomal dominant inheritance, Mary did not inherit the mutation from Susan. Thus, in this scenario, Mary's risk for ovarian cancer is probably closer to that of the general population and is based on her own risk factors, since her family history of ovarian cancer is attributable to a genetic mutation that she herself does not have. However, the second possibility is that Susan's and Jane's cancers are due to a mutation in a gene that has not yet been discovered. Since the gene has not been discovered, it is impossible to determine whether Mary has the same mutation. Therefore, in this scenario Mary remains at increased risk for ovarian cancer based on her genetically unexplained family history. Without genetically testing Susan, it is not possible to distinguish between these two possible explanations.

By contrast, if a genetic test were performed on Susan and a mutation were detected, one could reasonably attribute her ovarian cancer to the identified mutation. Determining whether Mary has this same mutation will then indicate whether she, too, is at increased risk for ovarian cancer. It also determines whether Mary's offspring have an increased risk for developing ovarian cancer.

Genetic analysis of the *BRCA1* and *BRCA2* genes is clinically available. For most families, full sequencing of both genes is required and is considered the most reliable method of gene analysis. However, an estimated 12% of deleterious mutations are large genomic deletions, duplications, or rearrangements, which are not always detectable with sequencing.[36] Therefore, additional technology, such as the BRAC Analysis Rearrangement Test (BART), may be necessary in families with a cancer pattern strongly suggestive of a hereditary component. If a woman with ovarian cancer undergoes full analysis of both genes and a mutation is identified, the mutation likely explains the most significant genetic component of her cancer. It also indicates that she is at increased risk for breast cancer, and, depending on her prognosis, increased screening or consideration of breast cancer risk-reducing options may be indicated. In addition, it is possible to offer predictive genetic testing to other interested family members to identify those who also have an increased risk of developing breast and ovarian cancer.

If no mutations are identified, the woman's ovarian cancer is genetically unexplained. Possible explanations are a *BRCA1* or *BRCA2* mutation that is not identifiable using current technology, a mutation in an undiscovered gene, or a combination of many genetic and environmental factors. The woman's risk for a future malignancy, and cancer risk to her relatives, is based on her family history.

A third possible result is a variant of uncertain significance, which is a change in the DNA sequence whose role in cancer development is not known. Through research, some variants are ultimately determined to be polymorphisms (normal genetic variation between individuals and populations), whereas others are ultimately classified as deleterious (cancer-causing). Until the significance of the variant is determined, genetic testing is generally not offered to unaffected relatives. Uncertain variants are detected in approximately 5% of samples tested from Caucasian individuals. In non-Caucasian populations, such as African Americans, the chance of an uncertain variant increases owing to less available genetic data in minority ethnicities.

In those of Ashkenazi Jewish descent, genetic testing usually begins with analysis of three founder mutations (Fig. 3-6). The 187delAG and 5385insC mutations in the *BRCA1* gene and the 6174delT mutation in the *BRCA2* gene account for approximately 90% of *BRCA1* and *BRCA2* mutations detected in the Ashkenazim. Because of the high detection rate with this three-mutation panel, full sequencing is generally considered only in Ashkenazi Jewish individuals who have a high pretest probability of a deleterious mutation and who are shown to be negative for the three founder mutations. Other populations known to have founder mutations include Icelanders (999del5 in *BRCA2*), as well as those from Finland, France, Russia, Denmark, Sweden, and Belgium.[37]

Once a mutation has been identified in a family, other relatives have the option of undergoing testing for that specific mutation. This is due to the rarity of *BRCA1* and *BRCA2* mutations, such that one seldom sees a family with more than one mutation. However, because these mutations are more common among Ashkenazi Jews and because a significant number of Ashkenazi families have more than one mutation, testing for the entire founder mutation panel is generally recommended even when only one founder mutation has been identified in the family.

Because of patent and licensing constraints, sequencing of *BRCA1* and *BRCA2* is clinically available only through Myriad Genetic Laboratories, a commercial laboratory in Salt Lake City, Utah. Peripheral blood is the preferred specimen, and turn-around time for the analysis is generally 2 to 3 weeks. Full sequencing costs more than $3000, whereas the Ashkenazi Jewish founder mutation panel is around $550 and mutation-specific testing is approximately $450. Most insurance companies cover a portion, if not all, of the cost for patients whose medical or family history is suggestive of an underlying mutation. Because of the expense, though, the laboratory offers insurance preauthorization services. These costs may change in the future.

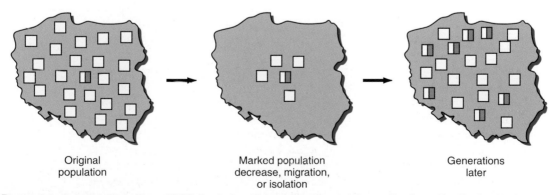

| Original population | Marked population decrease, migration, or isolation | Generations later |

Figure 3-6. Founder effect. (From ASCO Curriculum: Cancer Genetics and Cancer Predisposition Testing, 2nd ed, 2004, Slide 1-38.)

Management: Screening and Risk Reduction Options

Ovarian Cancer. Although there is no evidence that ovarian cancer screening is efficacious in *BRCA1* and *BRCA2* mutation carriers or in the general population, at present mutation-positive women who have not completed their family are recommended to have annual pelvic examination, transvaginal ultrasound, and serum CA-125 (see Chapter 6 for more details). Studies examining the ability of this surveillance to detect early-stage ovarian cancers have had mixed results, with one group finding four of five cancers detected at stage I or II[38] and a review of other studies finding that 63% of screen-detected ovarian cancers were stage IIC or greater.[39] The authors of the latter study suggest that the features of *BRCA*-related ovarian tumors—primarily serous and endometrioid—progress relatively rapidly to an advanced stage, making early detection difficult. Oral contraceptives as chemoprevention for ovarian cancer in *BRCA* mutation carriers have been suggested by studies showing significant reduction of risk. However, their use is not routinely recommended because of a possible increased risk of breast cancer.

For those who have completed childbearing, prophylactic bilateral salpingo-oophorectomy is the standard of care. Such surgery, when compared with increased surveillance, reduces the risk of ovarian cancer by 80% to 90%.[40,41] The majority of the remaining risk is attributed to primary peritoneal cancer, although a small proportion may arise in the remnant of fallopian tube remaining in the uterus. There is also some suggestion of an association between uterine papillary serous carcinoma and *BRCA1* mutations, although this is primarily based on case reports in the literature rather than large numbers of patients. For these reasons, some women also consider concurrent hysterectomy; however, this is not a standard recommendation for all mutation-positive women. In addition, up to 4% of mutation-positive women undergoing prophylactic oophorectomy have an occult cancer identified.[42] For this reason, it is generally recommended that a gynecologic oncologist either perform the surgery or be available for staging, if necessary. So far, a survival benefit has been shown in the short term but not long term.[43]

Timing of prophylactic oophorectomy after childbearing may differ depending on the underlying gene mutation and the family history. It is typically recommended that *BRCA1/2* mutation-positive women pursue surgery in their mid to late 30s or early 40s. An added benefit of bilateral oophorectomy, particularly when it occurs before menopause, is a reduction in breast cancer risk of up to 50%.[40] What is unknown at this time is whether the reduction in breast cancer risk conferred by prophylactic bilateral salpingo-oophorectomy is of the same magnitude in *BRCA1* compared with *BRCA2* carriers. Recently, it was reported that bilateral salpingo-oophorectomy resulted in a 72% reduction in breast cancer risk in *BRCA2* mutation carriers, with only a 45% risk reduction in *BRCA1* mutation carriers,[44] suggesting an age-dependent benefit.[45] Ultimately, timing of the surgery depends on a combination of factors, including the gene, and the woman's own medical and psychosocial history.

Hormone replacement therapy is often an issue of concern for mutation-positive women, since they are usually premenopausal at the time of prophylactic oophorectomy. Thus, entry into menopause is sudden, and severity of symptoms varies. Short-term hormone replacement for severe menopausal side effects (e.g., vasomotor symptoms, insomnia) is an option to provide improvement in quality of life, particularly with the use of estrogen alone if the uterus has been removed. Current views on hormone replacement therapy in this high-risk population vary considerably, ranging from no hormone replacement therapy to use of hormone replacement therapy until the age at which menopause would have naturally occurred. Data on hormone replacement therapy in *BRCA1* and *BRCA2* carriers have been extrapolated from data from the general population, and there is a need to evaluate its use in this population prospectively. Long-term hormone replacement is not generally recommended because of the already greatly increased risk of breast cancer due to mutation status, but further studies on the long-term effects of ovarian removal on the brain, bone, and cardiovascular system are needed.

Breast Cancer. Screening and risk reduction strategies for the breast in female *BRCA1* and *BRCA2* mutation carriers fall into three general categories: intensive cancer screening, chemoprevention, and prophylactic surgery. According to recommendations of the National Comprehensive Cancer Network, women with *BRCA1* or *BRCA2* mutations should have a clinical breast examination by a healthcare provider at least every 6 months, beginning at age 25 years (www.nccn.org). Mammograms generally begin at age 25 years, but can be adjusted based on the cancer pattern in the family. Adjuvant ultrasound is also a consideration for women with dense breast tissue; studies are ongoing to determine its effectiveness.

Recently, magnetic resonance imaging (MRI) has become a more routine part of breast screening for mutation carriers. The American Cancer Society recommends that women with a high risk for breast cancer (greater than 20% lifetime risk) should get an MRI and a mammogram every year. The optimal interval between these procedures (i.e., staggered with one of the two every 6 months, or both at the same time each year) has not yet been established.[46] A review of the effectiveness of MRI as an addition to mammography and ultrasound in screening high-risk young women found consistent evidence that MRI as a screening strategy provides high sensitivity compared with mammography alone or mammography and ultrasound, with or without clinical breast examination.[47] Whether this higher sensitivity translates to detection of earlier stage disease or a reduction in patient mortality compared with mammography alone is presently unclear. Based on the high sensitivity of MRI compared with mammography, particularly in younger women, it is possible that these recommendations may change as more data are obtained on MRI as a screening tool.

Risk reduction options include chemoprevention and prophylactic bilateral mastectomy. Data on the effectiveness of chemoprevention with tamoxifen in *BRCA1* and *BRCA2* carriers have been extrapolated from large trials within the general population. The National Surgical Adjuvant Breast and Bowel Project (NSABP) prevention trials showed a 62% decrease in the risk of breast cancer in *BRCA2*-positive women who received tamoxifen for 5 years, versus no reduction in breast cancer incidence among *BRCA1*-positive women.[48] However, another study examined the effects of tamoxifen on prevention of contralateral breast cancer in mutation carriers and found that the drug did provide protection overall; however, the protection reached significance only in *BRCA1* mutations carriers.[49] This is interesting in light of the lack of hormone receptor expression seen in *BRCA1* relative to BRCA2 cancers.

Another risk-reduction option is prophylactic bilateral mastectomy, which reduces the risk of breast cancer by at least 90% in unaffected mutation carriers.[50,51] For women with breast cancer who opt for contralateral prophylactic mastectomy, the rate of a contralateral malignancy is also reduced by 90%.[52] However, therapeutic and/or contralateral mastectomy does not reduce the risk of chest wall or distant recurrence. Furthermore, although such surgery results in the greatest reduction in breast cancer risk, it is often an emotionally difficult choice for women. Although expected to decrease mortality, the efficacy of bilateral prophylactic mastectomy in prolonging survival has not yet been shown.

Hereditary Nonpolyposis Colorectal Cancer

Features and Cancer Risks

Hereditary nonpolyposis colorectal cancer (HNPCC), also known as Lynch syndrome, was first identified in families with a significant history of young-onset colorectal cancer. The lifetime risk of this malignancy ranges from 25% to 75%, with an average age at diagnosis of colorectal cancer of 44 years. Almost 75% of HNPCC-associated colorectal cancers present in the ascending (right) colon, and the risk of a metachronous colorectal cancer ranges from 1% to 4% per year.

Although colorectal cancer is the predominant feature in HNPCC, this syndrome is associated with an increased risk of other malignancies as well. The second most common cancer is endometrial or uterine, with a lifetime risk of 30% to 60%, followed by ovarian cancer with a lifetime risk of 10%. Other associated cancers, with a lifetime risk generally of less than 10%, are stomach, small bowel, urinary tract, and biliary tract cancers. Synchronous primary endometrial and ovarian cancers are suggestive of HNPCC if the woman also has a personal history of colorectal cancer or a family history suggestive of HNPCC.[53]

As with hereditary breast and ovarian cancer, the precise factors that determine which mutation-positive individuals will and will not develop which cancers are unknown. It is suspected that cancer development is due to a combination of the specific mutation location along one of four DNA mismatch repair genes, other coinherited genetic factors, and environmental interactions. Therefore, it is not currently possible to provide personalized risk estimates to a specific person.

Genetic Testing

The Bethesda and Amsterdam criteria are used to identify affected persons who are most likely to benefit from additional genetic evaluation (Boxes 3-2 and 3-3). Diagnostic testing of the tumor is conducted in those who meet one or more of these criteria. Compared with most hereditary cancer syndromes, genetic testing for HNPCC is generally a two-step process. The first step is to analyze the tumor itself. Two analyses are performed, the first of which is microsatellite instability (MSI)

Box 3-2. The Revised Bethesda Guidelines for Testing Colorectal Tumors for Microsatellite Instability (MSI)

Tumors should be tested for MSI in the following situations:
- Colorectal cancer diagnosed in a patient who is less than 50 years of age.
- Presence of synchronous, metachronous colorectal, or other HNPCC-associated tumors,* regardless of age.
- Colorectal cancer with tumor infiltrating lymphocytes, Crohn's-like lymphocytic reaction, mucinous/signet-ring differentiation, or medullary growth pattern diagnosed in a patient who is less than 60 years of age.
- Colorectal cancer diagnosed in one or more first-degree relatives with an HNPCC-related tumor, with one of the cancers being diagnosed under age 50 years.
- Colorectal cancer diagnosed in two or more first- or second-degree relatives with HNPCC-related tumors, regardless of age.

*Hereditary nonpolyposis colorectal cancer (HNPCC)-related tumors include colorectal, endometrial, stomach, ovarian, pancreas, ureter and renal pelvis, biliary tract, and brain (usually glioblastoma as seen in Turcot syndrome) tumors, sebaceous gland adenomas and keratoacanthomas in Muir–Torre syndrome, and carcinoma of the small bowel.
Data from Umar A, Boland CR, Terdiman JP, et al: Revised Bethesda Guidelines for Hereditary Nonpolyposis Colorectal Cancer (Lynch Syndrome) and Microsatellite Instability. JNCI J Nat Cancer Inst 96(4):261–268, 2004.

Box 3-3. Amsterdam-I and Amsterdam-II Criteria for Clinical Diagnosis of Hereditary Nonpolyposis Colorectal Cancer (HNPCC)

Amsterdam-I Criteria
- **Three** relatives with colorectal cancer (one must be a first-degree relative of the other two)
- **Two** or more generations of colorectal cancer
- **One** or more relatives diagnosed with colorectal cancer before age 50 years
- Exclude Familial Adenomatous Polyposis (FAP)

Amsterdam-II Criteria
- **Three** relatives with an HNPCC-associated* cancer (one must be a first-degree relative of the other two)
- **Two** or more generations of HNPCC-associated* cancer
- **One** or more relatives diagnosed with HNPCC-associated* cancer before age 50 years
- Exclude FAP

---

*HNPCC-associated cancers include colorectal, endometrial, small bowel, ureter or renal pelvis.
Data from Vasen HF, Mecklin JP, Khan PM, Lynch HT: The International Collaborative Group on Hereditary Nonpolyposis Colorectal Cancer (ICG-HNPCC). Dis Colon Rectum 34:424–425, 1991; Vasen HF, Watson P, Mecklin JP, Lynch HT: New clinical criteria for hereditary nonpolyposis colorectal cancer (HNPCC, Lynch syndrome) proposed by the International Collaborative Group on HNPCC. Gastroenterology 116:1453–1456, 1999.

testing. Microsatellite instability testing evaluates numbers of repeats within specific DNA markers in the tumor and is performed in specific situations suggestive of HNPCC. Because the HNPCC-associated genes are involved in DNA mismatch repair, instability within the microsatellite repeats is suggestive of an underlying problem within the DNA repair process. Although microsatellite instability is detected in 90% to 95% of HNPCC-associated colorectal tumors, it is also present in 10% to 20% of sporadic colorectal tumors, generally due to acquired changes in the *MLH1* gene. Thus, microsatellite instability testing is not diagnostic of HNPCC, but increases the probability of having a DNA mismatch-repair germline mutation.

In addition to microsatellite instability testing, immunohistochemistry (IHC) analysis of the HNPCC-associated proteins is also performed. Immunohistochemistry currently assesses production of four mismatch repair proteins: MLH1, MSH2, MSH6, and PMS2. Absence of expression of any of these proteins, along with microsatellite instability, is strongly suggestive of HNPCC, and indicates that germline testing is warranted. By comparison, lack of instability and normal production of all HNPCC-associated gene products suggest that HNPCC is less likely, and germline testing is apt to be inconclusive.

Germline testing is available for all four of the HNPCC-associated genes, and as with *BRCA1* and *BRCA2* testing, peripheral blood is the preferred specimen.

Several different laboratories perform the testing, but the cost is still over $1000 per gene. The results of the immunohistochemistry help to guide the germline testing. Analysis generally begins with the gene whose protein product was absent on immunohistochemistry analysis, since it is the most likely site of mutation. Of all mutations detected, thus far approximately 90% have been found in *MLH1* and *MSH2*.

If a woman with ovarian cancer and a family history suggestive of HNPCC undergoes germline testing and a mutation is identified, the mutation likely genetically explains her cancer. It also indicates that she has an increased risk of colorectal cancer and other HNPCC-associated malignancies, including endometrial carcinoma, and her risk is modestly increased for cancer of the stomach, urinary tract, hepatobiliary tract, brain, and small intestine and for certain skin neoplasms.[54] Depending on her prognosis, increased screening or consideration of cancer risk-reducing options may

14. Antoniou A, Pharoah PD, Narod S, et al: Average risks of breast and ovarian cancer associated with BRCA1 or BRCA2 mutations detected in case series unselected for family history: a combined analysis of 22 studies. Am J Hum Genet 72:1117–1130, 2003.

15. Ford D, Easton DF, Bishop DT, et al: Risks of cancer in BRCA1-mutation carriers. Breast Cancer Linkage Consortium. Lancet 343:692–695, 1994.

16. Easton DF, Ford D, Bishop DT: Breast and ovarian cancer incidence in BRCA1-mutation carriers. Breast Cancer Linkage Consortium. Am J Hum Genet 56:265–271, 1995.

17. Chen S, Parmigiani G: Meta-analysis of BRCA1 and BRCA2 penetrance. J Clin Oncol 25:1329–1333, 2007.

18. Narod SA, Dube MP, Klijn J, et al: Oral contraceptives and the risk of breast cancer in BRCA1 and BRCA2 mutation carriers. J Natl Cancer Inst 94:1773–1779, 2002.

19. Gayther SA, Warren W, Mazoyer S, et al: Germline mutations of the BRCA1 gene in breast and ovarian cancer families provide evidence for a genotype-phenotype correlation. Nat Genet 11:428–433, 1995.

20. Risch HA, McLaughlin JR, Cole DE, et al: Prevalence and penetrance of germline BRCA1 and BRCA2 mutations in a population series of 649 women with ovarian cancer. Am J Hum Genet 68:700–710, 2001.

21. Aziz S, Kuperstein G, Rosen B, et al: A genetic epidemiological study of carcinoma of the fallopian tube. Gynecol Oncol 80:341–345, 2001.

22. Meijers-Heijboer EJ, Verhoog LC, Brekelmans CT, et al: Presymptomatic DNA testing and prophylactic surgery in families with a BRCA1 or BRCA2 mutation. Lancet 355:2015–2020, 2000.

23. Claus EB, Schildkraut JM, Thompson WD, et al: The genetic attributable risk of breast and ovarian cancer. Cancer 77:2318–2324, 1996.

24. Hwang ES, McLennan JL, Moore DH, et al: Ductal carcinoma in situ in BRCA mutation carriers. J Clin Oncol 25:642–647, 2007.

25. Claus EB, Petruzella S, Matloff E, et al: Prevalence of BRCA1 and BRCA2 mutations in women diagnosed with ductal carcinoma in situ. JAMA 293:964–969, 2005.

26. Metcalfe K, Lynch HT, Ghadirian P, et al: Contralateral breast cancer in BRCA1 and BRCA2 mutation carriers. J Clin Oncol 22:2328–2335, 2004.

27. Stratton MR and the Breast Cancer Linkage Consortium: Pathology of familial breast cancer: differences between breast cancers in carriers of BRCA1 or BRCA2 mutations and sporadic cases. Lancet 349:1505–1510, 1997.

28. Weber F, Shen L, Fukino K, et al: Total-genome analysis of BRCA1/2-related invasive carcinomas of the breast identifies tumor stroma as potential landscaper for neoplastic initiation. Am J Hum Genet 78:961–972, 2006.

29. Easton D and the Breast Cancer Linkage Consortium: Cancer risks in BRCA2 mutation carriers. J Natl Cancer Inst 91:1310–1316, 1999.

30. Risch HA, McLaughlin JR, Cole DE, et al: Population BRCA1 and BRCA2 mutation frequencies and cancer penetrances: a kin-cohort study in Ontario, Canada. J Natl Cancer Inst 98:1694–1706, 2006.

31. Risch HA, Weiss NS, Lyon JL, et al: Events of reproductive life and the incidence of epithelial ovarian cancer. Am J Epidemiol 117:128–139, 1983.

32. Narod SA, Risch H, Moslehi R, et al: Oral contraceptives and the risk of hereditary ovarian cancer. Hereditary Ovarian Cancer Clinical Study Group. N Engl J Med 339:424–428, 1998.

33. Modan B, Hartge P, Hirsh-Yechezkel G, et al: Parity, oral contraceptives, and the risk of ovarian cancer among carriers and noncarriers of a BRCA1 or BRCA2 mutation. N Engl J Med 345:235–240, 2001.

34. McLaughlin JR, Risch HA, Lubinski J, et al: Reproductive risk factors for ovarian cancer in carriers of BRCA1 or BRCA2 mutations: a case-control study. Lancet Oncol 8:26–34, 2007.

35. Phelan CM, Rebbeck TR, Weber BL, et al: Ovarian cancer risk in BRCA1 carriers is modified by the HRAS1 variable number of tandem repeat (VNTR) locus. Nat Genet 12:309–311, 1996.

36. Walsh T, Casadei S, Coats KH, et al: Spectrum of mutations in BRCA1, BRCA2, CHEK2, and TP53 in families at high risk of breast cancer. JAMA 295:1379–1388, 2006.

37. Szabo CI, King MC: Population genetics of BRCA1 and BRCA2. Am J Hum Genet 60:1013–1020, 1997.

38. Scheuer L, Kauff N, Robson M, et al: Outcome of preventive surgery and screening for breast and ovarian cancer in BRCA mutation carriers. J Clin Oncol 20:1260–1268, 2002.

39. Hogg R, Friedlander M: Biology of epithelial ovarian cancer: implications for screening women at high genetic risk. J Clin Oncol 22:1315–1327, 2004.

40. Rebbeck TR, Lynch HT, Neuhausen SL, et al: Prophylactic oophorectomy in carriers of BRCA1 or BRCA2 mutations. N Engl J Med 346:1616–1622, 2002.

41. Kauff ND, Satagopan JM, Robson ME, et al: Risk-reducing salpingo-oophorectomy in women with a BRCA1 or BRCA2 mutation. N Engl J Med 346:1609–1615, 2002.

42. Laki F, Kirova YM, This P, et al: Prophylactic salpingo-oophorectomy in a series of 89 women carrying a BRCA1 or a BRCA2 mutation. Cancer 109:1784–1790, 2007.

43. Domchek SM, Friebel TM, Neuhausen SL, et al: Mortality after bilateral salpingo-oophorectomy in BRCA1 and BRCA2 mutation carriers: a prospective cohort study. Lancet Oncol 7:223–229, 2006.

44. Kauff ND, Domchek SM, Friebel TM, et al: Multi-center prospective analysis of risk-reducing salpingo-oophorectomy to prevent BRCA-associated breast and ovarian cancer. J Clin Oncol 24:49s, 2006.

45. Chen S, Iversen ES, Friebel T, et al: Characterization of BRCA1 and BRCA2 mutations in a large United States sample. J Clin Oncol 24:863–871, 2006.

46. Saslow D, Boetes C, Burke W, et al: American Cancer Society guidelines for breast screening with MRI as an adjunct to mammography. CA Cancer J Clin 57:75–89, 2007.

47. Lord SJ, Lei W, Craft P, et al: A systematic review of the effectiveness of magnetic resonance imaging (MRI) as an addition to mammography and ultrasound in screening young women at high risk of breast cancer. Eur J Cancer 43:1905–1917, 2007.

48. King MC, Wieand S, Hale K, et al: Tamoxifen and breast cancer incidence among women with inherited mutations in BRCA1 and BRCA2: National Surgical Adjuvant Breast and Bowel Project (NSABP-P1) breast cancer prevention trial. JAMA 286:2251–2256, 2001.

49. Narod SA, Brunet JS, Ghadirian P, et al: Tamoxifen and risk of contralateral breast cancer in BRCA1 and BRCA2 mutation carriers: a case-control study. Hereditary Breast Cancer Clinical Study Group. Lancet 356:1876–1881, 2000.

50. Meijers-Heijboer H, van Geel B, van Putten WL, et al: Breast cancer after prophylactic bilateral mastectomy in women with a BRCA1 or BRCA2 mutation. N Engl J Med 345:159–164, 2001.

51. Rebbeck TR, Friebel T, Lynch HT, et al: Bilateral prophylactic mastectomy reduces breast cancer risk in BRCA1 and BRCA2 mutation carriers: the PROSE study group. J Clin Oncol 22:1055–1062, 2004.

52. van Sprundel TC, Schmidt MK, Rookus MA, et al: Risk reduction of contralateral breast cancer and survival after contralateral prophylactic mastectomy in BRCA1 or BRCA2 mutation carriers. Br J Cancer 93:287–292, 2005.

53. Soliman PT, Broaddus RR, Schmeler KM, et al: Women with synchronous primary cancers of the endometrium and ovary: do they have Lynch syndrome? J Clin Oncol 23:9344–9350, 2005.

54. Lindor NM, Petersen GM, Hadley DW, et al: Recommendations for the care of individuals with an inherited predisposition to Lynch syndrome: a systematic review. JAMA 296:1507–1517, 2006.

4

Ovarian Cancer Prevention: Chemoprevention and Prophylactic Surgery

Robert L. Giuntoli II, Teresa Diaz-Montes, and Robert E. Bristow

---

KEY POINTS

- There is no effective screening test for ovarian cancer.
- Both pregnancy and oral contraceptive use reduce the risk of ovarian cancer in the general population.
- In the general population, the benefits of prophylactic oophorectomy are modest and must be considered against the implications of surgical menopause.
- Approximately 10% of ovarian cancers are hereditary.
- The majority of studies support the use of oral contraceptives for the prevention of ovarian cancer in women with a high risk for developing ovarian cancer.
- Prophylactic oophorectomy should be considered in women at high risk for ovarian cancer after the age of 35 or once childbearing is complete.

Introduction

Ovarian cancer remains a highly lethal disease. Effective screening for ovarian cancer is lacking. Both prophylactic and surgery chemoprevention with oral contraceptives have been advocated. Oral contraceptive pills are believed to reduce risk both in the general population and in women without an increased risk for ovarian cancer. Prophylactic bilateral salpingectomy results in surgical menopause, but significantly reduces risk in the high-risk group. Although bilateral salpingo-oophorectomy is traditionally recommended to surgically reduce risk of ovarian cancer, hysterectomy and bilateral tubal ligation also appear to decrease this risk. Effective screening and chemopreventive measures are awaited.

Epidemiology

In the United States, ovarian cancer ranks fifth as a cause of cancer-related deaths among women. In 2008, this malignancy was diagnosed in 21,560 women and resulted in 15,520 deaths.[1] Unfortunately, most cases of ovarian cancer are diagnosed at an advanced stage. Despite optimal cytoreductive surgery and primary chemotherapy, 5-year survival rates for women with advanced ovarian cancer remain less than 30%.[2] Effective, durable therapies for ovarian cancer remain elusive. Current screening tests for the early detection of ovarian cancer do not possess sufficient sensitivity and specificity to be adopted into general practice. Given existing limitations of the treatment and early detection of ovarian cancer, disease prevention may represent a viable option for certain populations.

signed consent forms for additional procedures including hysterectomy and full surgical staging, since there is a 4% chance of detecting an occult malignancy at the time of the procedure.[21,22] Prophylactic bilateral salpingo-oophorectomy can be performed by laparotomy or laparoscopy (minimally invasive surgery). A methodical survey of the abdomen, pelvis, and entire peritoneum should be performed. All ovarian tissue and as much fallopian tube as possible should be removed. Any suspicious area that is noted at the time of the procedure should be excised and submitted for frozen-section evaluation. If adhesions between the ovary and other peritoneal structures are present, they should be resected to ensure that all ovarian tissue has been removed. The infundibulopelvic ligament should be clamped and cut at least 2 cm proximal to the ovary to prevent leaving any ovarian tissue behind. Although the intramural portion of the fallopian tube is left behind after the bilateral salpingo-oophorectomy, there have no reports of malignant transformation in the tubal remnant after prophylactic surgery.[23] See Figure 4-1.

A hysterectomy may be performed along with the bilateral salpingo-oophorectomy. The major disadvantage is that it converts a minor procedure into a major one with greater morbidity and requires admission to the hospital for postoper-

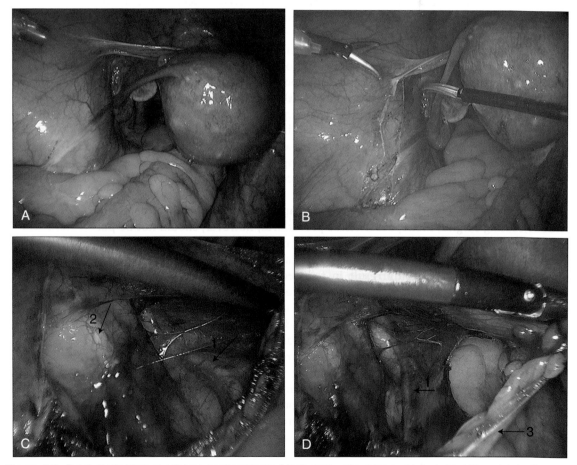

Figure 4-1. Prophylactic bilateral salpingo-oophorectomy. Manipulation of ovaries and tubes should be minimized. Infundibulopelvic vessels should be ligated approximately 2 cm proximal to the ovary. As much fallopian tube as possible should be excised. The pathology evaluation should include the entire specimen to rule out an occult malignancy. **A,** Laparoscopic view of the pelvis. Note location of uterus, left fallopian tube and ovary, left round ligament, and sigmoid colon. **B,** Divide broad ligament. **C,** Laparoscopic view of the left retroperitoneum. Note course of left ureter (1) on the medial leaf of the broad ligament. Left external iliac artery (2) is also visible. **D,** To mobilize the ureter away from the ovarian vessels, a defect is created between the left ureter (1) and the infundibulopelvic vessels (3).

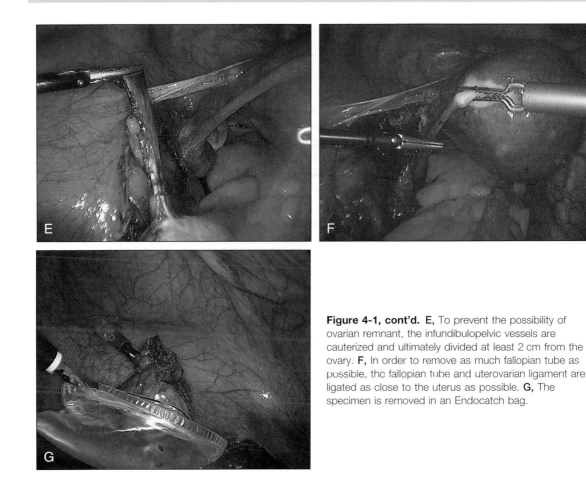

Figure 4-1, cont'd. E, To prevent the possibility of ovarian remnant, the infundibulopelvic vessels are cauterized and ultimately divided at least 2 cm from the ovary. **F,** In order to remove as much fallopian tube as possible, the fallopian tube and uterovarian ligament are ligated as close to the uterus as possible. **G,** The specimen is removed in an Endocatch bag.

ative care. Hysterectomy has been advocated as part of prophylactic surgery for several proposed benefits. Since the risk of endometrial carcinoma is no longer present, hormone replacement therapy with unopposed estrogen can be given to control menopausal symptoms. Normally, women with *BRCA1* mutations may carry an increased risk of endometrial and fallopian tube cancer. Hysterectomy would address this risk. Finally, *BRCA* mutation carriers undergoing hysterectomy are not at an increased risk for endometrial cancer if they opt to use the selective estrogen-receptor modulator tamoxifen for chemoprophylaxis of breast cancer.

Several investigations have demonstrated an association between prophylactic bilateral salpingo-oophorectomy and a reduction in the risk of gynecologic cancers. Rebbeck and associates[24] evaluated whether prophylactic bilateral salpingo-oophorectomy reduced the risk of cancers of the coelomic epithelium and breast in women who carry such mutations. A total of 551 women with disease-associated germline *BRCA1* or *BRCA2* gene mutations were identified from registries and studied for the occurrence of ovarian and breast cancer. The incidence of ovarian cancer was determined in 259 women who underwent prophylactic bilateral salpingo-oophorectomy and in 292 matched controls who did not undergo the procedure. In the subgroup of 241 women with no history of breast cancer or prophylactic mastectomy, the incidence of breast cancer was determined in 99 women who underwent prophylactic bilateral salpingo-oophorectomy and in 142 matched controls. The length of postoperative follow-up for both groups was at least 8 years. Six women (2.3%) who underwent prophylactic bilateral salpingo-oophorectomy were diagnosed with stage I ovarian cancer at the time of the procedure; two women (0.8%) were

10. John EM, Whittemore AS, Harris R, Itnyre J: Characteristics relating to ovarian cancer risk: collaborative analysis of seven U.S. case-control studies. Epithelial ovarian cancer in black women. Collaborative Ovarian Cancer Group. J Natl Cancer Inst 85(2):142–147, 1993.

11. La Vecchia C, Franceschi S: Oral contraceptives and ovarian cancer. Eur J Cancer Prev 8(4):297–304, 1999.

12. Rosenberg L, Palmer JR, Zauber AG, et al: A case-control study of oral contraceptive use and invasive epithelial ovarian cancer. Am J Epidemiol 139(7):654–661, 1994.

13. Stanford JL: Oral contraceptives and neoplasia of the ovary. Contraception 43(6):543–556, 1991.

14. Bosetti C, Negri E, Trichopoulos D, et al: Long-term effects of oral contraceptives on ovarian cancer risk. Int J Cancer 102(3):262–265, 2002.

15. Narod SA, Risch H, Moslehi R, et al: Oral contraceptives and the risk of hereditary ovarian cancer. Hereditary Ovarian Cancer Clinical Study Group. N Engl J Med 339(7):424–428, 1998.

16. Modan B, Hartge P, Hirsh-Yechezkel G, et al: Parity, oral contraceptives, and the risk of ovarian cancer among carriers and noncarriers of a BRCA1 or BRCA2 mutation. N Engl J Med 345(4):235–240, 2001.

17. Whittemore AS, Balise RR, Pharoah PD, et al: Oral contraceptive use and ovarian cancer risk among carriers of BRCA1 or BRCA2 mutations. Br J Cancer 91(11):1911–1915, 2004.

18. Walker GR, Schlesselman JJ, Ness RB: Family history of cancer, oral contraceptive use, and ovarian cancer risk. Am J Obstet Gynecol 186(1):8–14, 2002.

19. Averette HE, Nguyen HN: The role of prophylactic oophorectomy in cancer prevention. Gynecol Oncol 55(3 Pt 2):S38–S41, 1994.

20. Hankinson SE, Hunter DJ, Colditz GA, et al: Tubal ligation, hysterectomy, and risk of ovarian cancer. A prospective study. JAMA 270(23):2813–2818, 1993.

21. Finch A, Shaw P, Rosen B, et al: Clinical and pathologic findings of prophylactic salpingo-oophorectomies in 159 BRCA1 and BRCA2 carriers. Gynecol Oncol 100(1):58–64, 2006.

22. Powell CB: Occult ovarian cancer at the time of risk-reducing salpingo-oophorectomy. Gynecol Oncol 100(1):1–2, 2006.

23. Kauff ND, Barakat RR: Surgical risk-reduction in carriers of BRCA mutations: where do we go from here? Gynecol Oncol 93(2):277–279, 2004.

24. Rebbeck TR, Lynch HT, Neuhausen SL, et al: Prophylactic oophorectomy in carriers of BRCA1 or BRCA2 mutations. N Engl J Med 346(21):1616–1622, 2002.

25. Kauff ND, Satagopan JM, Robson ME, et al: Risk-reducing salpingo-oophorectomy in women with a BRCA1 or BRCA2 mutation. N Engl J Med 346(21):1609–1615, 2002.

26. Rutter JL, Wacholder S, Chetrit A, et al: Gynecologic surgeries and risk of ovarian cancer in women with BRCA1 and BRCA2 Ashkenazi founder mutations: an Israeli population-based case-control study. J Natl Cancer Inst 95(14):1072–1078, 2003.

27. Olivier RI, van Beurden M, Lubsen MA, et al: Clinical outcome of prophylactic oophorectomy in BRCA1/BRCA2 mutation carriers and events during follow-up. Br J Cancer 90(8):1492–1497, 2004.

28. Parazzini F, La Vecchia C, Negri E: Oral contraceptive use and the risk of ovarian cancer: an Italian case-control study. Eur J Cancer 27(5):594–598, 1991.

5

Imaging of Ovarian Cancer

Jingbo Zhang and Hedvig Hricak

KEY POINTS

- For women with known risk factors for ovarian cancer, transvaginal ultrasound continues to be the initial and the most promising imaging modality for ovarian cancer screening.
- Ultrasound (both gray-scale and Doppler) is considered the modality of choice for initial evaluation of an ovarian mass.
- The features suggestive of ovarian malignancy on all cross-sectional imaging modalities (ultrasound, computed tomography, and MRI) include septations greater than 3 mm in thickness, mural nodularity, and the presence of papillary projections. Unilocular or multilocular ovarian cystic lesions without solid parts are more likely to be benign.
- MR imaging is considered to be a problem-solving technique in the characterization of adnexal masses.
- CT is the modality of choice in staging and preoperative planning for ovarian cancer.
- The role of FDG-PET in combination with CT in the evaluation of ovarian cancer has been growing rapidly, with recognized advantages in the evaluation of tumor recurrence.

Overview of the Roles of Imaging in Ovarian Cancer

Imaging is an integral part of ovarian cancer detection, diagnosis, management, and treatment follow-up. A number of imaging modalities are available, and a variety of new techniques, especially molecular imaging approaches, are being developed. Each imaging modality has its unique advantages and limitations; therefore, evidence-based use of imaging is essential for achieving the greatest possible benefit without over- or underuse of specific modalities. Since imaging is a continuously advancing field, it is important for clinicians to keep abreast of new developments and revise aspects of their clinical practice in line with these developments.

Briefly, ultrasound, computed tomography (CT) and magnetic resonance imaging (MRI) are established imaging modalities in the evaluation of ovarian cancer, and positron emission tomography (PET) is an emerging modality. In terms of screening for ovarian cancer, established clinical guidelines are available to guide the selection of appropriate modalities. Transvaginal ultrasound has consistently been the most promising imaging modality for routine screening for ovarian cancer among the imaging modalities that have been tested. When it comes to lesion detection and characterization, for patients presenting with pertinent symptoms, the imaging workup generally includes an ultrasound or contrast-enhanced CT of the abdomen and pelvis in addition to a complete physical examination and appropriate laboratory tests.[1] MRI of the pelvis or abdomen may be used for problem solving when imaging findings on ultrasound are equivocal, or in patients who have contraindications to iodinated CT contrast. Chest x-ray is typically obtained as part of the overall evaluation before surgical staging. Other diagnostic studies, such as gastrointestinal tract evaluation, are not routinely recommended, unless indicated in specific clinical situations.

After the completion of primary surgery and chemotherapy in patients with ovarian cancer, imaging plays an important role in follow-up. The most frequently used imaging modalities include CT of the abdomen and pelvis, PET, and PET/CT. Again, MRI is reserved as a problem-solving tool or is used for patients with contra-indications to CT scanning. For patients with borderline epithelial ovarian cancer (also known as epithelial ovarian cancer of low malignant potential [LMP]) who chose fertility-sparing surgery, close monitoring with ultrasound examinations should be considered.

This chapter discusses the roles of different modalities, including ultrasound, CT, MRI, and PET in ovarian cancer screening, detection, and characterization, as well as pretreatment staging and post-treatment follow-up.

Screening for Ovarian Cancer

Ovarian cancer is the fifth most common cancer in women and is the most common cause of gynecologic cancer mortality. Approximately 1 in 70 women will develop ovarian cancer in their lifetime. Many risk factors have been identified in the carci-nogenesis of ovarian cancer, and patients with varying levels of risk can be further stratified into different groups. Recommendations for ovarian cancer screening vary according to the patient's level of risk. Advancing age, infertility, endometriosis, and postmenopausal hormone replacement therapy typically lead to a mildly increased risk of ovarian cancer in individuals compared with that of the general female popula-tion (relative risk [RR] < 3),[2-5] whereas inherited mutations in the cancer susceptibil-ity genes such as BRCA1, BRCA2, and mismatch repair genes associated with hereditary nonpolyposis colon cancer (HNPCC) syndrome lead to much higher RRs of approximately 30 to 45, 6 to 20, and 6 to 9, respectively, compared with RRs of the general population.[6-13] In the absence of genetic testing information, a family history of ovarian cancer or early-onset breast cancer has been associated with inter-mediately increased risk of ovarian cancer with a RR of approximately 3 to 5 com-pared with the general population,[14-16] but it is not clear how much of this increased risk is accounted for by mutations in the known ovarian cancer susceptibility genes.

A number of tests have been evaluated as potential methods of screening for ovarian cancer. Screening tests with the greatest evidence base include serum CA-125 and transvaginal ultrasound. Although a number of imaging modalities have been evaluated for possible use in ovarian cancer screening, transvaginal ultrasound has consistently been the most promising imaging modality for routine screening for ovarian cancer. In the largest study to date evaluating ultrasound as a screening method for ovarian cancer, 14,469 women predominantly with an average risk of ovarian cancer were followed up with annual transvaginal ultrasounds.[17] In this study, ultrasound was found to have 81% sensitivity and 98.9% specificity, resulting in a positive predictive value of 9.4%. The authors also suggested that transvaginal ultra-sound was associated with an early detection of ovarian cancer, with 11 of 17 screen-detected ovarian cancers being diagnosed at stage I. Critics, however, have pointed out that only 2 of the 11 stage I screen-detected cancers were high grade, compared with all six of the screen-detected advanced-stage ovarian cancers.

Several studies have evaluated the simultaneous use of transvaginal ultrasound and testing for CA-125. These studies have suggested that the combination of these tests results in a higher sensitivity for ovarian cancer detection, but at the cost of an increased rate of false-positive results. In the ongoing Prostate, Lung, Colorectal and

Ovarian Cancer (PLCO) Screening Trial, 28,816 women were randomized to receive annual transvaginal ultrasound and CA-125. At baseline, 1338 (4.7%) ultrasounds and 402 (1.4%) CA-125 tests were abnormal. Workup of these abnormalities led to the diagnoses of 20 invasive ovarian cancers. The positive predictive values of abnormal tests were 1.0% for transvaginal ultrasound and 3.7% for CA-125. When both tests were abnormal, however, their combined positive predictive value was 23.5%.[18] Final results comparing this screened cohort to a control group of 39,000 women randomized to usual care are expected in 2015.

Several national organizations, including the American Cancer Society, the American College of Obstetricians and Gynecologists/Society of Gynecologic Oncologists, the United States Preventive Services Task Force, and the National Cancer Institute, have stated that there is inadequate evidence to determine whether routine screening for ovarian cancer will result in decreased mortality rates and that therefore transvaginal ultrasound and CA-125 blood tests are generally not recommended for ovarian cancer screening of women without known strong risk factors, although genetic counseling may be helpful for women with intermediately increased risk (RR 3–5) to clarify the risk of ovarian and related cancers. For women with inherited risk (i.e., documented mutations in *BRCA1* or *BRCA2*), the Cancer Genetics Studies Consortium recommended screening with CA-125 and transvaginal ultrasound one to two times per year, starting between ages 25 and 35 years. The National Comprehensive Cancer Network recommends risk-reducing salpingo-oophorectomy in these high-risk individuals ideally between the ages of 35 and 40 years. For patients who do not choose to undergo risk-reducing salpingo-oophorectomy, ovarian cancer screening is recommended with transvaginal ultrasound and CA-125 twice a year starting at age 35 or 5 to 10 years earlier than the earliest ovarian cancer diagnosis in the family.

Detection and Characterization of Ovarian Tumors

Role of Ultrasound

Ultrasound is considered the modality of choice for initial evaluation of an ovarian mass.[19] It has been reported that in a setting similar to day-to-day clinical practice, in which the readers were given a brief clinical history of the patients (i.e., age, menstrual status, family history of ovarian cancer, previous pelvic surgery, and presenting symptoms), the experienced readers reached a prospective diagnostic accuracy of 92%, with excellent interobserver agreement (κ 0.85). The less experienced observers obtained an accuracy that ranged between 82% and 87%, with moderate to good interobserver agreement (κ 0.52 to 0.76).[20]

The features suggestive of ovarian malignancy on ultrasound include septations greater than 3 mm, mural nodularity, and papillary projections. Unilocular or multilocular ovarian cystic lesions without solid parts are more likely to be benign.[21,22] In other words, the most significant feature predictive of ovarian malignancy is the presence of solid components within the mass.[23] When solid excrescences or solid portions of the tumor demonstrate vascular flow with color Doppler sonography (conventional or power), the likelihood of malignancy is even greater.[23,24] Some benign lesions, such as endometriomas and hemorrhagic cysts, may mimic ovarian neoplasms on ultrasound (Fig. 5-1). Therefore, for premenopausal women, it may be prudent to obtain short-term follow-up on ovarian lesions to exclude transient physiologic changes.[22]

The role of spectral Doppler analysis using parameters such as resistive index (RI), pulsatility index (PI), and peak systolic velocity (PSV) in the evaluation of ovarian masses has been controversial. On spectral Doppler, ovarian cancer often

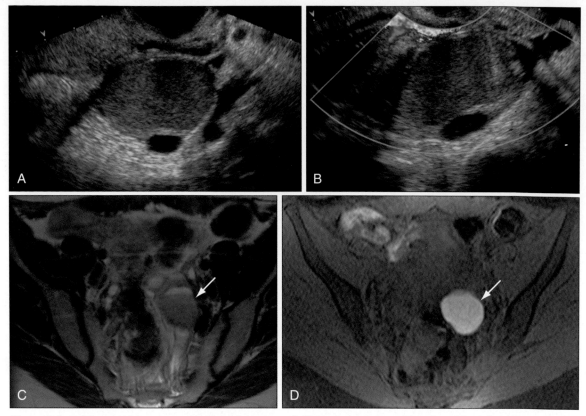

Figure 5-1. A 38-year-old woman with thyroid cancer.   A, Transverse ultrasound imaging of the left ovary demonstrates a mass of relatively homogeneous internal echoes. **B,** Color Doppler ultrasound image of this mass demonstrates no obvious internal flow. **C,** Axial T2-weighted MRI demonstrates "shading" phenomenon within this mass (*arrow*), a finding frequently seen in endometriomas. **D,** Axial T1-weighted fat-saturated MRI demonstrates high signal intensity within the left ovarian mass (*arrow*) consistent with a blood-containing lesion. The patient underwent subsequent left ovarian cystectomy, which revealed an endometrioma.

demonstrates low-resistance waveforms because tumor neovasculature lacks smooth muscle and arteriovenous shunting often occurs.[25] Lower RI, lower PI, and higher PSV are thought to be associated with lower impedance flow and higher vascularity in the adnexal mass and thus may be indicative of malignancy. Early research suggested high sensitivity and specificity using an RI less than 0.4 and a PI less than 1 as cut-off values for diagnosing malignant ovarian masses.[26–28] However, a later study by Levine and colleagues[29] showed that although use of the RI might improve specificity in the assessment of possibly malignant lesions, a significant number of malignant lesions could be miscategorized on the basis of the RI.[29] Other studies found that although PI and RI tended to be lower in malignant ovarian masses, they overlapped considerably in benign and malignant lesions, and no discriminatory cut-off value could be found.[21,30] Therefore, Doppler sonography has severe limitations in the differentiation of benign from malignant adnexal disease on the basis of low-impedance flow alone, although combining the flow velocity patterns obtained at pulsed Doppler ultrasound with a detailed analysis of the internal architectural appearance of the adnexal mass may increase the specificity and overall accuracy of the diagnosis.[31–36] In addition, lack of detectable flow on color Doppler ultrasound does not exclude ovarian malignancy.[36] It should be noted, however, that benign lesions such as corpora lutea with low-impedance flow are more common in premenopausal women; in a postmenopausal woman, low-impedance flow in an ovarian lesion is highly suggestive of malignancy.[22]

A study by Buy and colleagues[37] compared the accuracy of three ultrasonographic techniques in characterizing adnexal masses: conventional gray-scale sonography, conventional sonography combined with color Doppler, and spectral Doppler analysis only using RI, PI, or PSV as diagnostic criteria for malignancy. They showed that conventional sonography alone had an accuracy of 83%, sensitivity of 88%, and specificity of 82%. Using conventional ultrasound combined with color Doppler ultrasound, accuracy was 95%, sensitivity was 88%, and specificity was 97%. Using spectral Doppler analysis only with RI less than or equal to 0.4 as the indication for malignancy, accuracy was 77%, sensitivity was 18%, and specificity was 98%. Using PI less than or equal to 1 as the criterion for malignancy, accuracy was 68%, sensitivity was 71%, and specificity was 67%. For a PSV greater than or equal to 15 cm/s, accuracy was 72%, sensitivity was 47%, and specificity was 81% in diagnosing ovarian malignancy. These results indicated that adding color Doppler to conventional sonography produced higher specificity and positive predictive value than did conventional sonography alone, whereas RI, PI, and PSV were of limited value as stand-alone diagnostic tests.[37] A meta-analysis of 89 studies using receiver operating characteristic curve analysis found that accuracy (as measured by the area under the ROC curve [AUC]) was significantly higher for the combination of gray-scale ultrasound and Doppler ultrasound (0.92) than for morphologic information (0.85), Doppler ultrasound indexes (0.82), or color-flow Doppler imaging alone (0.73) ($P < .01$ for all).[38]

It is worth mentioning that technologic advances in diagnostic ultrasonography have led to the development of three-dimensional transvaginal gray-scale volume imaging and power Doppler imaging by ultrasound, which reportedly allows better visualization of the internal architecture of adnexal masses than does conventional two-dimensional transvaginal imaging.[39,40] A few studies have demonstrated that three-dimensional power Doppler imaging better defines the morphologic and vascular characteristics of ovarian lesions and significantly improves specificity in the diagnosis of ovarian malignancy.[39,41]

Role of Magnetic Resonance Imaging

MRI is considered a problem-solving technique in the assessment of adnexal masses.[19] For adequate evaluation of adnexal masses, T1- and T2-weighted images of the pelvis are fundamental in the delineation of pelvic anatomy and tumor, and subsequent gadolinium-enhanced sequences, typically done with fat saturation, can be helpful.[22] Fat saturation technique enables the reader to distinguish between fat and blood products. Gadolinium-enhanced MRI further improves characterization of the internal architecture of ovarian lesions and has been shown to be more accurate than ultrasound in the assessment of adnexal masses.[42–45] Transvaginal ultrasound cannot reliably differentiate blood products, debris, or fibrofatty tissue from neoplastic projections, whereas on gadolinium-enhanced MRI, neoplastic tissue enhances, and clot or debris do not. Gadolinium-enhanced MRI has been shown to have sensitivity, specificity, and accuracy up to 100%, 98%, and 99%, respectively, in the identification of solid components within an adnexal mass, and just as on ultrasound the presence of enhancing solid tissue on MRI is highly sensitive and specific in predicting malignancy.[44] A study by Hricak and colleagues[46] showed that gadolinium-enhanced MRI was highly accurate in the detection and characterization of complex adnexal masses, with excellent inter- and intraobserver agreement. Gadolinium-enhanced MRI depicted 94% of adnexal masses, with an overall accuracy of 93% for the diagnosis of malignancy.[46] The MRI imaging findings that were most predictive of malignancy were necrosis in a solid lesion (odds ratio 107) and vegetations in a cystic lesion (odds ratio 40).[46,47] Use of gadolinium-based contrast material contributed significantly to lesion characterization. Other features suggestive of malignancy on

MRI include enhancing septations thicker than 3 mm and septal nodularity, wall irregularity, large lesion size, early tumor enhancement on dynamic contrast-enhanced images, and the presence of ascites, peritoneal disease, or adenopathy.[47] The accuracy of MRI (AUC 0.91) has been shown to be superior to that of Doppler ultrasound (AUC 0.78) and of CT (AUC 0.87) in the diagnosis of malignant ovarian masses.[45] In addition, a meta-analysis showed that for women with an indeterminate ovarian mass at gray-scale ultrasound, MRI results contributed more to a change in the probability of ovarian cancer in both pre- and postmenopausal women than did CT or combined gray-scale and Doppler ultrasound results.[48]

Role of Computed Tomography

The advent of multislice CT, which allows faster acquisition times and higher spatial resolution, has led to a great increase in the number of CT examinations performed. For a number of clinical indications such as renal colic, appendicitis, and diverticulitis, CT has become a primary imaging approach. However, although CT has been shown to be the modality of choice in staging and preoperative planning for ovarian cancer,[49,50] it is generally not considered helpful for primary characterization of adnexal masses. When an adnexal mass is detected on CT, it is common practice not to characterize the mass based on its appearance on CT, but to refer patients to ultrasound or MRI for further characterization of the mass and management guidance.

As a matter of fact, CT can probably yield more diagnostic information than is generally believed.[51] One study found that the rates of detection of ovarian tumors were comparable for CT and ultrasound (87% and 86%). The study also found that CT had a higher accuracy than ultrasound in characterizing tumors as benign or malignant (94% versus 80%) and that there was no significant difference in specificity (99% for CT versus 92% for US).[52] Another study from the same group found no significant difference in the overall accuracy levels of CT (92%) and MRI (86%) in characterizing tumors as benign or malignant.[53] Another study showed that preoperative CT in patients with ovarian abnormalities had an accuracy of 87%, a sensitivity of 90%, and a specificity of 85% for predicting malignant disease.[50]

Role of FDG-PET

PET scanning with 2-[fluorine 18] fluoro-2-deoxy-D-glucose ([18]fluorodeoxyglucose; FDG) is based on uptake of FDG by functionally active tissue such as neoplasm, which has a higher glucose metabolism. The role of FDG-PET in combination with CT in the evaluation of pelvic malignancies has been growing rapidly in recent years. FDG-PET has proved valuable in the evaluation of a variety of pelvic malignancies, including colorectal cancer, uterine cervical cancer, and endometrial cancer.[54] Fusion of PET and CT images obtained simultaneously allows combined anatomic and functional imaging[55] and offers higher specificity than PET alone. It has been suggested that CT images of optimal diagnostic quality can be obtained using both oral and intravenous contrast material without interfering with PET, thus offering a "one-stop shopping" imaging protocol.[56,57] In addition, CT images can be used for attenuation correction for PET, thus decreasing the overall cost and acquisition time.[55]

PET, however, has recognized limitations. The major disadvantages include misinterpretation of normal physiologic activity in the abdomen or pelvis, and limited intrinsic image resolution leading to a failure to detect small lesions (less than 0.5 cm).[55] Since FDG-PET does not have the resolution needed to characterize the primary adnexal mass, the sensitivity and specificity of FDG-PET for diagnosis and assessment of adnexal masses are inferior to those of ultrasound, CT, and MRI; therefore, PET has a limited role in the evaluation of primary ovarian cancer.[58]

Physiologic uptake of FDG in ovaries during different phases of the menstrual cycle may hinder detection of primary ovarian cancer.[54] In addition, a variety of benign lesions, such as serous and mucinous cystadenomas, corpus luteum cysts, and dermoid cysts, are known to accumulate FDG and cannot be reliably differentiated from malignant lesions[22,58] (Fig. 5-2). Generally speaking, increased FDG uptake in a solid component of an ovary that does not correspond to one of the above-mentioned benign lesions should be considered suggestive of malignancy. The suggestion of malignancy is stronger when ovarian FDG uptake is present in a postmenopausal woman.

In addition, misregistration cannot be completely eliminated because the acquisition time is relatively long for PET and because physiologic patient activity, such as respiratory motion, bowel peristalsis, and bladder distention, occur during it.[55] It also should be noted that both physiologic uptake and tumor activity may appear larger on PET than on the corresponding CT image owing to the "blooming" effect if the uptake activity is intense on PET.[55]

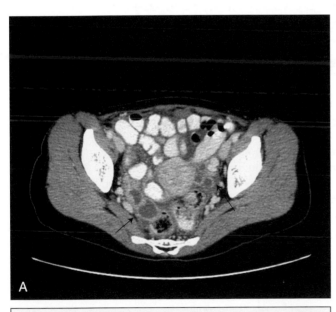

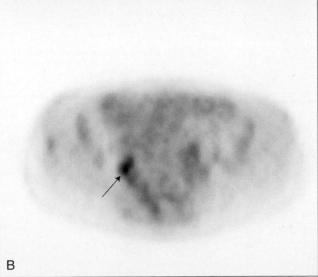

Figure 5-2. A 43-year-old woman referred to FDG-PET for suspicion of ovarian tumor. **A,** Axial contrast-enhanced CT image of the pelvis demonstrates complicated cystic structures in bilateral adnexae (*arrows*). **B,** Transverse PET image of the pelvis demonstrates increased metabolic activity in the adnexae up to 3.5 in maximum standardized uptake value (SUV) on the right (*arrow*) and 2.9 on the left (not shown). Subsequent surgical pathology showed acute–on-chronic salpingitis bilaterally. (We thank Dr. Pek Lan Khong at the Department of Diagnostic Radiology, University of Hong Kong for providing these images.)

Specific Tumor Characterization with Imaging

Preoperative characterization of an ovarian mass is of substantial clinical value for treatment planning. Although ovarian tumors may overlap in their clinical and radiologic features, certain specific imaging features may be present in certain types of ovarian tumors, and identification of these features may enable the reader to indicate a specific diagnosis or at least narrow the differential diagnosis considerably.[59]

Imaging findings for specific tumor characterization follow gross pathologic features. For example, *epithelial tumors* typically are primarily cystic—either unilocular or multilocular—and when malignant, they are associated with varying proportions of solid tissue.[51] Although the two most common types of epithelial tumors—serous and mucinous tumors—cannot always be differentiated based on their imaging appearances, certain features may suggest one diagnosis over the other. For example, a unilocular or multilocular cystic mass with a thin regular wall and septum, no soft tissues vegetations, and homogeneous CT attenuation or MRI signal intensity of the locules is most likely a benign serous cystadenoma.[59] A benign mucinous cystadenoma can be similar in appearance to a benign serous cystadenoma except that the mucinous tumor may contain liquids of different CT attenuation or MRI signal intensity, thus giving a "mosaic" pattern.[59] Mucinous cystadenomas also tend to be larger than their serous counterparts at presentation.

Although it has been suggested that lesions smaller than 4 cm in diameter are more likely to be benign,[60] a significant overlap in size exists between benign and malignant lesions, limiting the value of size criteria. Large benign ovarian tumors are occasionally seen and can remain clinically silent as they grow,[52] whereas the primary serous cystadenocarcinomas can be quite small and manifest as peritoneal carcinomatosis. Generally speaking, a greater amount of soft tissue components (e.g., irregular cystic wall and septum greater than 3 mm in thickness, or endocystic or exocystic vegetations) is suggestive of a greater likelihood of malignancy. A large soft tissue component with necrosis is also suggestive of malignancy.[46] However, benign masses such as cystadenofibromas could contain solid components and cannot be differentiated from malignant tumors by either the size of the solid portion or the intensity of contrast enhancement, and occasionally an ovarian epithelial tumor of low malignant potential may appear purely cystic on imaging[53,61] (Fig. 5-3).

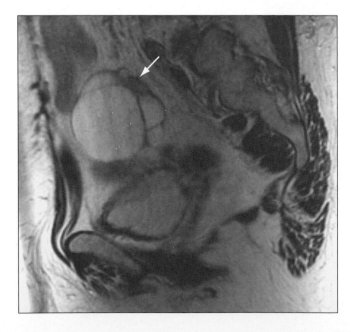

Figure 5-3. A 57-year-old woman with lymphoma.   Sagittal T2-weighted MRI demonstrates a multiloculated cystic mass with internal soft tissue nodularity (*arrow*) and multiple septations. Subsequent surgical pathology demonstrated a serous cystadenofibroma.

Papillary projections found on an imaging study are thought to constitute an important predictor of the diagnosis of epithelial ovarian tumors and may even correlate with the aggressiveness of the tumor.[59] These projections are usually absent in benign epithelial tumors, and, if present, they are generally small. Papillary projections can be profuse in epithelial tumors with low malignant potential. Although they can be in invasive epithelial carcinomas, their gross appearance is often dominated by a solid component.[59] However, these features do not allow confident differentiation of epithelial tumors with low malignant potential from invasive tumors.[62]

Ancillary findings such as ascites, tumor implants in the abdomen or pelvis, adenopathy, and adjacent organ invasion further increase confidence in the diagnosis of an ovarian malignancy. Bilateral primary ovarian tumors with peritoneal carcinomatosis are seen more frequently in serous than in mucinous cystadenocarcinomas, whereas mucinous adenocarcinomas can rupture and lead to pseudomyxoma peritonei.[59]

Endometrioid and clear cell carcinomas are the most common malignant neoplasms arising from endometriosis. Therefore, an endometrioma with solid components suggests malignancy and must be removed.[52,63,64] The imaging features of endometrioid ovarian carcinomas are nonspecific and include a large complex cystic mass with solid components.[59] However, 15% to 30% of endometrioid carcinomas are associated with synchronous endometrial carcinoma or hyperplasia, which manifests as concurrent endometrial thickening on imaging.[51,52,63] The imaging features of clear cell carcinomas are also nonspecific; however, clear cell carcinoma commonly presents as a large unilocular cystic lesion with solid protrusions, which tend to be round and sparse[65] (Fig. 5-4). Although benign endometriomas are typically T1 hyperintense and T2 hypointense on MRI, the signal intensity of clear cell carcinomas is variable.[65]

Fat in an adnexal mass is typically diagnostic of a **mature teratoma**. On ultrasound, the sebaceous material in a mature teratoma typically manifests as diffuse or partial echogenicity within the mass. However, increased echogenicity is not specific, and the presence of fat should be definitively confirmed with CT or MRI. On CT, a negative attenuation is indicative of fat. On MRI, fat is hyperintense on T1-weighted images and suppressed in signal on chemically selective fat suppression sequences. Mature teratomas often contain a protuberance projecting into the cystic cavity known as the Rokitansky nodule, which may contain hair, bone, or teeth[66] (Fig. 5-5). Rokitansky nodules are typically densely echogenic on ultrasound and may be associated with calcifications on CT. In addition, calcifications may also be present in the septations or wall of the mass. However, benign mature teratomas have a broad

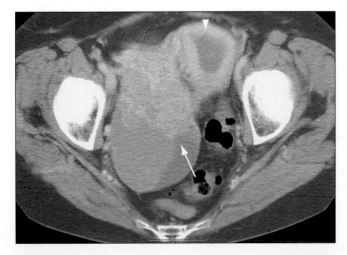

Figure 5-4. A 62-year-old woman with a history of breast cancer, presenting with an adnexal mass.   Axial contrast-enhanced CT image demonstrates a large complex cystic mass in the right adnexa, with large heterogeneous and irregular soft tissue components (*arrow*). In addition, the endometrial stripe also appears thickened on CT (*arrowhead*). Subsequent surgical pathology demonstrated a clear cell carcinoma of the right ovary, and endometrial polyp in the uterus.

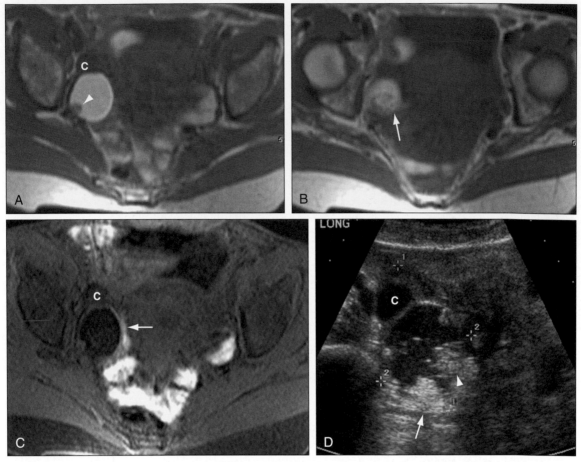

Figure 5-5. A 52-year-old woman with a history of breast cancer. **A,** Unenhanced axial T1-weighted MRI demonstrates a T1-hyperintense mass in the right ovary with a small mural nodule (*arrowhead*). **B,** Unenhanced axial T1-weighted MR image through the lower portion of the mass demonstrates amorphous material at the dependent portion of the mass (*arrow*). **C,** Axial unenhanced T1-weighted fat-saturated image demonstrates suppression of the signal within the right ovarian mass (*arrow*), indicating that this is a fat-containing lesion. **D,** Transverse ultrasound image of the right ovary illustrates the cystic mass in the right ovary with mural nodule (*arrowhead*) and echogenic material in the dependent portion (*arrow*). Subsequent surgical pathology confirmed that this was a mature cystic teratoma. C, an incidental simple cyst in the right ovary.

spectrum of imaging findings, which may overlap with those of a malignant mass. For example, a mature teratoma may manifest as a mixed mass with all the components of the three germ cell layers and demonstrate a complex appearance, or it may be purely cystic in nature, containing locules of fluid with septations, mimicking an epithelial tumor.[59]

A malignant *immature teratoma* may contain mature tissue elements similar to those seen in mature cystic teratomas, including small foci of fat. However, unlike mature teratomas, immature teratomas typically have prominent solid components with internal necrosis or hemorrhage, may contain scattered (rather than localized) calcifications, may demonstrate rapid growth, and may have a capsule that is not well defined, or may be perforated or ruptured.[66,67]

Dysgerminoma is the ovarian counterpart of seminoma of the testis.[67] Characteristic findings such as multilobulated solid ovarian masses with fibrovascular septa that demonstrate prominent flow on ultrasound or significant enhancement on CT or MR have been reported.[68,69] Calcification may be present in a speckled pattern. Necrotic and hemorrhagic areas may also be in the tumor.[59]

In addition to endometrioid carcinomas, sex cord-stromal tumors may also be associated with endometrial abnormality due to their estrogen-producing capabilities. The hyperestrogenemia may produce combined endometrial hyperplasia, polyps, or carcinoma.[59] The most common malignant sex cord-stromal tumors are *granulosa cell tumors* of the ovary, which have variable appearances on imaging, ranging from homogeneous solid masses, to heterogeneous tumors with varying degrees of hemorrhagic or fibrotic changes, to multilocular cystic lesions, to thick-walled or thin-walled unilocular cystic tumors.[59,70] In contrast to epithelial tumors, granulosa cell tumors do not have endocystic papillary projections, are less likely to cause peritoneal seeding, and are more likely to be confined to the ovary at the time of diagnosis.[59] The associated estrogenic effects on the uterus may manifest as uterine enlargement or as endometrial thickening or hemorrhage.[71,72]

Ovarian masses with fibrous components include fibroma, fibrothecoma, cystadenofibroma, Brenner tumor, and Sertoli-Leydig cell tumor.[59] Sertoli-Leydig cell tumor is rare and occurs most often in young adults. Approximately one third of female patients with Sertoli-Leydig cell tumors present with progressive masculinization owing to excess testosterone secreted by the tumor (Fig. 5-6). *Fibroma* is the most

Figure 5-6. A 15-year-old girl presenting with amenorrhea, obesity, and hirsutism.
A, Transverse ultrasound image of the pelvis demonstrates a heterogeneous mass that is mostly solid in the right ovary. **B,** Color Doppler image demonstrates blood flow within the solid components of the ovarian mass. Subsequent surgical pathology showed a right ovarian Sertoli-Leydig cell tumor. (We thank Dr. Pek Lan Khong at the Department of Diagnostic Radiology, University of Hong Kong for providing these images.)

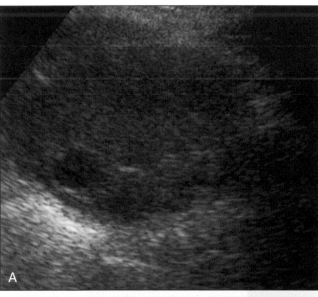

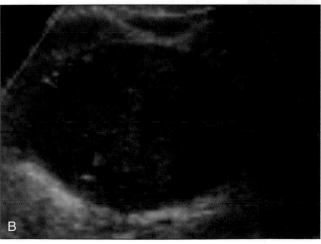

there is no difference in the detection of abdominal disease with these two modalities.[89] Similar to CT, MRI is highly accurate in predicting inoperable tumor and suboptimal debulking preoperatively in newly diagnosed ovarian cancer, with reported positive and negative predictive values higher than 90%.[89,92] This suggests that imaging may help to select patients who might be more appropriately managed by neoadjuvant chemotherapy.[92] For disease in the greater omentum and lesser sac, MRI is less accurate.[85]

Fused PET-CT is particularly helpful when implants are present on or near bowel loops.[55] Metastatic lesions from ovarian cancer including peritoneal implants and metastatic lymph nodes are FDG-avid,[55] although necrosis within a tumor and/or lymph node can appear as a photopenic area.[55] Standardized uptake values (SUV) should be routinely measured and reported. It is generally accepted that a standardized uptake value of less than 2 to 3 indicates malignancy.

When thoracic metastases are present, increased uptake may be seen in the pleural effusions and thoracic adenopathy.[55] However, one pitfall is that metastases from mucinous adenocarcinoma of the ovary may not be associated with increased metabolic activity and could be underdiagnosed by PET (Fig. 5-11). In the abdomen, FDG-PET was found to be more sensitive in the retroperitoneal than in the intraperitoneal region.[93] The data regarding combined FDG-PET/CT in the evaluation of ovarian malignancy are still emerging. In a study by Yoshida and colleagues[94] on preoperative tumor staging, CT alone had an accuracy of 53%, whereas FDG-PET evaluated in conjunction with CT had an accuracy of 87%. Another study demonstrated that FDG-PET and CT had a relatively low sensitivity for the detection of peritoneal metastases, indicating that surgical staging should remain the gold standard. Nevertheless, FDG-PET had a higher specificity and may be useful for evaluating residual or recurrent disease after surgery.

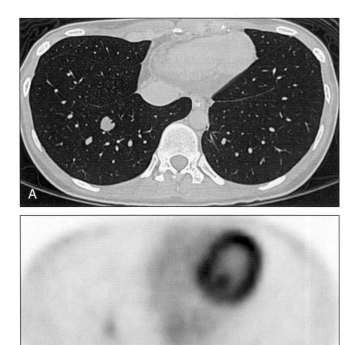

Figure 5-11. A 22-year-old woman with metastatic mucinous adenocarcinoma of the ovary. A, Axial contrast-enhanced CT image of the thorax displayed in lung window demonstrates a lobulated nodule in the right lower lobe. Multiple additional nodules are present in the lungs (not shown). **B,** Axial FDG-PET image of the thorax shows a maximum standardized uptake value of only 1.0 in the right lower lobe nodule. Subsequent surgical pathology confirmed this nodule to be a metastasis from the ovarian mucinous adenocarcinoma. (We thank Dr. Pek Lan Khong at the Department of Diagnostic Radiology, University of Hong Kong for providing these images.)

Follow-up

A number of approaches are used to detect recurrent disease after initial surgery and chemotherapy for ovarian cancer. These approaches include physical examination, determination of serum CA-125 levels, and imaging. CT, MRI, and PET all have been used to evaluate ovarian cancer recurrence.[55]

Recurrent ovarian malignancy may manifest as pelvic masses, peritoneal seeding, malignant ascites, and nodal recurrence (Fig. 5-12). Occasionally recurrent disease may present as pleuropulmonary lesions and liver metastasis.[95] Pelvic recurrence may involve the vaginal stump, parametria, urinary bladder, and/or bowel adjacent to the surgical bed. Peritoneal seeding presents as nodules on the peritoneal surface, most commonly around the liver or cul-de-sac, and mesenteric infiltration. Unusual manifestations include metastasis in the extrahepatic abdominal solid organs, bone metastasis, and an abdominal wall lesion involving subcutaneous fat or muscle.[95] Accurate detection of recurrent ovarian malignancy by imaging facilitates accurate diagnosis and prompt treatment.

CT is the primary imaging modality to prove macroscopic disease recurrence and can spare patients from the invasive restaging of second-look laparotomy.[96] Patients treated for ovarian cancer can be followed up with serial CT of the abdomen and pelvis. CT of the chest is generally not indicated, unless no sites of recurrence are

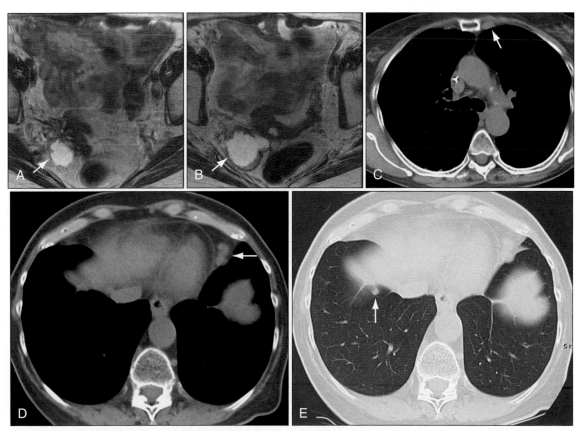

Figure 5-12. A 69-year-old woman with recurrent ovarian cancer after surgery. A and B, Axial T2-weighted MRI images demonstrate a complex cystic mass in the right pelvis with tethering of adjacent bowel loops (*arrow*). C and D, Unenhanced axial CT images of the thorax also demonstrate new adenopathy (*arrows*) in the left internal mammary and supradiaphragmatic regions suspicious for metastases. E, Axial unenhanced CT image of the chest in lung window demonstrates a new nodule (*arrow*) at the right lung base, also suspicious for metastasis.

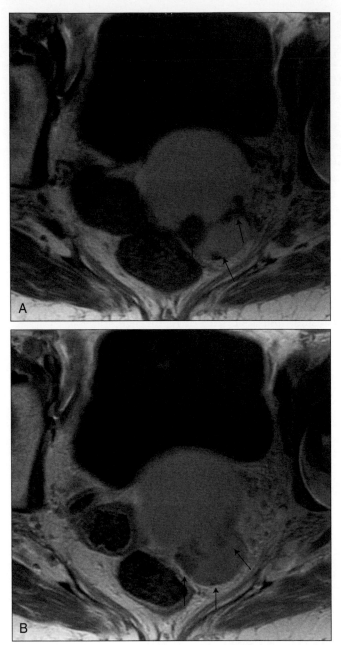

Figure 5-13. A 50-year-old woman with recurrent ovarian mullerian carcinoma after surgery.   A, Axial T1-weighted unenhanced MRI of the pelvis demonstrates a complex cystic lesion containing moderately T1-hyperintense fluid and multiple mural nodules (*arrows*) between the bladder and rectum. **B,** Axial T1-weighted contrast-enhanced MR image of the pelvis demonstrates increased signal in the mural nodules (*arrows*) compared with the unenhanced images, indicative of the presence of solid enhancing soft tissue.

detected on CT in the presence of elevated tumor marker.[88,97] Gadolinium-enhanced MRI is also a valuable diagnostic tool in patients with ovarian cancer (Fig. 5-13). An abnormal MRI examination result with a normal CA-125 value is a strong indication of residual or recurrent tumor.[98] It has been reported that gadolinium-enhanced spoiled gradient-echo MRI depicts residual tumor in women with treated ovarian cancer, with an accuracy, positive predictive value, and negative predictive value that are comparable to those of laparotomy and superior to those of serum CA-125 values alone.[99] However, neither CT nor MRI can confidently exclude microscopic disease.[96]

Usually patients with the bulk of the tumor burden in the pelvis are selected for secondary cytoreduction. Two types of pelvic recurrence may be present: central recurrence and pelvic sidewall recurrence.[22] The size of a pelvic mass is not an indicator of surgical outcome; however, the extension of a mass to the pelvic sidewall is. MRI may be superior to CT in the assessment of pelvic wall extension because of its high soft tissue contrast and multiplanar capability. The presence of a fat plane at least 3 mm thick on imaging between the tumor and pelvic sidewall is considered necessary for resection.[22] Pelvic sidewall invasion and large bowel obstruction are significant indicators of tumor nonresectability, although invasion of the bladder and rectum by itself is not a contraindication to definitive surgical therapy (pelvic exenteration may be considered in select cases). Preoperative imaging is essential in patients considered for potential secondary cytoreductive surgery, so that the presence of tumor elsewhere and any indicators of nonresectability can be identified.[22]

Multiple standard uptake value comparisons may be helpful for evaluation of tumor response to treatment, although variations in measurement are sometimes attributed to the difference in scanners, scanner dose, and postinjection imaging time. Mixed results have been reported regarding the value of FDG-PET in evaluating recurrent ovarian cancer.[54] One preliminary study suggested that in the follow-up of patients with ovarian cancer, FDG-PET could detect recurrence with higher accuracy than CT, and even with higher sensitivity than the tumor marker CA-125, with the additional advantage of being able to localize the site of recurrence.[100] However, other studies found that in the diagnosis of recurrent ovarian cancer, FDG-PET had a limited ability to detect small tumors and did not yield higher overall accuracy than CT.[101-103] Nevertheless, FDG-PET/CT has been found to have a higher accuracy in identifying recurrent ovarian tumor nodules that are at least 1 cm in size among patients with biochemical evidence of recurrence and negative or equivocal conventional CT findings, thus facilitating timely surgical cytoreduction.[104]

The sensitivity of PET is low in patients with clinically occult recurrence of ovarian cancer.[105] However, the sensitivity of FDG-PET in detecting recurrent ovarian cancer is higher in patients with clinically suspected relapse than in patients judged clinically disease-free. Therefore, FDG-PET may be useful in patients with clinically suspected recurrence but with negative or equivocal anatomic imaging findings.[55,106,107] When combined with clinical parameters such as CA-125 level, the sensitivity of FDG-PET can be as high as 97.8% in detecting recurrent ovarian cancer.[108] The combination of FDG-PET and CA-125 titer is therefore useful for an accurate detection of recurrence.

The reported specificity of PET in the detection of recurrent ovarian cancer ranges widely—from 42% up to 100%.[101,103,105,106,109,110] Physiologic activity in the abdomen and pelvis is one of the factors that can potentially affect the specificity of PET.[55] Physiologic uptake of FDG can be seen in the gastrointestinal tract, liver, and spleen, in addition to the urinary tract, since FDG is excreted by the kidneys. Therefore, digital fusion of PET and CT scan images allows for better differentiation between physiologic and pathologic activity on PET, and for lesions that are truly pathologic, enables accurate localization for treatment planning[111] (Fig. 5-14). Although Drieskens and associates[93] demonstrated that FDG-PET and CT have relatively low sensitivity for the detection of peritoneal metastases compared with surgical staging, FDG-PET has a higher specificity and may be useful for evaluating residual or recurrent disease after surgery. Overall, it appears that FDG-PET has the advantages of a high positive predictive value in detecting recurrent or residual disease after treatment.[102,104]

Such mixed results may be partially attributable to the fact that non-neoplastic hypermetabolic lesions are frequently present in post-treatment patients. These lesions include granulomatous disease, abscess, surgical changes, radiation changes, inflammation, and foreign body reaction. Therefore, consultation with the simultaneously obtained CT images, especially contrast-enhanced CT images, may help to reveal the nature of these FDG-avid non-neoplastic processes. It may be prudent to

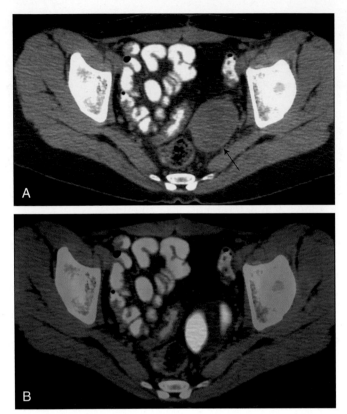

Figure 5-14. A 29-year-old woman with endometrioid adenocarcinoma arising from an endometriotic cyst, presented with elevated CA-125 after surgery and chemotherapy. A, Axial unenhanced CT image of the pelvis demonstrates a heterogeneous oval mass (arrow) in the left pelvis. **B,** Axial FDG-PET image fused with the CT image demonstrates increased metabolic activity in the mass with standardized uptake values of up to 7.7. Subsequent surgical pathology showed adenocarcinoma with clear cell and endometrioid components. (We thank Dr. Pek Lan Khong at the Department of Diagnostic Radiology, University of Hong Kong for providing these images.)

wait at least 6 weeks before PET/CT is performed to evaluate the surgical or irradiated bed. Integration of clinical information in the interpretation process may further increase specificity.

Overall FDG-PET has been shown to have a prognostic value similar to that of second-look laparotomy, and can substitute for second-look laparotomy in the follow-up of patients who have had ovarian carcinoma, especially when there is a high risk of recurrence.[112] Therefore, FDG-PET can reduce unnecessary invasive staging procedures and save health care costs when used appropriately in the management of patients with recurrent ovarian cancer.[113] Furthermore, precise localization of recurrent tumor during surgical treatment is often difficult, owing to limited tumor size and postsurgical anatomic modifications. It has been reported that the use of an FDG-sensitive surgical gamma probe combined with preoperative PET/CT image fusion can help to detect occult metastasis and guide laparoscopic excision in the patient with recurrent ovarian cancer.[114]

Conclusion

Imaging is essential for ovarian cancer detection, diagnosis, management, and treatment follow-up. Transvaginal ultrasound is the most promising imaging modality for routine screening for ovarian cancer in patients with inherited high risk. For patients presenting with pertinent symptoms, imaging workup generally includes ultrasound or CT of the abdomen and pelvis for lesion detection and characterization. MRI of the pelvis or abdomen is often reserved as a problem-solving tool. CT, PET, and PET/CT are the imaging modalities most frequently used for treatment follow-up.

References

1. Im SS, Gordon AN, Buttin BM, et al: Validation of referral guidelines for women with pelvic masses. Obstet Gynecol 105(1):35–41, 2005.
2. Ries LAG, Harkins D, Krapcho M, et al: SEER Cancer Statistics Review, 1975–2003. Bethesda, MD: National Cancer Institute. http://seer.cancer.gov/csr/1975_2003/ (Accessed August 2006).
3. Brinton LA, Lamb EJ, Moghissi KS, et al: Ovarian cancer risk associated with varying causes of infertility. Fertil Steril 82(2):405–414, 2004.
4. Rossing MA, Tang MT, Flagg EW, et al: A case-control study of ovarian cancer in relation to infertility and the use of ovulation-inducing drugs. Am J Epidemiol 160(11):1070–1078, 2004.
5. Rossouw JE, Anderson GL, Prentice RL, et al: Risks and benefits of estrogen plus progestin in healthy postmenopausal women: principal results from the Women's Health Initiative randomized controlled trial. JAMA 288(3):321–333, 2002.
6. Rubin SC, Blackwood MA, Bandera C, et al: BRCA1, BRCA2, and hereditary nonpolyposis colorectal cancer gene mutations in an unselected ovarian cancer population: relationship to family history and implications for genetic testing. Am J Obstet Gynecol 178(4):670–677, 1998.
7. Risch HA, McLaughlin JR, Cole DE, et al: Prevalence and penetrance of germline BRCA1 and BRCA2 mutations in a population series of 649 women with ovarian cancer. Am J Hum Genet 68(3):700–710, 2001.
8. Pal T, Permuth-Wey J, Betts JA, et al: BRCA1 and BRCA2 mutations account for a large proportion of ovarian carcinoma cases. Cancer 104(12):2807–2816, 2005.
9. Struewing JP, Hartge P, Wacholder S, et al: The risk of cancer associated with specific mutations of BRCA1 and BRCA2 among Ashkenazi Jews. N Engl J Med 336(20):1401–1408, 1997.
10. Ford D, Easton DF, Stratton M, et al: Genetic heterogeneity and penetrance analysis of the BRCA1 and BRCA2 genes in breast cancer families. The Breast Cancer Linkage Consortium. Am J Hum Genet 62(3):676–689, 1998.
11. Antoniou A, Pharoah PD, Narod S, et al: Average risks of breast and ovarian cancer associated with BRCA1 or BRCA2 mutations detected in case series unselected for family history: a combined analysis of 22 studies. Am J Hum Genet 72(5):1117–1130, 2003.
12. Dunlop MG, Farrington SM, Carothers AD, et al: Cancer risk associated with germline DNA mismatch repair gene mutations. Hum Mol Genet 6(1):105–110, 1997.
13. Aarnio M, Sankila R, Pukkala E, et al: Cancer risk in mutation carriers of DNA-mismatch-repair genes. Int J Cancer 81(2):214–218, 1999.
14. Kerlikowske K, Brown JS, Grady DG: Should women with familial ovarian cancer undergo prophylactic oophorectomy? Obstet Gynecol 80(4):700–707, 1992.
15. Stratton JF, Pharoah P, Smith SK, et al: A systematic review and meta-analysis of family history and risk of ovarian cancer. Br J Obstet Gynaecol 105(5):493–499, 1998.
16. Bergfeldt K, Rydh B, Granath F, et al: Risk of ovarian cancer in breast-cancer patients with a family history of breast or ovarian cancer: a population-based cohort study. Lancet 360(9337):891–894, 2002.
17. van Nagell JR, Jr, DePriest PD, Reedy MB, et al: The efficacy of transvaginal sonographic screening in asymptomatic women at risk for ovarian cancer. Gynecol Oncol 77(3):350–356, 2000.
18. Buys SS, Partridge E, Greene MH, et al: Ovarian cancer screening in the Prostate, Lung, Colorectal and Ovarian (PLCO) cancer screening trial: findings from the initial screen of a randomized trial. Am J Obstet Gynecol 193(5):1630–1639, 2005.
19. Rieber A, Nussle K, Stohr I, et al: Preoperative diagnosis of ovarian tumors with MR imaging: comparison with transvaginal sonography, positron emission tomography, and histologic findings. AJR Am J Roentgenol 177(1):123–129, 2001.
20. Timmerman D, Schwarzler P, Collins WP, et al: Subjective assessment of adnexal masses with the use of ultrasonography: an analysis of interobserver variability and experience. Ultrasound Obstet Gynecol 13(1):11–16, 1999.
21. Valentin L: Gray scale sonography, subjective evaluation of the color Doppler image and measurement of blood flow velocity for distinguishing benign and malignant tumors of suspected adnexal origin. Eur J Obstet Gynecol Reprod Biol 72(1):63–72, 1997.
22. Mironov S, Akin O, Pandit-Taskar N, Hann LE: Ovarian cancer. Radiol Clin North Am 45(1):149–166, 2007.
23. Brown DL, Doubilet PM, Miller FH, et al: Benign and malignant ovarian masses: selection of the most discriminating gray-scale and Doppler sonographic features. Radiology 208(1): 103–110, 1998.
24. Guerriero S, Alcazar JL, Coccia ME, et al: Complex pelvic mass as a target of evaluation of vessel distribution by color Doppler sonography for the diagnosis of adnexal malignancies: results of a multicenter European study. J Ultrasound Med 21(10):1105–1111, 2002.
25. Salem S, Wilson SR: Gynecologic ultrasound. In Rumack CM, Wilson SR, Charboneau JW, et al (eds): Diagnostic Ultrasound, 2nd ed. Philadelphia: Mosby, 2005.
26. Fleischer AC, Rodgers WH, Rao BK, et al: Assessment of ovarian tumor vascularity with transvaginal color Doppler sonography. J Ultrasound Med 10(10):563–568, 1991.
27. Bourne T, Campbell S, Steer C, et al: Transvaginal colour flow imaging: a possible new screening technique for ovarian cancer. BMJ 299(6712):1367–1370, 1989.
28. Kurjak A, Zalud I, Alfirevic Z: Evaluation of adnexal masses with transvaginal color ultrasound. J Ultrasound Med 10(6):295–297, 1991.
29. Levine D, Feldstein VA, Babcook CJ, Filly RA: Sonography of ovarian masses: poor sensitivity of resistive index for identifying malignant lesions. AJR Am J Roentgenol 162(6):1355–1359, 1994.
30. Stein SM, Laifer-Narin S, Johnson MB, et al: Differentiation of benign and malignant adnexal masses: relative value of gray-scale, color Doppler, and spectral Doppler sonography. AJR Am J Roentgenol 164(2):381–386, 1995.
31. Salem S, White LM, Lai J: Doppler sonography of adnexal masses: the predictive value of the pulsatility index in benign and malignant disease. AJR Am J Roentgenol 163(5):1147–1150, 1994.
32. Jain KA: Prospective evaluation of adnexal masses with endovaginal gray-scale and duplex and color Doppler US: correlation with pathologic findings. Radiology 191(1):63–67, 1994.
33. Schelling M, Braun M, Kuhn W, et al: Combined transvaginal B-mode and color Doppler sonography for differential diagnosis of ovarian tumors: results of a multivariate logistic regression analysis. Gynecol Oncol 77(1):78–86, 2000.
34. Hamper UM, Sheth S, Abbas FM, et al: Transvaginal color Doppler sonography of adnexal masses: differences in blood flow impedance in benign and malignant lesions. AJR Am J Roentgenol 160(6):1225–1228, 1993.
35. Rehn M, Lohmann K, Rempen A: Transvaginal ultrasonography of pelvic masses: evaluation of B-mode technique and Doppler ultrasonography. Am J Obstet Gynecol 175(1):97–104, 1996.
36. Brown DL, Frates MC, Laing FC, et al: Ovarian masses: can benign and malignant lesions be differentiated with color and pulsed Doppler US? Radiology 190(2):333–336, 1994.
37. Buy JN, Ghossain MA, Hugol D, et al: Characterization of adnexal masses: combination of color Doppler and conventional sonography compared with spectral Doppler analysis alone and conventional sonography alone. AJR Am J Roentgenol 166(2):385–393, 1996.
38. Kinkel K, Hricak H, Lu Y, et al: US characterization of ovarian masses: a meta-analysis. Radiology 217(3):803–811, 2000.
39. Cohen LS, Escobar PF, Scharm C, et al: Three-dimensional power Doppler ultrasound improves the diagnostic accuracy for ovarian cancer prediction. Gynecol Oncol 82(1):40–48, 2001.
40. Kurjak A, Kupesic S, Sparac V, Bekavac I: Preoperative evaluation of pelvic tumors by Doppler and three-dimensional sonography. J Ultrasound Med 20(8):829–840, 2001.
41. Kurjak A, Kupesic S, Sparac V, et al: The detection of stage I ovarian cancer by three-dimensional sonography and power Doppler. Gynecol Oncol 90(2):258–264, 2003.
42. Medl M, Kulenkampff KJ, Stiskal M, et al: Magnetic resonance imaging in the preoperative evaluation of suspected ovarian masses. Anticancer Res 15(3):1123–1125, 1995.

43. Yamashita Y, Torashima M, Hatanaka Y, et al: Adnexal masses: accuracy of characterization with transvaginal US and precontrast and postcontrast MR imaging. Radiology 194(2):557–565, 1995.

44. Komatsu T, Konishi I, Mandai M, et al: Adnexal masses: transvaginal US and gadolinium-enhanced MR imaging assessment of intratumoral structure. Radiology 198(1):109–115, 1996.

45. Kurtz AB, Tsimikas JV, Tempany CM, et al: Diagnosis and staging of ovarian cancer: comparative values of Doppler and conventional US, CT, and MR imaging correlated with surgery and histopathologic analysis—report of the Radiology Diagnostic Oncology Group. Radiology 212(1):19–27, 1999.

46. Hricak H, Chen M, Coakley FV, et al: Complex adnexal masses: detection and characterization with MR imaging–multivariate analysis. Radiology 214(1):39–46, 2000.

47. Sohaib SA, Sahdev A, Van Trappen P, et al: Characterization of adnexal mass lesions on MR imaging. AJR Am J Roentgenol 180(5):1297–1304, 2003.

48. Kinkel K, Lu Y, Mehdizade A, et al: Indeterminate ovarian mass at US: incremental value of second imaging test for characterization–meta-analysis and Bayesian analysis. Radiology 236(1):85–94, 2005.

49. Tempany CM, Zou KH, Silverman SG, et al: Staging of advanced ovarian cancer: comparison of imaging modalities—report from the Radiological Diagnostic Oncology Group. Radiology 215(3):761–767, 2000.

50. Byrom J, Widjaja E, Redman CW, et al: Can pre-operative computed tomography predict resectability of ovarian carcinoma at primary laparotomy? BJOG 109(4):369–375, 2002.

51. Kawamoto S, Urban BA, Fishman EK: CT of epithelial ovarian tumors. Radiographics Spec No:S85–S102; quiz S103–S104, 1999.

52. Buy JN, Ghossain MA, Sciot C, et al: Epithelial tumors of the ovary: CT findings and correlation with US. Radiology 178(3):811–818, 1991.

53. Ghossain MA, Buy JN, Ligneres C, et al: Epithelial tumors of the ovary: comparison of MR and CT findings. Radiology 181(3):863–870, 1991.

54. Subhas N, Patel PV, Pannu HK, et al: Imaging of pelvic malignancies with in-line FDG PET-CT: case examples and common pitfalls of FDG PET. Radiographics 25(4):1031–1043, 2005.

55. Pannu HK, Bristow RE, Cohade C, et al: PET-CT in recurrent ovarian cancer: initial observations. Radiographics 24(1):209–223, 2004.

56. Antoch G, Freudenberg LS, Stattaus J, et al: Whole-body positron emission tomography-CT: optimized CT using oral and IV contrast materials. AJR Am J Roentgenol 179(6):1555–1560, 2002.

57. Dizendorf EV, Treyer V, Von Schulthess GK, Hany TF: Application of oral contrast media in coregistered positron emission tomography-CT. AJR Am J Roentgenol 179(2):477–481, 2002.

58. Fenchel S, Grab D, Nuessle K, et al: Asymptomatic adnexal masses: correlation of FDG PET and histopathologic findings. Radiology 223(3):780–788, 2002.

59. Jung SE, Lee JM, Rha SE, et al: CT and MR imaging of ovarian tumors with emphasis on differential diagnosis. Radiographics 22(6):1305–1325, 2002.

60. Occhipinti KA: Computed tomography and magnetic resonance imaging of the ovary. In Anderson JC (eds) Gynecologic Imaging. London: Churchill Livingstone, 1999, pp 345–359.

61. Fukuda T, Ikeuchi M, Hashimoto H, et al: Computed tomography of ovarian masses. J Comput Assist Tomogr 10(6):990–996, 1986.

62. Exacoustos C, Romanini ME, Rinaldo D, et al: Preoperative sonographic features of borderline ovarian tumors. Ultrasound Obstet Gynecol 25(1):50–59, 2005.

63. Wagner BJ, Buck JL, Seidman JD, McCabe KM: From the archives of the AFIP. Ovarian epithelial neoplasms: radiologic-pathologic correlation. Radiographics 14(6):1351–1374; quiz 1375–1376, 1994.

64. Wu TT, Coakley FV, Qayyum A, et al: Magnetic resonance imaging of ovarian cancer arising in endometriomas. J Comput Assist Tomogr 28(6):836–838, 2004.

65. Matsuoka Y, Ohtomo K, Araki T, et al: MR imaging of clear cell carcinoma of the ovary. Eur Radiol 11(6):946–951, 2001.

66. Outwater EK, Siegelman ES, Hunt JL: Ovarian teratomas: tumor types and imaging characteristics. Radiographics 21(2):475–490, 2001.

67. Brammer HM III, Buck JL, Hayes WS, et al: From the archives of the AFIP. Malignant germ cell tumors of the ovary: radiologic-pathologic correlation. Radiographics 10(4):715–724, 1990.

68. Kim SH, Kang SB: Ovarian dysgerminoma: color Doppler ultrasonographic findings and comparison with CT and MR imaging findings. J Ultrasound Med 14(11):843–848, 1995.

69. Tanaka YO, Kurosaki Y, Nishida M, et al: Ovarian dysgerminoma: MR and CT appearance. J Comput Assist Tomogr 18(3):443–448, 1994.

70. Ko SF, Wan YL, Ng SH, et al: Adult ovarian granulosa cell tumors: spectrum of sonographic and CT findings with pathologic correlation. AJR Am J Roentgenol 172(5):1227–1233, 1999.

71. Outwater EK, Wagner BJ, Mannion C, et al: Sex cord-stromal and steroid cell tumors of the ovary. Radiographics 18(6):1523–1546, 1998.

72. Morikawa K, Hatabu H, Togashi K, et al:. Granulosa cell tumor of the ovary: MR findings. J Comput Assist Tomogr 21(6):1001–1004, 1997.

73. Bazot M, Ghossain MA, Buy JN, et al: Fibrothecomas of the ovary: CT and US findings. J Comput Assist Tomogr 17(5):754–759, 1993.

74. Troiano RN, Lazzarini KM, Scoutt LM, et al: Fibroma and fibrothecoma of the ovary: MR imaging findings. Radiology 204(3):795–798, 1997.

75. Kim SH, Sim JS, Seong CK: Interface vessels on color/power Doppler US and MRI: a clue to differentiate subserosal uterine myomas from extrauterine tumors. J Comput Assist Tomogr 25(1):36–42, 2001.

76. Torashima M, Yamashita Y, Matsuno Y, et al: The value of detection of flow voids between the uterus and the leiomyoma with MRI. J Magn Reson Imaging 8(2):427–431, 1998.

77. Kim SH, Kim YJ, Park BK, et al: Collision tumors of the ovary associated with teratoma: clues to the correct preoperative diagnosis. J Comput Assist Tomogr 23(6):929–933, 1999.

78. Demopoulos RI, Touger L, Dubin N: Secondary ovarian carcinoma: a clinical and pathological evaluation. Int J Gynecol Pathol 6(2):166–175, 1987.

79. Young RH, Scully RE: Metastatic tumors in the ovary: a problem-oriented approach and review of the recent literature. Semin Diagn Pathol 8(4):250–276, 1991.

80. Mazur MT, Hsueh S, Gersell DJ: Metastases to the female genital tract. Analysis of 325 cases. Cancer 53(9):1978–1984, 1984.

81. Cho KC, Gold BM: Computed tomography of Krukenberg tumors. AJR Am J Roentgenol 145(2):285–288, 1985.

82. Megibow AJ, Hulnick DH, Bosniak MA, Balthazar EJ: Ovarian metastases: computed tomographic appearances. Radiology 156(1):161–164, 1985.

83. Brown DL, Zou KH, Tempany CM, et al: Primary versus secondary ovarian malignancy: imaging findings of adnexal masses in the Radiology Diagnostic Oncology Group Study. Radiology 219(1):213–218, 2001.

84. Dvoretsky PM, Richards KA, Angel C, et al: Survival time, causes of death, and tumor/treatment-related morbidity in 100 women with ovarian cancer. Hum Pathol 19(11):1273–1279, 1988.

85. Ricke J, Sehouli J, Hach C, et al: Prospective evaluation of contrast-enhanced MRI in the depiction of peritoneal spread in primary or recurrent ovarian cancer. Eur Radiol 13(5):943–949, 2003.

86. Harisinghani MG, Saini S, Weissleder R, et al: MR lymphangiography using ultrasmall superparamagnetic iron oxide in patients with primary abdominal and pelvic malignancies: radiographic-pathologic correlation. AJR Am J Roentgenol 172(5):1347–1351, 1999.

87. Bellin MF, Roy C, Kinkel K, et al: Lymph node metastases: safety and effectiveness of MR imaging with ultrasmall superparamagnetic iron oxide particles—initial clinical experience. Radiology 207(3):799–808, 1998.

88. Sella T, Rosenbaum E, Edelmann DZ, et al: Value of chest CT scans in routine ovarian carcinoma follow-up. AJR Am J Roentgenol 177(4):857–859, 2001.

89. Forstner R, Hricak H, Occhipinti KA, et al: Ovarian cancer: staging with CT and MR imaging. Radiology 197(3):619–626, 1995.

90. Coakley FV, Choi PH, Gougoutas CA, et al: Peritoneal metastases: detection with spiral CT in patients with ovarian cancer. Radiology 223(2):495–499, 2002.

91. Stevens SK, Hricak H, Stern JL: Ovarian lesions: detection and characterization with gadolinium-enhanced MR imaging at 1.5 T. Radiology 181(2):481–488, 1991.

92. Qayyum A, Coakley FV, Westphalen AC, et al: Role of CT and MR imaging in predicting optimal cytoreduction of newly diagnosed primary epithelial ovarian cancer. Gynecol Oncol 96(2): 301–306, 2005.

93. Drieskens O, Stroobants S, Gysen M, et al: Positron emission tomography with FDG in the detection of peritoneal and retroperitoneal metastases of ovarian cancer. Gynecol Obstet Invest 55(3):130–134, 2003.

94. Yoshida Y, Kurokawa T, Kawahara K, et al: Incremental benefits of FDG positron emission tomography over CT alone for the preoperative staging of ovarian cancer. AJR Am J Roentgenol 182(1):227–233, 2004

95. Park CM, Kim SH, Kim SH, et al: Recurrent ovarian malignancy: patterns and spectrum of imaging findings. Abdom Imaging 28(3):404–415, 2003.

96. Prayer L, Kainz C, Kramer J, et al: CT and MR accuracy in the detection of tumor recurrence in patients treated for ovarian cancer. J Comput Assist Tomogr 7(4):626–632, 1993.

97. Dachman AH, Visweswaran A, Battula R, et al: Role of chest CT in the follow-up of ovarian adenocarcinoma. AJR Am J Roentgenol 176(3):701–705, 2001.

98. Low RN, Saleh F, Song SY, et al: Treated ovarian cancer: comparison of MR imaging with serum CA-125 level and physical examination—a longitudinal study. Radiology 211(2):519–528, 1999.

99. Low RN, Duggan B, Barone RM, et al: Treated ovarian cancer: MR imaging, laparotomy reassessment, and serum CA-125 values compared with clinical outcome at 1 year. Radiology 235(3):918–926, 2005.

100. Garcia Velloso MJ, Boan Garcia JF, Villar Luque LM, et al: [F-18-FDG positron emission tomography in the diagnosis of ovarian recurrence. Comparison with CT scan and CA 125]. Rev Esp Med Nucl 22(4):217–223, 2003.

101. Cho SM, Ha HK, Byun JY, et al: Usefulness of FDG PET for assessment of early recurrent epithelial ovarian cancer. AJR Am J Roentgenol 179(2):391–395, 2002.

102. Sironi S, Messa C, Mangili G, et al: Integrated FDG PET/CT in patients with persistent ovarian cancer: correlation with histologic findings. Radiology 233(2):433–440, 2004.

103. Kubik-Huch RA, Dorffler W, von Schulthess GK, et al: Value of (18F)-FDG positron emission tomography, computed tomography, and magnetic resonance imaging in diagnosing primary and recurrent ovarian carcinoma. Eur Radiol 10(5):761–767, 2000.

104. Bristow RE, del Carmen MG, Pannu HK, et al: Clinically occult recurrent ovarian cancer: patient selection for secondary cytoreductive surgery using combined PET/CT. Gynecol Oncol 90(3):519–528, 2003.

105. Rose PG, Faulhaber P, Miraldi F, Abdul-Karim FW: Positive emission tomography for evaluating a complete clinical response in patients with ovarian or peritoneal carcinoma: correlation with second-look laparotomy. Gynecol Oncol 82(1):17–21, 2001.

106. Zimny M, Siggelkow W, Schroder W, et al: 2-[Fluorine-18]-fluoro-2-deoxy-d-glucose positron emission tomography in the diagnosis of recurrent ovarian cancer. Gynecol Oncol 83(2):310–315, 2001.

107. Nanni C, Rubello D, Farsad M, et al: (18)F-FDG PET/CT in the evaluation of recurrent ovarian cancer: a prospective study on forty-one patients. Eur J Surg Oncol 31(7):792 797, 2005.

108. Murakami M, Miyamoto T, Iida T, et al: Whole-body positron emission tomography and tumor marker CA125 for detection of recurrence in epithelial ovarian cancer. Int J Gynecol Cancer 16 Suppl 1:99–107, 2006.

109. Torizuka T, Nobezawa S, Kanno T, et al: Ovarian cancer recurrence: role of whole-body positron emission tomography using 2-[fluorine-18]-fluoro-2-deoxy- D-glucose. Eur J Nucl Med Mol Imaging 29(6):797–803, 2002.

110. Yen RF, Sun SS, Shen YY, et al: Whole body positron emission tomography with 18F-fluoro-2-deoxyglucose for the detection of recurrent ovarian cancer. Anticancer Res 21(5):3691–3694, 2001.

111. Schaffler GJ, Groell R, Schoellnast H, et al: Digital image fusion of CT and PET data sets–clinical value in abdominal/pelvic malignancies. J Comput Assist Tomogr 24(4):644–647, 2000.

112. Kim S, Chung JK, Kang SB, et al: [18F]FDG PET as a substitute for second-look laparotomy in patients with advanced ovarian carcinoma. Eur J Nucl Med Mol Imaging 31(2):196–201, 2004.

113. Smith GT, Hubner KF, McDonald T, Thie JA: Cost analysis of FDG PET for managing patients with ovarian cancer. Clin Positron Imaging 2(2):63–70, 1999.

114. Barranger E, Kerrou K, Petegnief Y, et al: Laparoscopic resection of occult metastasis using the combination of FDG-positron emission tomography/computed tomography image fusion with intraoperative probe guidance in a woman with recurrent ovarian cancer. Gynecol Oncol 96(1):241–244, 2005.

screening program would identify those invasive, poorly differentiated serous tumors when confined to the ovary is unknown.

Second, except for patients with an increased risk of ovarian cancer based on family history, identification of the appropriate groups in the general population to target for screening is problematic. The prevalence of ovarian cancer in the general population is 40 per 100,000 postmenopausal women. Therefore, the detection of early-stage ovarian cancer requires tests with high sensitivity and specificity because of the low prevalence of ovarian cancer in the general population. In general, a positive predictive value (PPV) of 10% has been proposed as a clinical cut-point for screening tests for ovarian cancer. Clinically, a PPV of 10% means that there will be 10 operations for every one case of ovarian cancer detected. Screening tests must, therefore, achieve a sensitivity of at least 75% and a specificity of greater than 99.6% to achieve a PPV of 10%.

General Population Screening

Transvaginal Ultrasound

Transvaginal ultrasound (TVUS) has been evaluated for use in ovarian cancer screening in the general population. Because of the close proximity of the probe to the ovaries, TVUS offers excellent resolution of ovarian morphology. Volume, outline, papillations, and complexity of ovarian masses can be used to raise suspicion of cancer. Benign ovarian lesions are common, however, resulting in false-positives that may necessitate invasive surgery for asymptomatic women. In addition, TVUS as an initial screening test is expensive. Figure 6-1 shows an ultrasound image with color Doppler of the typical appearance of an involuting corpus luteal cyst.

Van Nagell and colleagues[14] conducted a screening study to examine whether TVUS could be used to detect ovarian cancer at an earlier stage and to decrease ovarian cancer mortality. They reported that between 1987 and 1999, 14,469 asymptomatic women underwent annual screening with TVUS. Women with an abnormal TVUS had a repeat TVUS in 4 to 6 weeks, and women with a persistently abnormal scan were advised to undergo surgery. Eligible women included all women 50 years of age and older and women 25 years or older with a first- or second-degree relative

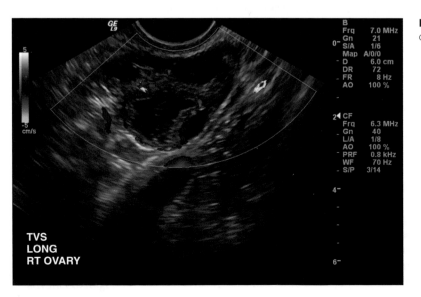

Figure 6-1. Typical appearance of an involuting corpus luteal cyst.

with ovarian cancer. One hundred eighty (1.2%) patients underwent surgery for suspicious findings on ultrasound, with 17 ovarian cancers detected: 11 stage I, 3 stage II, and 3 stage III. Sensitivity was 81%, and the negative predictive value was at 99.7%. The PPV was 9.4%, close to the clinically acceptable goal of a 10% PPV. These researchers also updated their data to include 25,327 women screened from 1987 to 2005. Three hundred sixty-four women (1.4%) underwent surgery, with 35 primary invasive ovarian cancers detected. Sensitivity for all stages was 85%, specificity was 98.7%, positive predictive value was 14% and negative predictive value was 99.9%.[15] Despite this encouraging outcome, interpretation of ultrasonography is observer dependent, and it is not certain that community-based trials could match the expertise of this group in eliminating false positives. In addition, the cost of annual TVUS would be prohibitive in our current health system.

CA-125 and Multimodal Approaches

CA-125 is the most extensively studied tumor marker for ovarian cancer. Figure 6-2 shows the genetic structure of the CA-125 marker. CA-125 is a high-molecular-weight mucin found in müllerian-derived epithelium, namely, fallopian tube, endometrium, and endocervix. Normal surface epithelium does not express CA-125, but it is elevated in 80% of patients with epithelial ovarian cancer and in over 90% of patients with advanced-stage disease.[16] CA-125 received FDA approval for use in monitoring patients with ovarian cancer for disease persistence and recurrence.[17] It is not approved as a screening tool for early detection of ovarian cancer.

Several issues limit the usefulness of CA-125 as a screening tool for ovarian cancer. First, although over 90% of advanced-stage patients display CA-125 elevations, only 50% to 60% of patients with stage I disease display elevations. Second, tumors with mucinous histologies are less likely to be associated with a CA-125 elevation.[18] Third, CA-125 has inadequate specificity, particularly in pre- and perimenopausal women. False-positive elevations are seen with benign ovarian cysts, endometriosis, adenomyosis, fibroids, diverticulitis, and liver cirrhosis, in addition to other benign and malignant conditions.

A Swedish study published by Einhorn and colleagues[19] in 1992 examined 5550 healthy asymptomatic women through the Stockholm Population Registry to determine whether CA-125 is a useful initial screening test for ovarian cancer. All participants had a CA-125 level drawn. Women with elevated CA-125 levels were age-matched to an equal number of women with normal CA-125 levels, and these women underwent pelvic examinations, transabdominal ultrasounds, and serial CA-125 levels. Six of the 175 women with elevated CA-125 levels were diagnosed with ovarian cancer; conversely, ovarian cancer was diagnosed in three of the controls, all of whom were younger than 50 years of age. Using a threshold of 35 μ/mL for the

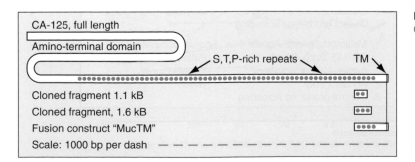

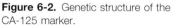

Figure 6-2. Genetic structure of the CA-125 marker.

Box 6-2. Tumor Markers That May Be Useful in Screening for Ovarian Carcinoma

Alpha-l-antitrypsin	Galactosyltransferase	M-CSF
BHCG	HE4	Mesothelin
CA15-3	HER-2/neu	Mucin-like carcinoma antigen
CA19-9	Human milk fat globule protein	Osteopontin
CA50	Human milk globule 2	Ovarian serum antigen
CA54-61	IL-2 receptor	OVXI
CA72-4	IL-6	p110 epidermal growth factor receptor
CA-125	IL-8	Placental alkaline phosphatase
CA-195	IL-10	Prostasin
Cathepsin L	Inhibin	Sialyl TN
Carcinoembryonic antigen	Kallekrein-6	Soluble Fas ligand
Ceruloplasmin	Kallekrein-10	Tetranectin
CRP	Lipid-associated sialic acid	Tumor-associated trypsin inhibitor
CYFRA21-1	Lysophosphatidic acid	Tumor necrosis factor receptor
Dianon marker 70/K	Matrix metaloproteinase 2	Urinary gonadotropin peptide

From Chu CS, Rubin SC: Screening for ovarian cancer in the general population. Best Pract Res Clin Obstet Gynaecol 20:307–320, 2006, page 312.

Over the past decade, novel markers have been discovered using monoclonal antibodies raised against ovarian cancer tissue, lipid analysis, gene expression arrays, and proteomic techniques. Mesothelin (soluble mesothelin-related protein, SMRP), an adhesion molecule found both on ovarian cancer and normal mesothelial cells, was originally detected empirically using monoclonal antibodies. Mesothelin is elevated in a majority of ovarian cancers and complements CA-125 for detecting early-stage disease.[30] Interestingly, SMRP can be detected in the urine, and, when corrected for glomerular filtration rate, urinary SMRP levels detect 40% of stage I patients.[31]

Lysophosphatidic acid (LPA) is a lipid of low molecular weight that is found in the ascites fluid and plasma of most patients with ovarian cancer. LPA stimulates calcium influx, proliferation, and drug resistance of ovarian cancer cells. Although there was initial enthusiasm about LPA for detecting women with stage I ovarian cancer,[32] confirming studies have not been published.

Overexpression of several potential biomarkers has been detected with gene expression arrays, including HE4, kallikreins, prostasin, osteopontin, vascular endothelial growth factor (VEGF), and interleukin 8 (IL-8). After CA-125, HE4, a human whey protein, has been the object of most intense study.[33] HE4 is slightly less sensitive than CA-125 for detecting early-stage disease but has greater specificity for distinguishing malignant from benign pelvic masses, particularly in premenopausal women. Kallikreins include a family of 15 secreted serine proteases of approximately 30 kD that include prostate-specific antigen (PSA). Several may prove useful as biomarkers for the prognosis or detection of ovarian cancer.[34,35] All the kallikreins are tandemly localized on chromosome 19q13.4 and were initially isolated by cloning the area. Kallikrein 6 and 10 are being investigated for usefulness as serum tumor markers for ovarian cancer.

Proteomic techniques have been used for early detection of ovarian cancer in two ways: to identify a distinctive pattern of peptide and protein expression in serum or

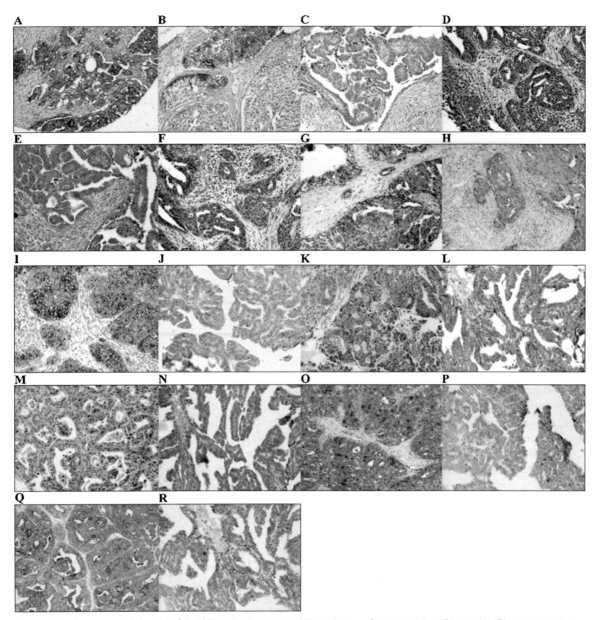

Figure 6-6. Immunostaining for CA-125 and other potential markers. Strong staining (**A**), patchy (**B**), and negative staining (**C**) for CA-125 (×20). Positive immunostainings for HK6 (**D**), HK10 (**E**), osteopontin (**F**), claudin 3 (**G**), and DF3 (**H**) (×20). Positive immunostaining for MUC1 (**I**), negative staining for MUC1 (**J**), positive immunostaining for VEGF (**K**), negative immunostaining for VEGF (**L**), positive immunostaining for mesothelin (**M**), negative immunostaining for mesothelin (**N**), positive immunostaining for HE4 (**O**), negative immunostaining for HE4 (**P**), positive immunostaining for CA-19-9 (**Q**), and negative immunostaining for CA-19-9 (**R**) (×20). (From Rosen DG, Wang L, Atkinson JN, et al: Potential markers that complement expression of CA125 in epithelial ovarian cancer. Gynecol Oncol 99:267–277, 2005: Fig. 1.)

in urine and to discover individual peptides or protein biomarkers and then to develop conventional immunoassays that can be performed in combination. A comparison of the proteomic techniques used for discovery and validation of markers is summarized in Table 6-3.

Surface-enhanced laser desorption and ionization time-of-flight mass spectrometry (SELDI-TOF) and matrix-assisted laser desorption and ionization time-of-flight mass spectrometry (MALDI-TOF) have been used to analyze the pattern of peptides in

7

Ovarian Cancer Surgery

Amer K. Karam, Christine Walsh, and Beth Y. Karlan

KEY POINTS

- Cytoreductive surgery is one of the cornerstones of therapy for advanced-stage ovarian cancer.
- Complete tumor removal and microscopic residual disease seem to offer the best survival outcomes.
- Secondary cytoreductive surgery should be reserved for patients with prolonged disease-free interval and localized disease.
- Second-look surgery does not result in improved survival.
- Accurate and complete surgical staging is the foundation of therapy for early-stage ovarian cancer.
- Fertility sparing and minimally invasive surgery are often practicable in young women with early-stage ovarian cancer without untoward effects on survival.
- Frozen-section analysis is accurate in the diagnosis of ovarian cancer but is less reliable in the diagnosis of borderline ovarian tumors.

Introduction

Surgery is a cornerstone of the diagnosis and treatment of ovarian carcinoma. The surgical goals differ based on the nature and stage of disease. The most commonly encountered scenario unfortunately is that of advanced epithelial ovarian cancer.

Advanced-Stage Epithelial Ovarian Cancer

Principles of Surgical Cytoreduction

Advanced epithelial ovarian cancer typically presents with widely disseminated intra-abdominal disease. The standard treatment of advanced epithelial ovarian cancer (EOC) includes primary cytoreductive or debulking surgery followed by adjuvant systemic chemotherapy. The goal of primary surgery for advanced epithelial ovarian cancer is to accurately establish a diagnosis and leave little or no residual disease. There are several potential benefits to the surgical removal of bulky tumor masses[1,2]:

- Removal of resistant clones of tumor cells decreases the likelihood of drug resistance according to the Goldie-Coldman hypothesis.
- Removal of large poorly vascularized and hypoxic tumors enhances chemotherapy delivery.
- The higher growth fraction in smaller, better-vascularized lesions increases cytotoxicity of chemotherapy.

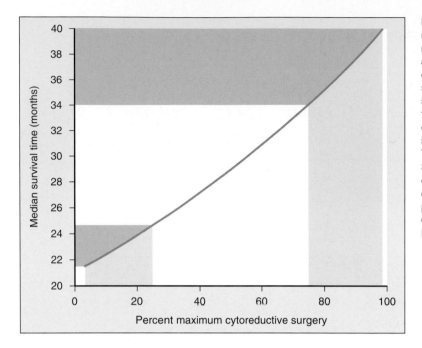

Figure 7-1. Simple linear regression analysis: de-logged median survival time plotted against percent maximal cytoreductive surgery. Light shaded area, maximal cytoreductive surgery less than 25% and more than 75%; dark shaded area, corresponding range of median survival times. (From Bristow RE, Tomacruz RS, Armstrong DK, et al: Survival effect of maximal cytoreductive surgery for advanced ovarian carcinoma during the platinum era: a meta-analysis. J Clin Oncol 20:1248–1259, 2002, Figure 2.)

- Smaller lesions require fewer cycles of chemotherapy, reducing development of drug resistance.
- Removal of bulk disease rapidly improves symptoms of advanced EOC resulting in improved quality of life, appetite, and immune status.

With regard to surgical debulking, there are no randomized controlled trials supporting its initial use. Nearly every retrospective and prospective study since Griffiths' seminal study in 1975 has demonstrated an inverse relationship between residual tumor diameter and patient survival,[3] including a recent meta-analysis by Bristow and colleagues,[4] which identified 6885 patients from previous publications. They found that each 10% increase in maximal cytoreduction was associated with a 5.5% increase in median survival (Fig. 7-1).

The definition of "optimal cytoreduction" continues to evolve. Since 1986, the Gynecologic Oncology Group (GOG) has defined optimal cytoreduction as leaving residual disease less than 1 cm in maximum tumor diameter based on their retrospective analysis and long-term follow-up of 726 patients with advanced epithelial ovarian cancer enrolled in two of their early adjuvant therapy trials.[5] Thus, defined optimal cytoreduction can be achieved in 75% or more of women explored by gynecologic oncologists.[6] The GOG has since performed two retrospective analyses of large chemotherapy trials, which again asserted the survival advantage of optimal debulking with residual tumor nodules less than 1 cm. They also suggested that cytoreduction that did not achieve optimal status or at least nodules less than 2 cm appears to have little benefit on survival[7,8] (Fig. 7-2).

Several studies have also shown that patients deriving the most survival benefit are those in whom tumors are primarily reduced to microscopic levels. For 348 patients from GOG 52 with stage III ovarian cancer cytoreduced to less than 1 cm of residual disease, Hoskins and colleagues[7] reported on the effect of diameter of the largest residual disease on survival. Five-year survival rates were greater for patients with microscopic residual disease (60%) even when compared with macroscopic disease less than 1 cm (35%). Chi and associates[9] recently analyzed survival rates at

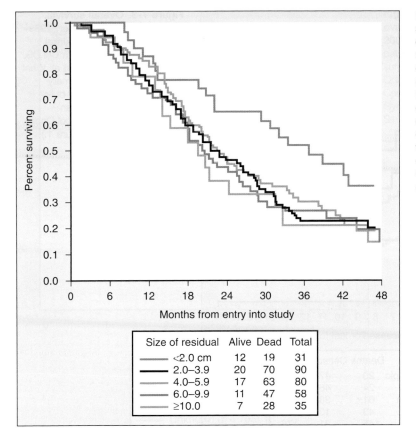

Size of residual	Alive	Dead	Total
<2.0 cm	12	19	31
2.0–3.9	20	70	90
4.0–5.9	17	63	80
6.0–9.9	11	47	58
≥10.0	7	28	35

Figure 7-2. Survival of women with suboptimal ovarian cancer entered on GOG protocol 97, according to maximal diameter of residual disease after debulking surgery. (From Hoskins WJ, McGuire WP, Brady MF, et al: The effect of diameter of largest residual disease on survival after primary cytoreductive surgery in patients with suboptimal residual epithelial ovarian carcinoma. Am J Obstet Gynecol 170:974–979, 1994; discussion 979–980, Figure 3.)

specific residual disease diameters to determine the optimal goal of primary cytoreduction for bulky stage IIIC disease. In this retrospective analysis of 465 patients, patients with no gross disease had longer overall median survival compared with patients with macroscopic residual disease of 1 to 5 mm (106 months versus 66 months)[9] (Fig. 7-3). Finally, the results of the two latest chemotherapy trials conducted by GOG seem to suggest a survival advantage for patients with microscopic residual disease when compared with those with macroscopic optimal disease.[10,11] The number of residual nodules may also influence prognosis. In their retrospective analysis of 78 patients left with residual disease less than 5 mm in maximum diameter, Farias-Eisner and colleagues[12] demonstrated a significant survival disadvantage for patients with extensive carcinomatosis. These studies provide compelling data supporting the benefit of macroscopic disease elimination when possible (Fig. 7-4).

Surgical Principles

A substantial number of patients with advanced-stage ovarian cancer present with bulky upper abdominal disease, malignant pleural effusions, or even intraparenchymal liver disease and may require diaphragmatic or intestinal procedures, splenectomy with or without a distal pancreatectomy, and peritoneal stripping to achieve an optimal cytoreduction. A survey of the Society of Gynecologic Oncologists (SGO) in 2000 revealed that up to 45% of patients deferred several procedures such as splenectomy with or without distal pancreatectomy, diaphragm stripping with or without full-thickness resection, and excision of grossly positive aortic nodes during

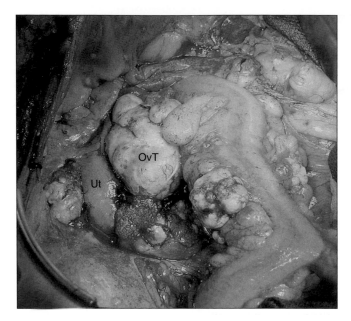

Figure 7-5. Locally advanced ovarian cancer with confluent extension to and encasement of the reproductive organs, pelvic peritoneum (including vesicouterine peritoneal reflection), cul-de-sac of Douglas, and rectosigmoid colon. OvT, ovarian tumor; Ut, uterus. (From Bristow RE, del Carmen MG, Kaufman HS, et al: Radical oophorectomy with primary stapled colorectal anastomosis for resection of locally advanced epithelial ovarian cancer. J Am Coll Surg 197:565–574, 2003, Figure 1.)

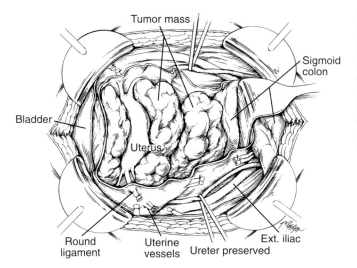

Figure 7-6. Radical oophorectomy. A circumscribing peritoneal incision encompasses all pan-pelvic disease, the round ligaments and ovarian vessels are divided, the ureters are mobilized, and the anterior pelvic peritoneal tumor is dissected from the bladder muscularis. (From Bristow RE, del Carmen MG, Kaufman HS, et al: Radical oophorectomy with primary stapled colorectal anastomosis for resection of locally advanced epithelial ovarian cancer. J Am Coll Surg 197:565–574, 2003, Figure 2.)

along the psoas muscles and then medially along the symphysis pubis. The infundibulopelvic and round ligaments are then secured retroperitoneally and the ureters detached from the medial leaf of the peritoneum and traced down to the ureteral canal. The uterine vessels are then skeletonized and ligated at the level of the ureters, allowing them to be mobilized off the specimen. The peritoneum overlying the bladder is detached sharply admitting access to the vesicouterine space, which is further developed (Fig. 7-6). The hysterectomy is completed in a retrograde fashion by first entering the vagina anteriorly and circumscribing the remaining anterior and lateral vagina along with the cardinal ligaments. The posterior vaginal wall is finally incised, exposing the rectovaginal space. The overlying cul-de-sac and attached tumor can then be mobilized off the rectosigmoid (Fig. 7-7).

Alternatively, the rectosigmoid can be resected en bloc with the specimen in the event of deep or extensive infiltrating disease. The proximal rectosigmoid is resected 2 to 3 cm above the uppermost extent of disease using a linear gastrointestinal stapler, and its mesentery is secured caudally. The distal rectosigmoid is then divided using thoracoabdominal stapler (Fig. 7-8). Once the specimen is removed, the continuity

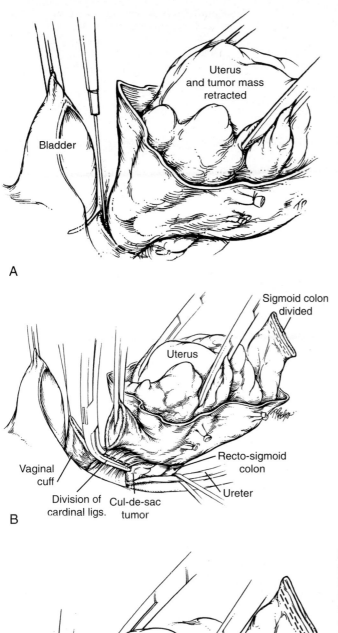

Figure 7-7. Radical oophorectomy. A, The anterior pelvic peritoneal tumor has been dissected from the bladder dome, the proximal vagina is exposed, and a transverse anterior colpotomy is created using electrocautery to enter the vagina. **B,** The remaining cardinal ligament attachments are divided between Heaney clamps working in a ventral-to-dorsal direction toward the cul-de-sac tumor mass. (From Bristow RE, del Carmen MG, Kaufman HS, et al: Radical oophorectomy with primary stapled colorectal anastomosis for resection of locally advanced epithelial ovarian cancer. J Am Coll Surg 197:565–574, 2003, Figure 3.)

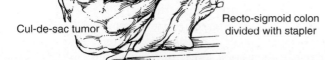

Figure 7-8. Radical oophorectomy. The rectovaginal space has been developed to a level 2 to 3 cm below the caudal-most extent of the cul-de-sac tumor mass, and the distal rectosigmoid colon is divided using an automated stapling device. (From Bristow RE, del Carmen MG, Kaufman HS, et al: Radical oophorectomy with primary stapled colorectal anastomosis for resection of locally advanced epithelial ovarian cancer. J Am Coll Surg 197:565–574, 2003, Figure 4.)

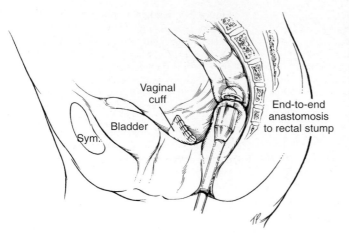

Figure 7-9. Radical oophorectomy.
Intestinal continuity is reestablished using a circular end-to-end anastomosis (CEEA) automated stapling device. Sym., symphysis pubis (From Bristow RE, del Carmen MG, Kaufman HS, et al: Radical oophorectomy with primary stapled colorectal anastomosis for resection of locally advanced epithelial ovarian cancer. J Am Coll Surg 197:565–574, 2003, Figure 7.)

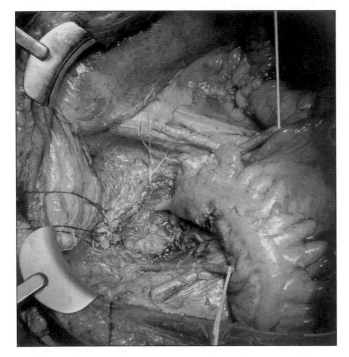

Figure 7-10. Radical oophorectomy. The pelvis is macroscopically tumor-free after en bloc resection. (From Bristow RE, del Carmen MG, Kaufman HS, et al: Radical oophorectomy with primary stapled colorectal anastomosis for resection of locally advanced epithelial ovarian cancer. J Am Coll Surg 197:565–574, 2003, Figure 6.)

of the bowel is restored using a circular end-to-end anastomotic stapler (Figs. 7-9 and 7-10).

In their series of 31 consecutive patients, Bristow and associates[17] encountered no postoperative deaths, but 4 of 31 (13%) of patients developed life-threatening postoperative complications with one patient undergoing a re-exploration for an anastomotic breakdown. This procedure should therefore not be undertaken in women with unresectable upper abdominal disease because of the procedure's high morbidity and low potential for cure.

Intestinal involvement in epithelial ovarian cancer frequently affects the rectosigmoid colon, and rectosigmoid resection represents the majority of gastrointestinal surgeries performed in patients with epithelial ovarian cancer. This surgery is often necessary to obtain optimal cytoreduction.[18] In one of the largest series, the morbidity associated with en bloc resection of ovarian carcinoma with low rectosigmoid resection and anastomosis was 6.7%. In a number of cases, superficial implants can simply be shaved off, but bulkier implants may require resection and anastomosis, particularly in the presence of obstruction.[19] As stated earlier, bowel resection should be carried out only when optimal cytoreduction is possible or when obstruction is present.

Diaphragm Resection

The bulk of disease is usually distributed among the pelvis, omentum, and right diaphragm. Diaphragm resection or stripping is often necessary to achieve optimal cytoreductive surgery. In a recent review of a single institution's experience, Aletti and associates[20] identified 181 patients with tumor involving the diaphragm. Patients who underwent diaphragm surgery (stripping of the diaphragmatic peritoneum, full- or partial-thickness diaphragm resection, excision of nodules or Cavitron ultrasonic surgical aspirator) had improved 5-year survival relative to those who did not (53% versus 15%). Furthermore, in multivariate analysis of patients with diaphragm disease, both residual disease and performance of diaphragm surgery were independent predictors of outcome.

In most instances, the right hemidiaphragm bears the largest volume of disease. To gain access to the entire right diaphragm, the abdominal incision is extended to the xiphoid process. A liver mobilization should then be completed by first dividing and ligating the infrahepatic portion of the falciform ligament, which is then incised superiorly to detach the liver from its anterior attachments to the abdominal wall. The anterior right coronary and right triangular ligaments are cautiously divided, being careful not to injure the right hepatic vein and inferior vena cava. Small implants can be excised or fulgurated using electrocautery, the argon beam coagulator, or the ultrasonic surgical aspirator. Larger-volume disease often requires a peritoneal resection, which is carried out by first mobilizing the anterior or lateral free edge of the diaphragm peritoneum and then separating it from the underlying musculature using a combination of sharp and blunt dissection proceeding ventrocaudally or lateromedially, respectively (Figs. 7-11 and 7-12). The integrity of the diaphragm is then confirmed by filling the ipsilateral space with water and observing for air bubbles at end inspiration. The defect is repaired by placing a catheter through the hole and aspirating at maximum inspiration as the edges of the opening are reapproximated using a purse string or a series of interrupted permanent sutures.

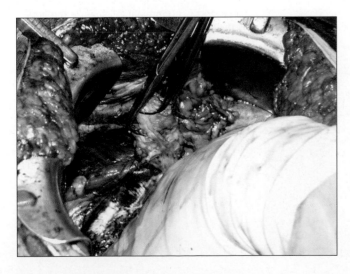

Figure 7-11. Diaphragm peritonectomy. (From Levine DA, Barakat RR, and Abu-Rustum NR: Atlas of Procedures in Gynecologic Oncology, 2nd ed. New York and London: Informa Healthcare, 2008. Reprinted courtesy of the authors.)

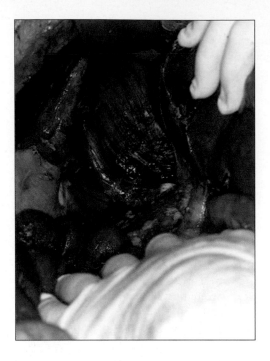

Figure 7-12. Peritonectomy completed. (From Levine DA, Barakat RR, and Abu-Rustum NR: Atlas of Procedures in Gynecologic Oncology, 2nd ed. New York and London: Informa Healthcare, 2008. Reprinted courtesy of the authors.)

Liver Resection

When parenchymal liver disease is present, a partial liver resection can be attempted. Hepatic resection is considered safe, with a mortality rate of less than 5%, but it is not yet regarded as standard of care for the treatment of ovarian cancer. Bristow and associates[22] identified a 50.1-month median survival in patients who were optimally cytoreduced of extrahepatic and parenchymal liver disease compared with 27.0 months in patients with optimal extrahepatic disease but suboptimal residual hepatic tumor. Patients with suboptimal extrahepatic and suboptimal hepatic residual disease had a median survival of only 7.6 months. Radiofrequency ablation has been explored as an alternative to conventional surgery for metastatic hepatic tumors. It allows the ablation of multiple lesions and is best suited for small lesions that are peripheral to major vascular structures[23] (Fig. 7-13).

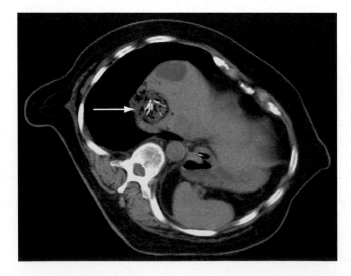

Figure 7-13. Abdominal CT scan at the time of the percutaneous radiofrequency ablation (RFA) of the liver metastasis. Note the tines that have been deployed from the RFA electrode into the tumor mass. The thermal necrosis of the tumor is seen acutely with gas and debris in the tumor bed (*arrow*). (From Bojalian MO, Machado GR, Swensen R, et al: Radiofrequency ablation of liver metastasis from ovarian adenocarcinoma: case report and literature review. Gynecol Oncol 93:557–560, 2004, Figure 2.)

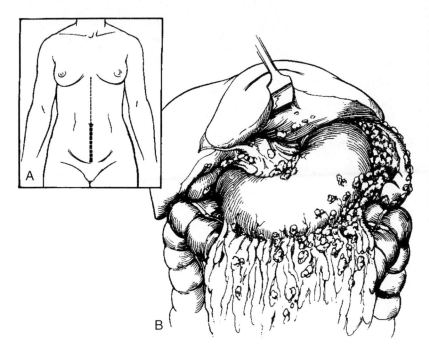

Figure 7-14. A, To ensure adequate exposure, a lower abdominal midline incision should be extended to the xiphoid process. **B,** Extensive tumor involvement of the omentum with extension to the greater curvature of the stomach and to the hilum and capsule of the spleen. (From Morris M, Gershenson DM, Burke TW, et al: Splenectomy in gynecologic oncology: indications, complications, and technique. Gynecol Oncol 43:118–122, 1991, Figure 2.)

Splenectomy

In the presence of extensive omental involvement, metastatic implants occasionally involve the splenic hilum, capsule, or parenchyma and may necessitate the removal of the spleen en bloc with the omentum. Magtibay and colleagues[24] described their center's experience with splenectomy as part of cytoreductive surgery in ovarian cancer and showed that splenectomy as part of primary or secondary cytoreductive surgery is associated with modest morbidity and mortality. Their data also confirmed that overall survival was substantially influenced by residual disease status after completion of primary surgical cytoreduction.

Before proceeding with the splenectomy, it is necessary to palpate the spleen and omentum to determine the extent of disease. Not infrequently one has to proceed with an en bloc resection of the omentum and spleen, since splenic involvement is often a result of direct extension from the omentum (Fig. 7-14). In such a case, a posterior approach is often preferred. The splenocolic, splenorenal, and spleno-phrenic ligamentous attachments of the spleen are first divided, allowing the spleen to be gently rotated anteriorly and medially (Fig. 7-15). The gastrosplenic ligament is then incised while carefully isolating and ligating the short gastric vessels and thus exposing the vascular supply, which can then be divided safely (Fig. 7-16). Care should be taken not to injure the tail of the pancreas. An anterior approach often limits blood loss in the event of a hilar injury or uncontrolled bleeding during the dissection. The gastrosplenic ligament is first divided and the short gastric vessels identified and ligated. The parietal peritoneum is incised, allowing the splenic vessels to be identified and secured (Fig. 7-17). The remaining attachments can then be incised and the specimen removed.

Because of the risk of postsplenectomy sepsis, patients undergoing elective splenectomy should be immunized against encapsulated organisms (meningococcus, pneumococcus, and *Haemophilus influenzae*) ideally a minimum of 10 days before surgery; alternatively, the vaccines can be given postoperatively.

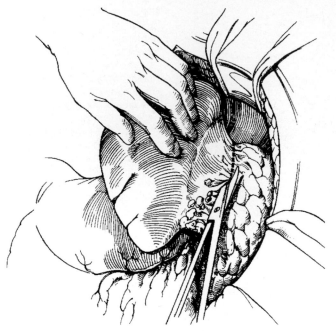

Figure 7-15. Division of the lateral ligamentous attachments allows early control of the vascular supply. (From Morris M, Gershenson DM, Burke TW, et al: Splenectomy in gynecologic oncology: indications, complications, and technique. Gynecol Oncol 43:118–122, 1991, Figure 4.)

Figure 7-16. The splenic vessels may be ligated by a posterior approach. (From Morris M, Gershenson DM, Burke TW, et al: Splenectomy in gynecologic oncology: indications, complications, and technique. Gynecol Oncol 43:118–122, 1991, Figure 5.)

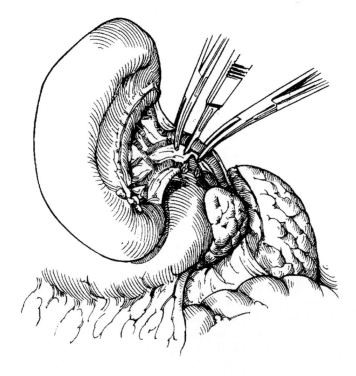

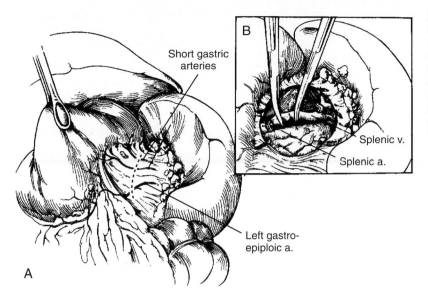

Short gastric arteries

B

Splenic v.

Splenic a.

Left gastro-epiploic a.

A

Figure 7-17. An anterior approach to the splenic vessels allows early control of the vascular supply. (From Morris M, Gershenson DM, Burke TW, et al: Splenectomy in gynecologic oncology: indications, complications, and technique. Gynecol Oncol 43:118–122, 1991, Figure 3.)

Lymph Node Resection

A bilateral pelvic and periaortic lymph node sampling must be done when the tumor nodules outside the pelvis are less than or equal to 2 cm (presumed stage IIIB) and in apparent stage I disease to exclude the possibility of microscopic nodal metastasis, which can occur in up to one third of patients with apparent early-stage disease. The role of lymph node resection has not been fully defined in advanced epithelial ovarian cancer. In their analysis of 93 patients who underwent lymph node assessment, Aletti and associates[26] showed that removing obviously involved lymph nodes in patients with residual disease near 1 cm appears to offer a survival advantage. The role of systematic aortic and pelvic lymphadenectomy in patients with optimally debulked advanced ovarian cancer has been addressed by a randomized clinical trial in which 427 eligible patients with optimally debulked FIGO stage IIIB-C and IV epithelial ovarian carcinoma were randomly assigned to undergo systematic pelvic and para-aortic lymphadenectomy or resection of bulky nodes only. The authors of the study did confirm the high prevalence of both pelvic and para-aortic lymph node metastases in patients with advanced ovarian cancer, but they were unable to detect any difference in overall survival between the two treatment arms[27] (Fig. 7-18). Therefore, patients with stage IV disease and those with tumor nodules outside the pelvis that are greater than 2 cm do not require pelvic or periaortic lymph node biopsies unless a clinically enlarged lymph node is discovered—in which case it must be resected.

Predictors of Optimal Cytoreduction

Predicting which patients can be optimally debulked remains difficult. Chi and associates[28] and subsequently Brockbank and associates[29] demonstrated in their small series that optimal cytoreduction, defined as residual disease of 1 cm or less, was achieved in 73% and 83% of patients with a preoperative CA-125 level of less than 500 U/mL, whereas optimal tumor cytoreduction could be accomplished in only 22% and 18% of patients with CA-125 level above 500 U/mL, respectively. Scoring systems that are based on imaging studies are complex and difficult to apply clinically and have not been validated in large series.[30–32] Axtell and colleagues,[33] in their review of a cohort of patients at one institution, were able to identify the three strongest CT predictors of optimal cytoreduction with an accuracy of 80%. However, when this

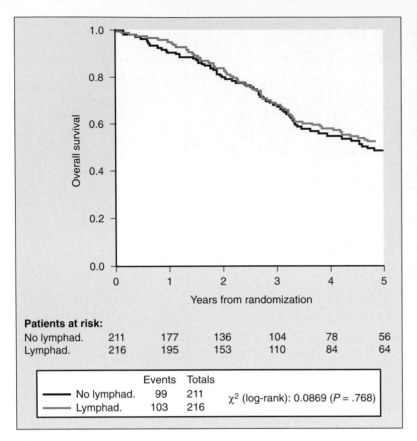

Figure 7-18. Overall survival (OS) for patients with optimally debulked advanced ovarian carcinoma undergoing systematic aortic and pelvic lymphadenectomy (Lymphad.) versus resection of bulky nodes only (No lymphad.).   Median OS times were 62.1 months (interquartile range = 30.9 months to still not reached) in the systematic lymphadenectomy arm and 56.3 months (interquartile range = 31.3 to 123.6 months) in the no-lymphadenectomy arm. (From Panici PB, Maggioni A, Hacker N, et al: Systematic aortic and pelvic lymphadenectomy versus resection of bulky nodes only in optimally debulked advanced ovarian cancer: a randomized clinical trial. J Natl Cancer Inst 97:560–566, 2005, Figure 3.)

model was applied to two previously published patient cohorts, the accuracy rates dropped to 27% and 60%, respectively. Reciprocally, when the CT models derived from the latter two studies were applied to the initial group of patients, the rates of accuracy fell from 93% and 79% to 65% and 69%, respectively. Some authors have used laparoscopy to establish the diagnosis and assess the resectability in patients with advanced epithelial ovarian cancer. Using diagnostic open laparoscopy, Angioli and colleagues[34] were able to identify 53 patients who were deemed operable among 87 patients with advanced epithelial ovarian cancer. Optimal debulking, which was defined as complete absence of disease after cytoreduction, was achieved in 96% of these patients.

Interval Cytoreduction

Since complete tumor resection is achieved in only 40% to 60% of advanced ovarian cancers and in an effort to increase the proportion of patients with advanced ovarian cancer that are ultimately left with an optimal volume of residual disease, the concept of a second attempt at debulking, or interval cytoreductive, surgery following an initial suboptimal effort and several cycles of systemic chemotherapy has been proposed by some clinicians. The European Organization for Research and Treatment of Cancer evaluated interval debulking surgery in a randomized trial. They evaluated 278 patients with residual disease greater than 1 cm after primary surgery. After three cycles of cyclophosphamide and cisplatin, patients were randomized to debulking surgery and no surgery, followed by additional chemotherapy. After adjustment for other prognostic factors, surgery reduced the risk of death by 33%.[35]

Table 7-1. Comparison of GOG 152 and EORTC Studies of Secondary/Interval Debulking Surgery after Three Doses of Chemotherapy

	GOG 152	EORTC Study
No. of eligible patients	424	319
Maximal surgical effort at initial surgery	Yes	No
Chemotherapy regimen	Cisplatin and paclitaxel	Cisplatin and cyclophosphamide
Serous cancers (%)	76	57
Stage IV disease (%)	6	22
Disease >5 cm after initial surgery (%)	44	72
Optimal at start of secondary surgery (%)	44 (89/201)	35 (44/127)*
Optimal at end of secondary surgery (%)	84 (168/201)	64 (81/127)*
Median progression-free survival for secondary surgery group from study entry (months)	12.5	18
Median survival for secondary surgery group from study entry (months)	36.2	26

*Surgical data not available on three in EORTC study.
EORTC, European Organization for Research and Treatment of Cancer.
From Monk BJ, Disaia PJ: What is the role of conservative primary surgical management of epithelial ovarian cancer: the United States experience and debate. Int J Gynecol Cancer 15(Suppl 3):199-205, 2005.

Another study conducted by GOG randomized 550 patients with suboptimal primary cytoreduction, and three cycles of cisplatin and paclitaxel were randomized to interval debulking surgery and chemotherapy versus chemotherapy alone. Both groups had median survivals of 33 months, and the authors concluded that the addition of secondary cytoreductive surgery did not improve progression-free survival or overall survival.[36] The fact that the GOG trial involved initial "maximal surgical effort" and the use of a more active chemotherapy regimen may help explain this divergent conclusion[37] (Table 7-1).

Similarly, malnourished women, in whom the risk of postoperative morbidity and mortality is high, may be better served by upfront or neoadjuvant chemotherapy and later maximal surgical cytoreduction in chemotherapy responders.[16] The potential advantages of this approach include an increased rate of optimal debulking, less extensive surgery, reduced blood loss, lower morbidity, shortened hospital stay, and the avoidance of aggressive surgery in women with chemoresistant disease who have poor outcome regardless of treatment. Bristow and Chi[38] recently performed a meta-analysis of the published literature pertaining to neoadjuvant chemotherapy and identified 21 studies totaling 835 patients that met their inclusion criteria. They were again able to demonstrate that for each 10% increase in the percentage of patients undergoing maximal interval cytoreductive surgery, which was variably defined, there was an associated 1.9-month increase in median survival time. It is interesting that the investigators also found that within the range of three to six median cycles of chemotherapy before interval surgery, each additional cycle of chemotherapy was associated with an incremental decrease in median survival time of 4.1 months (Fig. 7-19).

However, without prospective, randomized trials, neoadjuvant chemotherapy followed by later cytoreduction cannot be considered to provide a superior outcome over that achieved by aggressive initial surgical debulking followed by combination chemotherapy with paclitaxel.

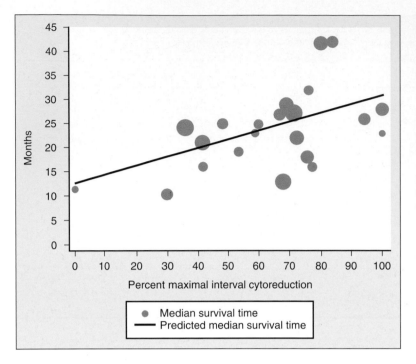

Figure 7-19. Simple linear regression analysis: median cohort survival time plotted against percent maximum interval cytoreductive surgery. Circle size is proportional to the number of subjects in each study and does not reflect the degree of statistical variation between studies. (From Bristow RE, Chi DS: Platinum-based neoadjuvant chemotherapy and interval surgical cytoreduction for advanced ovarian cancer: a meta-analysis. Gynecol Oncol 103:1070–1076, 2006, Figure 1.)

Second-Look Surgery

The role of second-look surgery was to assess the completeness of response and resect any residual tumor after the completion of initial chemotherapy in patients with advanced epithelial ovarian cancer. Initial enthusiasm for the procedure has been tempered by its lack of efficacy. GOG examined the role of second-look surgery as part of its GOG 158 trial. Patients were asked to choose whether they wanted to undergo second-look surgery after completing chemotherapy. The patients who received second-look surgery showed no improvement in progression-free or overall survival when compared with the group of patients who did not[39] (Fig. 7-20). Obermair and Sevelda[40] analyzed their group's experience with secondary cytoreductive surgery at the time of second-look laparotomy. There was no significant survival difference when those debulked to no residual disease were compared with women debulked to less than 2 cm or more than 2 cm residual disease. Nevertheless, second-look surgery continues to be the most accurate means of documenting the response to chemotherapy and providing prognostic information.

Recurrent Disease

Although complete clinical remission can be achieved in many patients with advanced epithelial ovarian cancer using a combination of cytoreductive surgery and chemotherapy, the disease will likely recur and require further intervention. Management of recurrent disease may then involve further chemotherapy, surgery, or radiation. Most of the studies that have examined surgical cytoreduction in recurrent ovarian cancer have demonstrated the technical feasibility of further resection, with optimal debulking in 39% to 87% of patients and demonstrate a survival advantage for those left with minimal residual disease.[41-45] Munkarah and Coleman[46] recently reviewed the role of secondary cytoreductive surgery in recurrent ovarian cancer. In their analysis of 12 publications, complete resection of the tumor recurrence was one of the most powerful determinants of prolonged survival. Harter and associates[47] recently reviewed the results of their DESKTOP-OVAR I exploratory multicenter

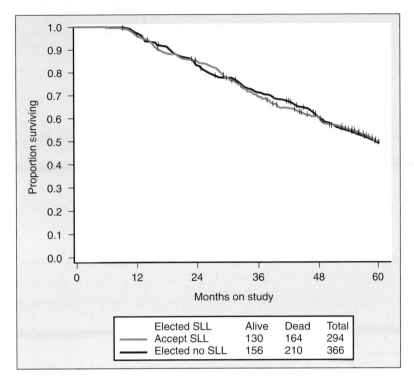

Figure 7-20. Survival (progression-free survival of less than 6 months removed). Accept second-look laparotomy (SLL) versus elected no SLL. (From Greer BE, Bundy BN, Ozols RF, et al: Implications of second-look laparotomy in the context of optimally resected stage III ovarian cancer: a non-randomized comparison using an explanatory analysis: a Gynecologic Oncology Group study. Gynecol Oncol 99:71–79, 2005, Figure 5.)

trial in Germany aimed at gathering evidence to help formulate a hypothesis for selection criteria and predictive factors for successful cytoreductive surgery in recurrent ovarian cancer. In their review of 267 patients, 87% of whom had a treatment-free interval of more than 6 months, the researchers found that the women with macroscopically completely resected tumors showed a significantly longer survival compared with patients who had any visible residual tumor, with a median survival of 45.2 and 19.7 months, respectively, and a hazard ratio for survival of 3.71 (Fig. 7-21). Multivariate analysis of their data suggest that good performance status, early FIGO stage initially, no residual tumor after first surgery, and the absence of ascites could predict complete resection in 79%. A longer disease-free interval has also been associated with an improved survival outcome. Salani and associates[18] identified 55 patients who underwent secondary cytoreductive surgery for recurrent epithelial ovarian cancer at their institution with 12 months or more between initial diagnosis and recurrence, and five recurrence sites or less on preoperative imaging. The median survival for patients with 18 months or more diagnosis-to-recurrence interval was 49 months compared with median survival of 3 months for those patients with a diagnosis-to-recurrence interval less than 18 months (Fig. 7-22). Surgery for recurrent epithelial ovarian carcinoma should therefore be considered for patients with a localized recurrence, an extended disease-free interval of at least 6 to 12 months, and a good performance status. The resection of isolated hepatic and extra-abdominal disease such as solitary lung or CNS lesions also seems to afford a similar survival advantage for the affected patients.[49]

Palliative Surgery

For many patients with recurrent ovarian cancer, the progressive encasement of the small and large bowel with tumor results in bowel obstruction. Palliative surgery to relieve the obstruction is often successful but fraught with complications. In a review of the published literature on surgery for intestinal obstruction in ovarian cancer, Pothuri and colleagues[50] analyzed 694 patients who underwent attempts at surgical

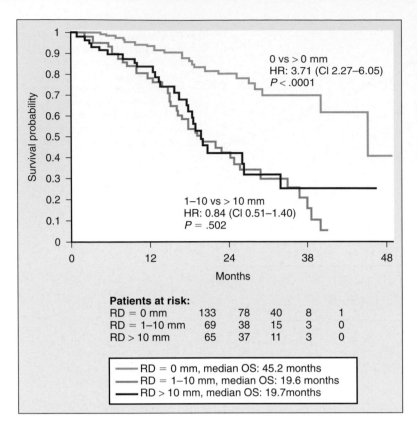

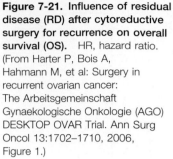

Figure 7-21. Influence of residual disease (RD) after cytoreductive surgery for recurrence on overall survival (OS). HR, hazard ratio. (From Harter P, Bois A, Hahmann M, et al: Surgery in recurrent ovarian cancer: The Arbeitsgemeinschaft Gynaekologische Onkologie (AGO) DESKTOP OVAR Trial. Ann Surg Oncol 13:1702–1710, 2006, Figure 1.)

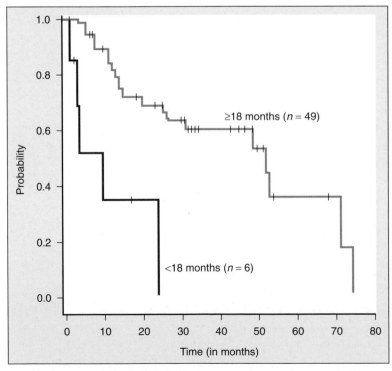

Figure 7-22. Survival according to the number of recurrence sites based on radiographic imaging. Patients who had one or two recurrence sites had a median survival of 50 months, and patients who had from three to five recurrence sites had a median survival of 12 months ($P = .026$). (From Salani R, Santillan A, Zahurak ML, et al: Secondary cytoreductive surgery for localized, recurrent epithelial ovarian cancer: analysis of prognostic factors and survival outcome. Cancer 109:685–691, 2007, Figure 4.)

palliation. Ninety percent of these were able to be surgically corrected. The perioperative mortality rate among these patients was 15.5%, and the rate of major operative complications was noted to be 32%. In addition, the median survival after surgery was 4.1 months and up to 50% of patients suffer from re-obstruction.[51] Jong and associates[52] have identified the presence of multiple obstructive sites, a preoperative weight loss of more than 9 kg, poor nutritional status, and a history of pelvic or abdominal radiation as indicative of a lower likelihood of successful palliation. For patients who are poor surgical candidates or who refuse palliative surgery, the placement of a percutaneous gastrostomy tube offers an option for palliation of nausea and vomiting due to intestinal obstruction.[53]

Early-Stage Epithelial Ovarian Cancer

At diagnosis, approximately one third of patients with epithelial ovarian cancer have early-stage disease that is confined to the ovary or pelvis. Although the 5-year survival for patients with early-stage ovarian cancer is much better than that for those with advanced disease, relapse rates ranging from 20% to 30% have been quoted for patients with poor prognostic factors. Classic clinical and pathologic prognostic factors, such as degree of differentiation, FIGO substage, histologic type, dense adhesions, large-volume ascites, rupture before or during surgery, bilaterality, positive peritoneal cytology extracapsular growth, and age of the patient have been identified as prognostic characteristics.[54,55] The main limitation of the conclusions derived from previous retrospective analyses is that the sample sizes of most were too small for some independent prognostic variables to be detectable with sufficient power.

Vergote and colleagues[56] conducted a large retrospective study of 1545 patients with stage I disease. In this study, the degree of differentiation was the most powerful prognostic indicator of disease-free survival (moderately versus well-differentiated hazard ratio 3.13, poorly versus well-differentiated hazard ratio 8.89). The study also confirmed that cyst rupture before surgery was an independent poor prognostic factor. Similarly, intraoperative cyst rupture also seemed to confer an unfavorable impact on survival, underscoring the importance of avoiding rupture during surgery (Table 7-2, Fig. 7-23).

Table 7-2. Significant Variables for Actuarial Disease-Free Survival in Final Multivariate Model

Characteristic	Hazard Ratio (95% CI) on Multivariate Analysis	P Value
Degree of differentiation		
Good*	1.00	—
Moderate	3.13 (1.68–5.85)	.0003
Poor	8.89 (4.96–15.9)	.0001
Rupture before surgery		
No*	1.00	—
Yes	2.65 (1.53–4.56)	.0005
Rupture during surgery		
No*	1.00	—
Yes	1.64 (1.07–2.51)	.022
FIGO stage 1973		
IA	1.00	—
IB	1.70 (1.01–2.85)	.046
Age (per year)	1.02 (1.00–1.03)	.053

Reference category.
From Vergote I, De Brabanter J, Fyles A, et al: Prognostic importance of degree of differentiation and cyst rupture in stage I invasive epithelial ovarian carcinoma. Lancet 357:176–182, 2001, Table 3.

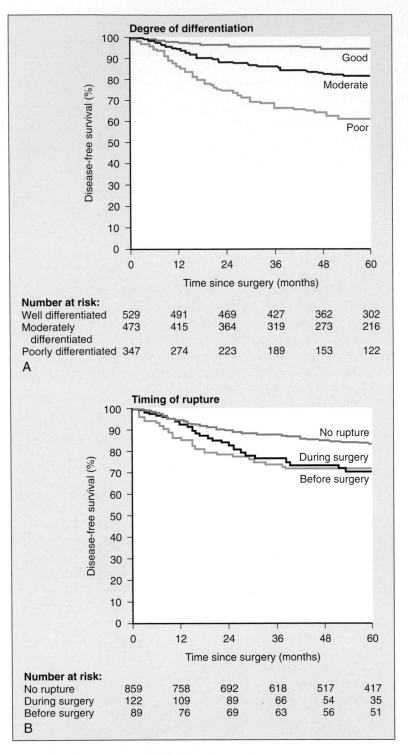

Figure 7-23. Actuarial disease-free survival according to degree of differentiation (**A**) and timing of cyst rupture (**B**) in stage I invasive epithelial ovarian carcinoma. (From Vergote I, De Brabanter J, Fyles A, et al: Prognostic importance of degree of differentiation and cyst rupture in stage I invasive epithelial ovarian carcinoma. Lancet, 357, 176–182, 2001, Figure 3.)

Surgical Staging

The importance of a thorough surgical staging was underscored by McGowan and colleagues[57] when they reported in 1983 the stage distribution of 157 patients properly staged in comparison with data from the FIGO annual report of the same period showing a reduction in stage I figures from 28% to 16%, in stage II figures from 17% to 4%, and a reallocation to stage III from 55% to 80% when a thorough staging procedure was adopted. Similarly, Young and colleagues and subsequently Helewa and associates and Buchsbaum and associates showed that an accurate staging procedure resulted in a reallocation to a more advanced disease (stage III) in 31% of early-stage ovarian cancer.[58-60] An analysis of surgeon specialty revealed that 97%, 52%, and 35% of gynecologic oncologists, obstetrician-gynecologists, and general surgeons, respectively, performed a comprehensive staging procedure for early-stage disease.[57] In addition, Le and colleagues,[61] in their retrospective chart review of patients with ovarian cancer macroscopically confined to the ovary at the time of laparotomy, found lack of proper surgical staging to be an important independent factor in predicting recurrence with an odds ratio of 2.62 (Fig. 7-24).

The primary procedure should include an abdominal incision that is adequate to explore the entire abdominal cavity. Care should be taken to remove the adnexal mass intact to prevent rupture, since this may impair prognosis. Any free peritoneal fluid is to be aspirated for cytology. If no free fluid is present, separate peritoneal

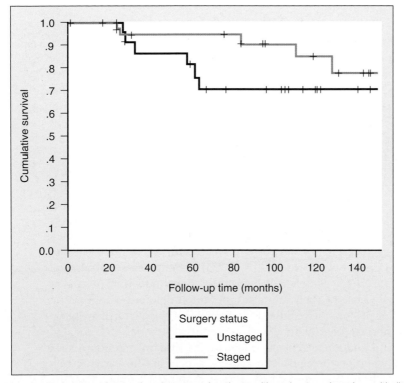

Figure 7-24. Survival status of staged and unstaged patients with early-stage invasive epithelial ovarian cancer treated expectantly. (From Le T, Adolph A, Krepart GV, et al: The benefits of comprehensive surgical staging in the management of early-stage epithelial ovarian carcinoma. Gynecol Oncol 85:351–355, 2002, Figure 1.)

washings should be obtained from the pelvis, paracolic gutters, and infradiaphragmatic area. These may be submitted separately or as a single specimen. All peritoneal surfaces, including the surface of both diaphragms and the serosa and mesentery of the entire gastrointestinal tract, should be visualized and palpated for evidence of metastatic disease. The omentum should be carefully inspected, and at minimum a biopsy of the omentum must be obtained.

If there is no evidence of disease beyond the ovary or the pelvis, peritoneal biopsies from the cul-de-sac, bladder peritoneum, right and left pelvic sidewalls, right and left paracolic gutters, and the right diaphragm should be carried out along with bilateral pelvic and periaortic lymphadenectomy with high para-aortic lymphadenectomy.

Controversies still exist as far as the extent of lymphadenectomy is concerned and, in particular, whether or not it has any therapeutic value. Benedetti Panici and associates[62] reported in the interim analysis of their multicenter, prospective, randomized Italian study comparing the feasibility and morbidity of systematic versus selective lymphadenectomy in early-stage ovarian cancer that the relapse rates for the two groups was comparable (21%). Moreover, even if the percentage of patients found to have retroperitoneal involvement was obviously higher in the "systematic lymphadenectomy" group (14% versus 8%), no differences in disease-free or crude survival were seen. Cass and colleagues[63] reviewed 96 patients with disease clinically confined to one ovary. Fifty-four patients had bilateral lymph node sampling performed, 30% of patients with lymph node spread had isolated contralateral metastases, highlighting the need for bilateral pelvic and para-aortic node sampling for accurate staging.

Fertility Preservation

If possible, an extrafascial total abdominal hysterectomy and bilateral salpingo-oophorectomy should be performed. However, in young patients who desire to preserve fertility, several studies support conservative surgical staging when the disease is confined to one ovary. Schilder and collegues[64] in a multi-institutional retrospective investigation examined 52 women presenting with stage IA and IC epithelial ovarian carcinoma who were treated with fertility-sparing surgery. Five patients developed tumor recurrence 8 to 78 months after initial surgery, and two died of recurrent cancer. Of the five recurrences, three occurred in the contralateral ovary. Twenty-four patients attempted pregnancy and 17 (71%) conceived. These 17 patients had 26 full-term deliveries. Likewise in their retrospective analysis of 56 patients treated with fertility-sparing surgery and 43 treated with the removal of the internal genital apparatus, Zanetta and associates[65] reported a 9% recurrence rate in the group treated conservatively compared with 12% in those treated with conventional surgery after a median follow-up of 7 years. Benjamin and associates[66] identified 118 women who had undergone a full-staging laparotomy including bilateral salpingo-oophorectomy for stage I disease. In 3 out of 118 (2.5%) patients, the contralateral ovary was found to have histologic evidence of malignancy despite looking normal at the time of laparotomy. Because of their low yield, potential deleterious effects on ovarian reserve, and risk of postoperative adhesions, which can impair fertility, biopsies of the apparently normal contralateral ovary should be abandoned. Finally, because of the possibility of endometrial involvement by the disease, an endometrial biopsy may be indicated when performing a conservative procedure for early ovarian cancer. Some clinicians have also advocated for a systematic appendectomy owing to the presence of microscopic metastasis in up to 37% of patients and the possibility of an occult appendiceal primary in the presence of a mucinous tumor.[67]

Role of Laparoscopy

Historically, laparoscopy was indicated for patients with apparent early-stage disease who had been inadequately staged. In their report, Childers and associates[68] upstaged eight of their 14 patients with apparent early stage disease who underwent laparoscopic staging. Leblanc and associates[69] reported on a series of 29 patients with invasive epithelial ovarian tumors who underwent laparoscopic staging. Laparoscopic staging was successfully completed in all but one case. Four of 29 (13.7%) patients were upstaged after laparoscopic staging. With a median follow-up of 59 months, no long-term complications (including port site recurrences) were observed, and the 5-year disease-free and overall survival were 90.6% and 92.6% respectively.[69] Similarly in their series of 11 patients, Tozzi and colleagues[70] observed only two recurrences without any port site metastasis after a median follow-up of 46 months. Chi and associates[71] reported the first case-control study comparing 20 patients with early-stage ovarian cancer staged by laparoscopy versus 30 patients who were staged by laparotomy. The number of nodes and omentum size were similar in both groups with fewer complications and shorter postoperative stay in spite of a longer operative room time for the laparoscopic group. The series also included seven patients who were fully managed laparoscopically after the frozen-section analysis of the affected adnexa (Table 7-3).

Intraoperative Frozen-Section Analysis

The reliability and accuracy of frozen-section diagnosis are critical determinants in the selection of the appropriate surgical procedure. Medeiros and colleagues[72] performed a quantitative meta-analysis of 14 studies that estimate the accuracy of frozen

Table 7-3. Surgical Outcomes of 20 Patients Who Underwent Comprehensive Laparoscopic Surgical Staging for Apparent Stage I Ovarian Cancer and 30 Patients Who Underwent Laparotomy

Variables	Group 1 Laparoscopy Group (N = 20)	Group 2 Laparotomy Group (N = 30)	P Value
Number of nodes			
Left pelvic	5.8 ± 2.9	7.1 ± 4.3	.30
Right pelvic	6.5 ± 3.9	7.6 ± 3.8	.31
Left para-aortic	2.9 ± 1.7	4.8 ± 4.2	.08
Right para-aortic	3.8 ± 1.8	4.4 ± 2.8	.36
Omental specimen (cm^3)	186 ± 178	347 ± 378	.09
Site of metastasis (%)	2 (10)	3 (10)	1.00
Uterus	1 (5)	1 (3)	
Nodes	1 (5)	2 (7)	
Omentum	0	0	
Other surgery (%)			
Hysterectomy	12 (60)	25 (83)	.10
Adnexal	13 (65)	27 (90)	.07
Operating time (min)	321 ± 64	276 ± 68	.04
Estimated blood loss (mL)	235 ± 138	367 ± 208	.003
Hospital stay (days)	3.1 ± 0.7	5.8 ± 2.6	<.001
Complications (%)	0 (0)	2 (7)	1.00

From Chi DS, Abu-Rustum NR, Sonoda Y, et al: The safety and efficacy of laparoscopic surgical staging of apparent stage I ovarian and fallopian tube cancers. Am J Obstet Gynecol 192:1614–1619, 2005, Table II.

section in the diagnosis of ovarian tumors. Among the broad sample of ovarian tumors in this systematic review, 71% were benign, 5.9% were borderline, and 22.7% were malignant. The pooled sensitivity rates for benign and malignant ovarian tumors were 99% and 94%. The positive frozen-section results for malignancy increased the probability of ovarian cancer to 98%, whereas a negative result reduced the probability of cancer to 1.6%. The pooled sensitivity for borderline ovarian tumors, however, was low at 66% owing to the greater incidence of false-negative results. Insufficient tumor removal, technical problems in sampling, and the range of experience of pathologist may have contributed to the reduced sensitivity among borderline cases, resulting in a post-test probability of borderline tumors that was only 51% when compared with malignant tumors.[72] Thus, in patients in whom the result is a diagnosis of borderline tumor in the frozen section, the surgeon should still consider performing comprehensive staging.

Risk-Reducing Surgery

Approximately 10% of patients with epithelial ovarian cancer carry a deleterious mutation of the *BRCA1*, *BRCA2*, or the DNA mismatch repair genes. The presence of these mutations carries a lifetime risk of ovarian cancer ranging from 15% to 54%.[73,74] Women who carried these mutations were asked to undergo intensive surveillance or to consider prophylactic salpingo-oophorectomy at age 35 or following the completion of their childbearing. Kauff and associates[75] prospectively analyzed 170 *BRCA* mutation carriers. In the 98 women who underwent prophylactic salpingo-oophorectomy, early-staged tumors were identified in three patients at the time of surgery (3.1%), and primary peritoneal cancer developed in 1 patient during follow-up (1.0%). Of the 72 women who underwent surveillance only, epithelial ovarian or primary peritoneal cancer developed in five (6.9%). The time to breast cancer or *BRCA*-related gynecologic cancer was also significantly longer in the salpingo-oophorectomy group, with a hazard ratio for subsequent breast cancer or *BRCA*-related gynecologic cancer of 0.25 (Fig. 7-25). In another multicenter study, Rebbeck and associates[76] determined the incidence of ovarian cancer among 259 patients who had undergone prophylactic surgery and compared them with 292 matched controls who had not undergone the risk-reducing procedures. Six patients

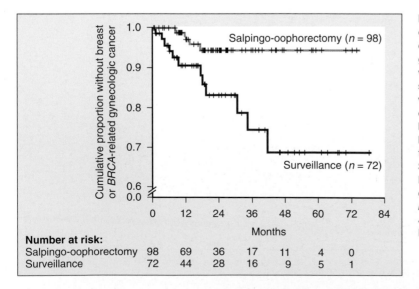

Figure 7-25. Kaplan-Meier estimates of the time to breast cancer or *BRCA*-related gynecologic cancer among women electing risk-reducing salpingo-oophorectomy and women electing surveillance for ovarian cancer. *P* = .006 by the log-rank test for the comparison between the actuarial mean times to cancer. (From Kauff ND, Satagopan JM, Robson ME, et al: Risk-reducing salpingo-oophorectomy in women with a *BRCA1* or *BRCA2* mutation. N Engl J Med 346:1609–1615, 2002, Figure 1.)

were diagnosed with cancer at the time of surgery. After excluding these patients, the authors found that prophylactic surgery reduced the risk of epithelial ovarian cancer by 96%. Finch and associates,[77] in the largest multicenter prospective study of patients carrying a deleterious BRCA1 or BRCA2 mutation, evaluated 1273 women with intact ovaries at the inception of the study. Four hundred ninety patients underwent an oophorectomy during the follow-up period; of these, 11 (2.2%) were diagnosed with a malignancy at the time of surgery and a further 7 patients developed primary peritoneal carcinoma following surgery. On the other hand, 32 malignancies were observed among the 783 patients with intact ovaries. The adjusted reduction in risk of malignancy associated with prophylactic oophorectomy was 80%. It is interesting that 3 of the 11 patients diagnosed with an occult malignancy at the time of risk-reducing surgery had a cancer that originated from the fallopian tubes, thus emphasizing the need to remove all of the ovarian tissue and as much of the fallopian tubes as possible. Although some authors have suggested that the intramural portion of the tubes may undergo malignant transformation, there have been no reported cases of such an occurrence.[78] The surgery at a minimum should also include a careful survey of all the peritoneal surfaces, a peritoneal cytology, and liberal biopsies of any suspicious area including the omentum to rule out an occult carcinoma. The ovaries and fallopian tubes should be step-sectioned and carefully surveyed for an occult malignancy as well.

Ovarian Tumors of Low Malignant Potential

Ovarian epithelial tumors of low malignant potential or borderline ovarian tumors account for approximately 15% of ovarian epithelial tumors.[13] Borderline ovarian tumors with serous or mucinous histologies are the most commonly observed (65% and 32%, respectively). Patients with these lesions tend to be younger than those with invasive ovarian carcinoma (average age at diagnosis: 49 years), and a large portion of these tumors occurs in the 15- to 29-year-old age group.[79]

Surgery is required for diagnosis, and staging is approached in the same fashion as for invasive ovarian carcinoma. In review of the literature, Tinelli and colleagues[80] showed 70% of cases presented as stage I and an additional 10% presented as stage II. Borderline tumors have an excellent prognosis with 5-year survival ranging between 85% and 97% and 10-year survival between 70% and 95% mainly owing to late recurrences[13] (Fig. 7-26).

The more frequent occurrence of ovarian tumors of low malignant potential among women of reproductive age and the overall excellent prognosis have cast doubt on the need for aggressive surgical staging in these patients. Lin and colleagues[81] compared traditional staging approaches with limited procedures in a cohort of 255 women diagnosed with serous borderline ovarian tumors. Forty-seven percent of patients were upstaged and women undergoing cystectomy alone were more likely to recur in either the ipsilateral or contralateral ovary. Morris and colleagues[82] reviewed the outcomes of 43 patients at a single institution who were diagnosed with borderline ovarian tumors and had undergone conservative surgery. Patients undergoing ovarian cystectomy were more likely to require additional surgery (63% versus 40%) in the future and were more likely to have recurrences (75% versus 24%) compared with women undergoing oophorectomy. In one of the largest series reported in the literature, Zanetta and colleagues[83] showed a recurrence rate of 19% in 189 cases treated conservatively versus 4.6% in 150 cases treated by hysterectomy and bilateral oophorectomy. Conservative surgery did not seem to impact survival, and all but one woman with recurrent disease were salvaged by further surgery. It seems reasonable to offer conservative surgery to women with borderline ovarian tumors desiring fertility preservation; however, they should be cautioned regarding the risk

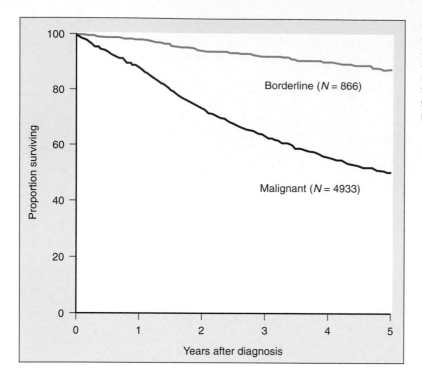

Figure 7-26. Carcinoma of the ovary: patients treated in 1999–2001. Survival by histology, N = 5799. (From Heintz A, Odicino F, Maisonneuve P, et al: Carcinoma of the ovary. Int J Gynaecol Obstet 95(Suppl 1):S161–S92, 2006, Figure 8.)

Histology	Patients (N)	Mean Age (yr)	Overall Survival (%) at					Hazard Ratio* (95% CI)
			1 Year	2 Years	3 Years	4 Years	5 Years	
Borderline	866	49.3	97.7	94.1	92.1	90.2	87.3	Reference
Malignant	4933	57.6	87.4	72.7	62.9	54.9	49.7	1.9 (1.5–2.3)

*Hazard ratios and 95% confidence intervals obtained from a Cox model adjusted for age, stage, and country.

of recurrence and the need for future surgery. The usefulness of lymph node sampling has also been called into question, Seidman and Kurman,[84] in their meta-analysis of over 4000 patients with serous borderline ovarian tumors, identified only 63 patients with lymph node lesions with a survival rate of 98%.

The need for complete surgical staging is justified, however, in the event that final pathologic analysis finds invasive disease missed on frozen section. Medeiros and associates[72] reported in their meta-analysis that the pooled sensitivity for borderline ovarian tumors was low at 66% due to the greater incidence of false-negative results, resulting in a post-test probability of borderline tumors that was only 51% compared with malignant tumors. Similarly, Geomini and associates[85] showed in their review of the literature on the accuracy of frozen-section diagnosis that sensitivity varied between 65% and 97% and the specificity between 97% and 100%. Factors that lower the sensitivity of frozen-section diagnosis included large neoplasms, mucinous tumors, and tumors exhibiting extraovarian disease.

Advanced-stage mucinous borderline ovarian tumors have a graver prognosis, and a number of studies show that these tumors may represent metastases from appendiceal primaries, especially in the setting of pseudomyxoma peritoneii.[86] An appendectomy should be considered if the appendix is present, and the frozen section suggests a mucinous histology. In the event of advanced-case disease, a total abdomi-

Table 7-4. Surgically Documented Complete Response Rates to Platinum-Based Chemotherapy According to Residual Disease in Patients with Advanced Serous Ovarian Tumors of Low Malignant Potential

Author	Complete Response	
	Macroscopic Disease	Microscopic Disease
Kliman et al[88]	0/1	—
Nation and Krepart[89]	0/2	2/2
Chambers et al[90]	0/1	1/1
Hopkins and Morley[91]	—	1/3
Gershenson and Silva[92]	2/4	2/5
Sutton et al[93]	2/8	4/6
Barakat et al[87]	2/7	7/8
Total	6/23 (26%)	17/25 (68%)

From Barakat RR, Benjamin I, Lewis JL Jr, et al: Platinum-based chemotherapy for advanced-stage serous ovarian carcinoma of low malignant potential. Gynecol Oncol 59:390–393, 1995.

nal hysterectomy, bilateral salpingo-oophorectomy, and maximal cytoreduction are advised. Barakat and associates[87] showed a higher rate of complete clinical response following platinum based chemotherapy among patients with advanced-stage borderline ovarian tumors who were left with microscopic residual disease (Table 7-4). Gershenson and colleagues[94] confirmed the latter results when they demonstrated that macroscopic residual disease was an independent adverse prognostic factor. Although recurrences are uncommon, 10% to 20% of patients are expected to have recurrences, with malignant transformation in 2% to 7% of cases.[95] As in epithelial ovarian cancer, Crispens and associates[96] demonstrated that for patients who underwent complete or optimal resection their recurrence had a better response to chemotherapy and better overall survival (92% versus 35%).

Malignant Germ Cell Tumors of the Ovary

Malignant germ cell tumors of the ovary, which include dysgerminomas, immature teratomas, embryonal carcinomas, endodermal sinus tumors, and ovarian choriocarcinomas, are uncommon and rare. Surgery is required for the diagnosis and staging of malignant germ cell ovarian tumors. The staging system for malignant ovarian germ cell tumors is identical with that used for epithelial ovarian cancer. In contrast to epithelial ovarian cancer, malignant germ cell tumors occur primarily in girls and young women. These tumors are now curable, mainly as a result of great advances in chemotherapy in the last two decades. Fertility-sparing surgery has increasingly been used in the management of these women. In a review of 281 patients with ovarian germ cell tumors, Kurman and Norris[97] first reported that the prognosis of patients with disease grossly confined to one ovary who were treated with unilateral salpingo-oophorectomy was not worse than that of patients undergoing more radical surgery (Table 7-5). Peccatori and colleagues[98] identified 129 patients with germ cell tumors, 108 of whom have been treated by fertility-sparing surgery. The overall survival was 96%, and conservative surgery did not affect the recurrence or survival rates. Zanetta and associates[99] reported on 169 women with malignant ovarian germ cell tumors. Fertility-sparing surgery was performed in 138 of these patients.

Table 7-5. Comparison of Survival after Unilateral Versus Bilateral Salpingo-oophorectomy in 182 Patients with Tumors Grossly Confined to One Ovary

Tumor	No. of Patients	Treatment	Actuarial Survival (%)
Dysgerminoma	46	SO	91
	21	BSO	90
			91*
Endodermal sinus tumor	27	SO	22
	22	BSO	9
			16†
Immature teratoma	34	SO	76
	6	BSO	66
			70*
Embryonal carcinoma	7	SO	57
	1	BSO	—
			50‡
Mixed germ cell tumors	13	SO	54
	5	BSO	40
			50‡

*At 10 years.
†At 3 years.
‡At 5 years.
BSO, bilateral salpingo-oophorectomy; SO, unilateral salpingo-oophorectomy.
From Kurman RJ, Norris HJ: Malignant germ cell tumors of the ovary. Hum Pathol 8:551–564, 1977.

Table 7-6. Status of Contralateral Ovary in 191 Patients with Stage I Tumors

Tumor	No. of Patients		No. of Grossly Normal Ovaries Examined Microscopically	No. Positive for Occult Tumor
	Stage IA	Stage IB		
Dysgerminoma	67	11	21	4*
Endodermal sinus tumor	51	0	24	0
Immature teratoma	40	0	6	0
Embryonal carcinoma	9	0	0	0
Mixed germ cell tumor	19	1	5	1†‡

*Dysgerminoma developed in two additional patients in a contralateral ovary that appeared normal at the time of operation, 6 and 15 months later.
†Dysgerminoma was one of the components of the tumor and was the only type of tumor in the opposite ovary.
‡Another neoplasm with the same histologic composition developed in the contralateral ovary of an additional patient with a mixed dysgerminoma and endodermal sinus tumor 22 months after the operation.
From Kurman RJ, Norris HJ: Malignant germ cell tumors of the ovary. Hum Pathol 8:551–564, 1977.

The survival rate for women who were treated conservatively was 98% for dysgerminomas, 90% for endodermal sinus tumors, and 100% for either mixed types or immature teratomas. Fifty-five conceptions and 40 term pregnancies were recorded, indicating a marginal effect of treatment on fertility. The contralateral ovary should not be biopsied if it appears grossly normal, unless the tumor is a dysgerminoma or a mixed germ cell tumor with a component of dysgerminoma because the risk of occult contralateral ovarian involvement is up to 20%[97] (Table 7-6).

The role of cytoreductive surgery for advanced-stage malignant germ cell tumors of the ovary is less well established. Nevertheless, the same principles of cytoreductive surgery that have been applied for epithelial ovarian cancer are generally recommended with maximum resection to achieve the smallest amount of residual disease. Slayton and colleagues[100] examined 76 patients with malignant germ cell tumors of the ovary who received vincristine, dactinomycin, and cyclophosphamide as part of the GOG 44 phase II protocol. Twenty-eight percent of the patients with completely resected disease failed vincristine, adriamycin, cyclophosphamide (VAC) therapy compared with 68% of patients with incompletely resected tumors. Similar findings were recorded in the follow-up GOG 45 study of the combination vinblastine, bleomycin, and cisplatin in which 83% of the patients with no measurable disease at the start of chemotherapy remained disease-free compared with 42% of patients with measurable disease[101] (Table 7-7). In their review of 33 patients with malignant germ cell tumors of the ovary, Bafna and associates[102]

Table 7-7. Disease-Free Survival by Pretreatment Characteristics in Patients with Tumors other than Dysgerminoma

Patient Characteristics	No. Disease-Free/Total (%)
Cell type	
Endodermal sinus	16/29 (55)
Embryonal	1/4 (25)
Mixed	14/27 (52)
Immature teratoma	14/26 (54)
Choriocarcinoma	2/3 (67)
Age	
<20	23/38 (61)
20–29	15/33 (45)
30–39	8/13 (62)
40–49	0/4 (0)
≥50	1/1 (100)
Stage	
II	5/5 (100)
III	22/37 (60)
IV	5/9 (56)
Recurrent	15/38 (40)
Measurable disease	
Yes	12/35 (34)
No	35/54 (65)
Previous therapy	
Yes*	14/35 (40)
No	33/54 (61)
Residual disease	
Optimal	
At initial surgery	10/12 (83)
After debulking surgery	17/29 (59)
Suboptimal	20/48 (42)
Markers	
Elevated	32/56 (57)
Normal	13/27 (48)
Not done	2/6 (33)

*Chemotherapy, radiation therapy, or both.
From Williams SD, Blessing JA, Moore DH, et al: Cisplatin, vinblastine, and bleomycin in advanced and recurrent ovarian germ-cell tumors. A trial of the Gynecologic Oncology Group. Ann Intern Med 111:22–27, 1989.

reported that 13 patients had bulky disease (larger than 10 cm) at the start of chemotherapy with bleomycin, etoposide, and cisplatin. Seven of the 13 patients had
dysgerminomas, and all of them achieved a sustained complete response, whereas
only 3 of the 6 patients with nondysgerminoma tumors achieved a sustained complete
response, indicating that aggressive cytoreductive surgery may be more important for
nondysgerminomatous tumors.

Despite the success of modern chemotherapy, a small number of patients will
present with persistent or recurrent disease. Munkarah and associates[103] reported on
the M.D. Anderson Cancer Center experience with salvage surgery for malignant
ovarian germ cell tumors. Twenty cases were identified, and 16 patients received
postoperative chemotherapy following salvage surgery. At the time of analysis, 11
patients were alive and disease-free, 1 was alive with tumor, 6 had died of tumor
progression, and 2 had died of treatment-related complications. Survival of patients
with immature teratoma who underwent salvage surgery was significantly better than
survival of those with other tumor cell types. A case report and review of the literature by Rezk and associates[104] again demonstrated that patients with recurrent or
persistent immature teratomas might benefit from salvage surgery. Immature teratomas may also become mature during chemotherapy, resulting in a growing teratoma
syndrome that is surgically unresectable or that may invade and/or obstruct neighbor-
ing structures and necessitate prompt surgical intervention.[105,106] Finally, unresected
mature teratomas can occasionally undergo malignant transformation and tend to be
resistant to traditional chemotherapies.[107]

Sex Cord-Stromal Tumors of the Ovary

Ovarian sex cord and stromal tumors represent a heterogeneous group of rare
tumors arising from the ovarian stroma and cells that surround the oocytes. Their
rarity precludes any definite recommendations regarding their management.
Surgery is the cornerstone of therapy and is required for definitive diagnosis. The
staging system is the same as that for epithelial ovarian cancer. Most malignant
ovarian sex cord-stromal tumors, however, tend to present at an earlier age and
stage and to follow an indolent course and recur late, and can thus be managed
more conservatively. In their review of 83 women with sex cord-stromal tumors of
the ovary, Chan and colleagues[108] reported that nearly 50% of their patients were
less than 50 years of age and over 70% presented with early-stage disease. They
were able to confirm that, similar to previous reports, tumor size (less than 10 cm)
and absence of residual disease improved prognosis with a nearly 8% decrease in
risk of death for every 1 cm decrease in size and an improvement of 66 months in
overall survival for patients left with no residual disease[108] (Fig. 7-27). Although
the investigators did not report a significant difference in overall survival between
unstaged and staged patients, the recurrence rate was significantly higher for
patients who were not staged (64% versus 28%). Since most sex cord-stromal
tumors tend to secrete sex steroids including estrogen, up to 55% of cases are
associated with concurrent endometrial hyperplasia and up to 10% with a synchronous uterine adenocarcinoma.[109] In postmenopausal women and women having
completed their childbearing, a total abdominal hysterectomy and bilateral salpingo-oophorectomy is recommended; if the patient desires to conserve fertility, a
unilateral salpingo-oophorectomy is acceptable treatment for early-stage disease as
long as a preoperative endometrial biopsy is performed to exclude the possibility
of a synchronous endometrial carcinoma. Treatment for recurrent or metastatic
disease is primarily surgical, with reports of long-term disease control with complete resection of localized recurrences[110] (Fig. 7-28), since these tumors tend to
be relatively chemotherapy- and radiation-resistant.[111]

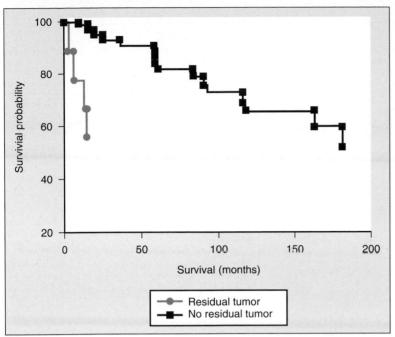

Figure 7-27. Kaplan-Meier survival analysis based on the residual tumor status for 83 patients with sex cord stromal tumors of the ovary. (From Chan JK, Zhang M, Kaleb V, et al: Prognostic factors responsible for survival in sex cord stromal tumors of the ovary—a multivariate analysis. Gynecol Oncol 96:204–209, 2005, Figure 4.)

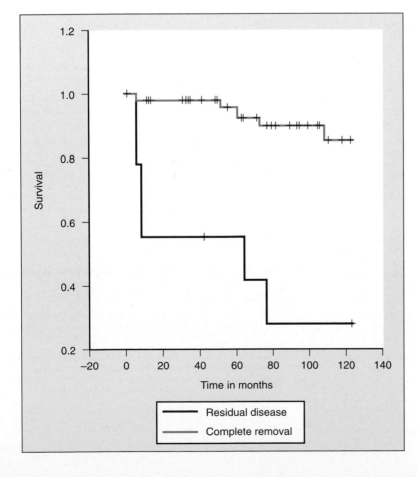

Figure 7-28. Kaplan-Meier survival analysis based on the residual tumor status of 65 patients with granulosa cell tumor of the ovary. (From Sehouli J, Drescher FS, Mustea A, et al: Granulosa cell tumor of the ovary: 10 years follow-up data of 65 patients. Anticancer Res 24:1223–1239, 2004, Figure 7.)

References

1. Covens AL: A critique of surgical cytoreduction in advanced ovarian cancer. Gynecol Oncol 78: 269–274, 2000.
2. Thigpen T:, The if and when of surgical debulking for ovarian carcinoma. N Engl J Med 351:2544–2546, 2004.
3. Griffiths CT: Surgical resection of tumor bulk in the primary treatment of ovarian carcinoma. Natl Cancer Inst Monogr 42:101–104, 1975.
4. Bristow RE, Tomacruz RS, Armstrong DK, et al: Survival effect of maximal cytoreductive surgery for advanced ovarian carcinoma during the platinum era: a meta-analysis. J Clin Oncol 20:1248–1259, 2002.
5. Omura GA, Brady MF, Homesley HD, et al: Long-term follow-up and prognostic factor analysis in advanced ovarian carcinoma: the Gynecologic Oncology Group experience. J Clin Oncol 9:1138–1150, 1991.
6. Chi DS, Franklin CC, Levine DA, et al: Improved optimal cytoreduction rates for stages IIIC and IV epithelial ovarian, fallopian tube, and primary peritoneal cancer: a change in surgical approach. Gynecol Oncol 94:650–654, 2004.
7. Hoskins WJ, Bundy BN, Thigpen JT, et al: The influence of cytoreductive surgery on recurrence-free interval and survival in small-volume stage III epithelial ovarian cancer: a Gynecologic Oncology Group study. Gynecol Oncol 47:159–166, 1992.
8. Hoskins WJ, McGuire WP, Brady MF, et al: The effect of diameter of largest residual disease on survival after primary cytoreductive surgery in patients with suboptimal residual epithelial ovarian carcinoma. Am J Obstet Gynecol 170:974–979, 1994; discussion 979–980.
9. Chi DS, Eisenhauer EL, Lang J, et al: What is the optimal goal of primary cytoreductive surgery for bulky stage IIIC epithelial ovarian carcinoma (EOC)? Gynecol Oncol 103:559–564, 2006.
10. Armstrong DK, Bundy B, Wenzel L, et al: Intraperitoneal cisplatin and paclitaxel in ovarian cancer. N Engl J Med 354:34–43, 2006.
11. Bookman MA: GOG0182-ICON5: 5-arm phase III randomized trial of paclitaxel (P) and carboplatin (C) vs combinations with gemcitabine (G), PEG-liposomal doxorubicin (D), or topotecan (T) in patients (pts) with advanced-stage epithelial ovarian (EOC) or primary peritoneal (PPC) carcinoma. J Clin Oncol 24:5002, 2006.
12. Farias-Eisner R, Teng F, Oliveira M, et al: The influence of tumor grade, distribution, and extent of carcinomatosis in minimal residual stage III epithelial ovarian cancer after optimal primary cytoreductive surgery. Gynecol Oncol 55:108–110, 1994.
13. Heintz A, Odicino F, Maisonneuve P, et al: Carcinoma of the ovary. Int J Gynaecol Obstet 95(Suppl 1):S161–S192, 2006.
14. Eisenkop SM, Spirtos NM: What are the current surgical objectives, strategies, and technical capabilities of gynecologic oncologists treating advanced epithelial ovarian cancer? Gynecol Oncol 82:489–497, 2001.
15. Akahira JI, Yoshikawa H, Shimizu Y, et al: Prognostic factors of stage IV epithelial ovarian cancer: a multicenter retrospective study. Gynecol Oncol 81:398–403, 2001.
16. Alphs HH, Zahurak ML, Bristow RE, et al: Predictors of surgical outcome and survival among elderly women diagnosed with ovarian and primary peritoneal cancer. Gynecol Oncol 103:1048–1053, 2006.
17. Bristow RE, del Carmen MG, Kaufman HS, et al: Radical oophorectomy with primary stapled colorectal anastomosis for resection of locally advanced epithelial ovarian cancer. J Am Coll Surg 197:565–574, 2003.
18. Obermair A, Hagenauer S, Tamandl D, et al: Safety and efficacy of low anterior en bloc resection as part of cytoreductive surgery for patients with ovarian cancer. Gynecol Oncol 83:115–120, 2001.
19. Tamussino KF, Lim PC, Webb MJ, et al: Gastrointestinal surgery in patients with ovarian cancer. Gynecol Oncol 80:79–84, 2001.
20. Aletti GD, Dowdy SC, Podratz KC, et al: Surgical treatment of diaphragm disease correlates with improved survival in optimally debulked advanced stage ovarian cancer. Gynecol Oncol 100:283–287, 2006.
21. Levine DA, Barakat RR, Hoskins WJ, et al: Procedures in Gynecologic Oncology. Informa Healthcare: New York and London, 2007, pp. 45–80.
22. Bristow RE, Montz FJ, Lagasse LD, et al: Survival impact of surgical cytoreduction in stage IV epithelial ovarian cancer. Gynecol Oncol 72:278–287, 1999.
23. Bojalian MO, Machado GR, Swensen R, et al: Radiofrequency ablation of liver metastasis from ovarian adenocarcinoma: case report and literature review. Gynecol Oncol 93:557–560, 2004.
24. Magtibay PM, Adams PB, Silverman MB, et al: Splenectomy as part of cytoreductive surgery in ovarian cancer. Gynecol Oncol 102:369–374, 2006.
25. Morris M, Gershenson DM, Burke TW, et al: Splenectomy in gynecologic oncology: indications, complications, and technique. Gynecol Oncol 43:118–122, 1991.
26. Aletti GD, Dowdy S, Podratz KC, et al: Role of lymphadenectomy in the management of grossly apparent advanced stage epithelial ovarian cancer. Am J Obstet Gynecol 195:1862–1868, 2005.
27. Panici PB, Maggioni A, Hacker N, et al: Systematic aortic and pelvic lymphadenectomy versus resection of bulky nodes only in optimally debulked advanced ovarian cancer: a randomized clinical trial. J Natl Cancer Inst 97:560–566, 2005.
28. Chi DS, Venkatraman ES, Masson V, et al: The ability of preoperative serum CA-125 to predict optimal primary tumor cytoreduction in stage III epithelial ovarian cancer. Gynecol Oncol 77:227–231, 2000.
29. Brockbank EC, Ind TE, Barton DP, et al: Preoperative predictors of suboptimal primary surgical cytoreduction in women with clinical evidence of advanced primary epithelial ovarian cancer. Int J Gynecol Cancer 14:42–50, 2004.
30. Bristow RE, Duska LR, Lambrou NC, et al: A model for predicting surgical outcome in patients with advanced ovarian carcinoma using computed tomography. Cancer 89:1532–1540, 2000.
31. Byrom J, Widjaja E, Redman CW, et al: Can pre-operative computed tomography predict resectability of ovarian carcinoma at primary laparotomy? BJOG 109:369–375, 2002.
32. Dowdy SC, Mullany SA, Brandt KR, et al: The utility of computed tomography scans in predicting suboptimal cytoreductive surgery in women with advanced ovarian carcinoma. Cancer 101:346–352, 2004.
33. Axtell A, Cass I, Li A, et al: Computed tomography predictors of primary suboptimal cytoreduction in patients with advanced ovarian cancer: a multi-institutional reciprocal validation study. [Abstract 57]. Gynecol Oncol 101:26, 2006.
34. Angioli R, Palaia I, Zullo MA, et al: Diagnostic open laparoscopy in the management of advanced ovarian cancer. Gynecol Oncol 100:455–461, 2006.
35. van der Burg ME, van Lent M, Buyse M, et al: The effect of debulking surgery after induction chemotherapy on the prognosis in advanced epithelial ovarian cancer. Gynecological Cancer Cooperative Group of the European Organization for Research and Treatment of Cancer. N Engl J Med 332:629–634, 1995.
36. Rose PG, Nerenstone S, Brady MF, et al: Secondary surgical cytoreduction for advanced ovarian carcinoma. N Engl J Med 351:2489–2497, 2004.
37. Monk BJ, Disaia PJ: What is the role of conservative primary surgical management of epithelial ovarian cancer: the United States experience and debate. Int J Gynecol Cancer 15(Suppl 3):199–205, 2005.
38. Bristow RE, Chi DS: Platinum-based neoadjuvant chemotherapy and interval surgical cytoreduction for advanced ovarian cancer: a meta-analysis. Gynecol Oncol 103:1070–1076, 2006.
39. Greer BE, Bundy BN, Ozols RF, et al: Implications of second-look laparotomy in the context of optimally resected stage III ovarian cancer: a non-randomized comparison using an explanatory analysis: a Gynecologic Oncology Group study. Gynecol Oncol 99:71–79, 2005.
40. Obermair A, Sevelda P: Impact of second look laparotomy and secondary cytoreductive surgery at second-look laparotomy in ovarian cancer patients. Acta Obstet Gynecol Scand 80:432–436, 2001.

41. Eisenkop SM, Friedman RL, Spirtos NM: The role of secondary cytoreductive surgery in the treatment of patients with recurrent epithelial ovarian carcinoma. Cancer 88:144–153, 2000.

42. Gadducci A, Iacconi P, Cosio S, et al: Complete salvage surgical cytoreduction improves further survival of patients with late recurrent ovarian cancer. Gynecol Oncol 79:344–349, 2000.

43. Morris M, Gershenson DM, Wharton JT, et al: Secondary cytoreductive surgery for recurrent epithelial ovarian cancer. Gynecol Oncol 34:334–338, 1989.

44. Segna RA, Dottino PR, Mandeli JP, et al: Secondary cytoreduction for ovarian cancer following cisplatin therapy. J Clin Oncol 11:434–439, 1993.

45. Zang RY, Li ZT, Tang J, et al: Secondary cytoreductive surgery for patients with relapsed epithelial ovarian carcinoma: who benefits? Cancer 100:1152–1161, 2004.

46. Munkarah AR, Coleman RL: Critical evaluation of secondary cytoreduction in recurrent ovarian cancer. Gynecol Oncol 95:273–280, 2004.

47. Harter P, Bois A, Hahmann M, et al: Surgery in recurrent ovarian cancer: the Arbeitsgemeinschaft Gynaekologische Onkologie (AGO) DESKTOP OVAR Trial. Ann Surg Oncol 13:1702–1710, 2006.

48. Salani R, Santillan A, Zahurak ML, et al: Secondary cytoreductive surgery for localized, recurrent epithelial ovarian cancer: analysis of prognostic factors and survival outcome. Cancer 109:685–691, 2007.

49. Tangjitgamol S, Levenback CF, Beller U, et al: Role of surgical resection for lung, liver, and central nervous system metastases in patients with gynecological cancer: a literature review. Int J Gynecol Cancer 14:399–422, 2004.

50. Pothuri B, Vaidya A, Aghajanian C, et al: Palliative surgery for bowel obstruction in recurrent ovarian cancer: an updated series. Gynecol Oncol 89:306–313, 2003.

51. Feuer DJ, Broadley KE, Shepherd JH, et al: Surgery for the resolution of symptoms in malignant bowel obstruction in advanced gynaecological and gastrointestinal cancer. Cochrane Database Syst Rev 2000: CD002764.

52. Jong P, Sturgeon J, Jamieson CG: Benefit of palliative surgery for bowel obstruction in advanced ovarian cancer. Can J Surg 38:454–457, 1995.

53. Pothuri B, Montemarano M, Gerardi M, et al: Percutaneous endoscopic gastrostomy tube placement in patients with malignant bowel obstruction due to ovarian carcinoma. Gynecol Oncol 96:330–334, 2005.

54. Dembo AJ, Davy M, Stenwig AE, et al: Prognostic factors in patients with stage I epithelial ovarian cancer. Obstet Gynecol, 75:263–273, 1990.

55. Sevelda P, Vavra N, Schemper M, et al: Prognostic factors for survival in stage I epithelial ovarian carcinoma. Cancer 65:2349–2352, 1990.

56. Vergote I, De Brabanter J, Fyles A, et al: Prognostic importance of degree of differentiation and cyst rupture in stage I invasive epithelial ovarian carcinoma. Lancet 357:176–182, 2001.

57. McGowan L, Lesher LP, Norris HJ, et al: Misstaging of ovarian cancer. Obstet Gynecol 65:568–572, 1985.

58. Buchsbaum HJ, Brady MF, Delgado G, et al: Surgical staging of carcinoma of the ovaries. Surg Gynecol Obstet 169:226–232, 1989.

59. Helewa ME, Krepart GV, Lotocki R: Staging laparotomy in early epithelial ovarian carcinoma. Am J Obstet Gynecol 154:282–286, 1986.

60. Young RC, Decker DG, Wharton JT, et al: Staging laparotomy in early ovarian cancer. JAMA 250:3072–3076, 1983.

61. Le T, Adolph A, Krepart GV, et al: The benefits of comprehensive surgical staging in the management of early-stage epithelial ovarian carcinoma. Gynecol Oncol 85:351–355, 2002.

62. Benedetti Panici P, et al: XVI FIGO World Congress of Gynecology and Obstetrics, Washington, September. Int J Gynecol Obstet 70(Suppl 1): A1–A147, 2000.

63. Cass I, Li AJ, Runowicz CD, et al: Pattern of lymph node metastases in clinically unilateral stage I invasive epithelial ovarian carcinomas. Gynecol Oncol 80:56–61, 2001.

64. Schilder JM, Thompson AM, DePriest PD, et al: Outcome of reproductive age women with stage IA or IC invasive epithelial ovarian cancer treated with fertility-sparing therapy. Gynecol Oncol 87:1–7, 2002.

65. Zanetta G, Chiari S, Rota S, et al: Conservative surgery for stage I ovarian carcinoma in women of childbearing age. Br J Obstet Gynaecol 104:1030–1035, 1997.

66. Benjamin I, Morgan MA, Rubin SC: Occult bilateral involvement in stage I epithelial ovarian cancer. Gynecol Oncol 72:288–291, 1999.

67. Ayhan A, Gultekin M, Taskiran C, et al: Routine appendectomy in epithelial ovarian carcinoma: is it necessary? Obstet Gynecol 105:719–724, 2005.

68. Childers JM, Lang J, Surwit EA, et al: Laparoscopic surgical staging of ovarian cancer. Gynecol Oncol 59:25–33, 1995.

69. Leblanc E, Querleu D, Narducci F, et al: Laparoscopic restaging of early stage invasive adnexal tumors: a 10-year experience. Gynecol Oncol 94:624–629, 2004.

70. Tozzi R, Kohler C, Ferrara A, et al: Laparoscopic treatment of early ovarian cancer: surgical and survival outcomes. Gynecol Oncol 93:199–203, 2004.

71. Chi DS, Abu-Rustum NR, Sonoda Y, et al: The safety and efficacy of laparoscopic surgical staging of apparent stage I ovarian and fallopian tube cancers. Am J Obstet Gynecol 192:1614–1619, 2005.

72. Medeiros LR, Rosa DD, Edelweiss MI, et al: Accuracy of frozen-section analysis in the diagnosis of ovarian tumors: a systematic quantitative review. Int J Gynecol Cancer 15:192–202, 2005.

73. Antoniou A, Pharoah PD, Narod S, et al: Average risks of breast and ovarian cancer associated with BRCA1 or BRCA2 mutations detected in case series unselected for family history: a combined analysis of 22 studies. Am J Hum Genet 72:1117–1130, 2003.

74. Risch HA, McLaughlin JR, Cole DE, et al: Prevalence and penetrance of germline BRCA1 and BRCA2 mutations in a population series of 649 women with ovarian cancer. Am J Hum Genet 68:700–710, 2001.

75. Kauff ND, Satagopan JM, Robson ME, et al: Risk-reducing salpingo-oophorectomy in women with a BRCA1 or BRCA2 mutation. N Engl J Med 346:1609–1615, 2002.

76. Rebbeck TR, Lynch HT, Neuhausen SL, et al: Prophylactic oophorectomy in carriers of BRCA1 or BRCA2 mutations. N Engl J Med 346:1616–1622, 2002.

77. Finch A, Beiner M, Lubinski J, et al: Salpingo-oophorectomy and the risk of ovarian, fallopian tube, and peritoneal cancers in women with a BRCA1 or BRCA2 mutation. JAMA 296:185–192, 2006.

78. Kauff ND, Barakat RR: Surgical risk-reduction in carriers of BRCA mutations: where do we go from here? Gynecol Oncol 93:277–279, 2004.

79. Harlow BL, Weiss NS, Lofton S: Epidemiology of borderline ovarian tumors. J Natl Cancer Inst 78:71–74, 1987.

80. Tinelli R, Tinelli A, Tinelli FG, et al: Conservative surgery for borderline ovarian tumors: a review. Gynecol Oncol 100:185–191, 2006.

81. Lin PS, Gershenson DM, Bevers MW, et al: The current status of surgical staging of ovarian serous borderline tumors. Cancer 85:905–911, 1999.

82. Morris RT, Gershenson DM, Silva EG, et al: Outcome and reproductive function after conservative surgery for borderline ovarian tumors. Obstet Gynecol 95:541–547, 2000.

83. Zanetta G, Rota S, Chiari S, et al: Behavior of borderline tumors with particular interest to persistence, recurrence, and progression to invasive carcinoma: a prospective study. J Clin Oncol 19:2658–2664, 2001.

84. Seidman JD, Kurman, RJ: Ovarian serous borderline tumors: a critical review of the literature with emphasis on prognostic indicators. Hum Pathol 31:539–557, 2000.

85. Geomini P, Bremer G, Kruitwagen R, et al: Diagnostic accuracy of frozen section diagnosis of the adnexal mass: a metaanalysis. Gynecol Oncol 96:1–9, 2005.

86. Ronnett BM, Kajdacsy-Balla A, Gilks CB, et al: Mucinous borderline ovarian tumors: points of general agreement and persistent controversies regarding nomenclature, diagnostic criteria, and behavior. Hum Pathol 35:949–960, 2004.

87. Barakat RR, Benjamin I, Lewis JL Jr, et al: Platinum based chemotherapy for advanced-stage serous ovarian carcinoma of low malignant potential. Gynecol Oncol 59:390–393, 1995.

88. Kliman L, Rome RM, Fortune DW: Low malignant potential tumors of the ovary: a study of 76 cases. Obstet Gynecol 68:338–344, 1986.

89. Nation JG, Krepart GV: Ovarian carcinoma of low malignant potential: staging and treatment. Am J Obstet Gynecol 154:290–293, 1986.

90. Chambers JT, Merino MJ, Kohorn EI, et al: Borderline ovarian tumors. Am J Obstet Gynecol 159:1088–1094, 1988.

91. Hopkins MP, Morley GW: The second-look operation and tumors of the ovary: a study of 76 cases. Obstet Gynecol 74:375–378, 1989.

92. Gershenson DM, Silva EG: Serous ovarian tumors of low malignant potential with peritoneal implants. Cancer 65:578–585, 1990.

93. Sutton GP, Bundy BN, Omura GA, et al: Stage III ovarian tumors of low malignant potential treated with cisplatin combination therapy (a Gynecologic Oncology Group study). Gynecol Oncol 41:230–233, 1991.

94. Gershenson DM, Silva EG, Tortolero-Luna G, et al: Serous borderline tumors of the ovary with noninvasive peritoneal implants. Cancer 83:2157–2163, 1998.

95. Longacre TA, McKenney JK, Tazelaar HD, et al: Ovarian serous tumors of low malignant potential (borderline tumors): outcome-based study of 276 patients with long-term (> or =5-year) follow-up. Am J Surg Pathol 29:707–723, 2005.

96. Crispens MA, Bodurka D, Deavers M, et al: Response and survival in patients with progressive or recurrent serous ovarian tumors of low malignant potential. Obstet Gynecol 99:3–10, 2002.

97. Kurman RJ, Norris HJ: Malignant germ cell tumors of the ovary. Hum Pathol 8:551–564, 1977.

98. Peccatori F, Bonazzi C, Chiari S, et al: Surgical management of malignant ovarian germ-cell tumors: 10 years' experience of 129 patients. Obstet Gynecol 86:367–372, 1995.

99. Zanetta G, Bonazzi C, Cantu M, et al: Survival and reproductive function after treatment of malignant germ cell ovarian tumors. J Clin Oncol 19:1015–1120, 2001.

100. Slayton RE, Park RC, Silverberg SG, et al: Vincristine, dactinomycin, and cyclophosphamide in the treatment of malignant germ cell tumors of the ovary. A Gynecologic Oncology Group Study (a final report). Cancer 56:243–248, 1985.

101. Williams SD, Blessing JA, Moore DH, et al: Cisplatin, vinblastine, and bleomycin in advanced and recurrent ovarian germ-cell tumors. A trial of the Gynecologic Oncology Group. Ann Intern Med 111:22–27, 1989.

102. Bafna UD, Umadevi K, Kumaran C, et al: Germ cell tumors of the ovary: is there a role for aggressive cytoreductive surgery for nondysgerminomatous tumors? Int J Gynecol Cancer 11:300–304, 2001.

103. Munkarah A, Gershenson DM, Levenback C, et al: Salvage surgery for chemorefractory ovarian germ cell tumors. Gynecol Oncol 55:217–223, 1994.

104. Rezk Y, Sheinfeld J, Chi DS: Prolonged survival following salvage surgery for chemorefractory ovarian immature teratoma: a case report and review of the literature. Gynecol Oncol 96:883–887, 2005.

105. Andre F, Fizazi K, Culine S, et al: The growing teratoma syndrome: results of therapy and long-term follow-up of 33 patients. Eur J Cancer 36:1389–1394, 2000.

106. Zagame L, Pautier P, Duvillard P, et al: Growing teratoma syndrome after ovarian germ cell tumors. Obstet Gynecol 108:509–514, 2006.

107. Comerci JT Jr, Licciardi F, Bergh PA, et al: Mature cystic teratoma: a clinicopathologic evaluation of 517 cases and review of the literature. Obstet Gynecol 84:22–28, 1994.

108. Chan JK, Zhang M, Kaleb V, et al: Prognostic factors responsible for survival in sex cord stromal tumors of the ovary—a multivariate analysis. Gynecol Oncol 96:204–209, 2005.

109. Evans AT III, Gaffey TA, Malkasian GD Jr, et al: Clinicopathologic review of 118 granulosa and 82 theca cell tumors. Obstet Gynecol 55:231–238, 1980.

110. Sehouli J, Drescher FS, Mustea A, et al: Granulosa cell tumor of the ovary: 10 years follow-up data of 65 patients. Anticancer Res 24:1223–1239, 2004.

111. Gershenson DM, Morris M, Burke TW, et al: Treatment of poor-prognosis sex cord-stromal tumors of the ovary with the combination of bleomycin, etoposide, and cisplatin. Obstet Gynecol 87:527–531, 1996.

8

Chemotherapy for Ovarian Cancer

Jeffrey G. Bell and Christopher V. Lutman

KEY POINTS

- Early ovarian cancer can be divided into low-risk and high-risk groups.
- Complete surgical staging impacts treatment decisions.
- Patients with low-risk early-stage ovarian cancer do not require adjuvant chemotherapy.
- Adjuvant chemotherapy definitely benefits incompletely staged patients.
- The need for adjuvant chemotherapy for completely staged patients with high-risk, stage I non–clear cell histology is controversial.
- Carboplatin with paclitaxel is the preferred adjuvant regimen by extrapolation from treatment of advanced disease.
- Three cycles of adjuvant treatment are sufficient for completely staged high-risk ovarian cancer patients.
- Stage II patients should be treated as stage III.
- Clear cell histology requires special consideration.
- The standard, preferred chemotherapy regimen for advanced disease is six cycles of carboplatin and paclitaxel.
- Intraperitoneal chemotherapy is an alternative regimen that should be offered to patients with optimal residual stage III disease.
- Maintenance chemotherapy should be discussed with patients who have achieved a complete response to frontline therapy in advanced disease.
- Neoadjuvant chemotherapy is an option for patients with poor performance status and advanced disease.

EARLY OVARIAN CARCINOMA

Definition of Early Ovarian Cancer

Most authors and trials of early ovarian carcinoma have defined "early" stage as FIGO (International Federation of Gynecology and Obstetrics) stages I and II (Box 8-1). The subject of adjuvant chemotherapy for the early stages of ovarian carcinoma has been controversial for decades, and at this time some aspects remain unresolved.

Some of the earlier trials identified subgroups of stage I whose prognosis was excellent and therefore warranted a classification of "low-risk" for cancer recurrence and death. Subsequent studies often stratified the early-stage ovarian cancer populations into low-risk and high-risk groups (Box 8-2).

In 1994, the National Institutes of Health (NIH) convened a Consensus Development Conference on ovarian cancer for the purpose of identifying issues that had sufficiently confirmed data at that time.[1] Box 8-3 summarizes the conference's statement on management of stage I cancer. The conference panel could not reach consensus on the need for adjuvant therapy in the subsets of stage I not listed in the

Box 8-1. Early-Stage Epithelial Carcinoma: FIGO (International Federation of Gynecology and Obstetrics) Stages I and II

Stage I: Growth limited to the ovaries
IA   Growth limited to one ovary; no malignant ascites; no tumor on external surface; capsule intact
IB   Growth limited to both ovaries; no malignant ascites; no tumor on external surface; capsules intact
IC   Growth involving one or both ovaries with malignant ascites or peritoneal washings; or with tumor on external surface; or with ruptured capsule.

Stage II: Growth involving one or both ovaries with pelvic extension
IIA   Extension or metastases to uterus and/or tubes
IIB   Extension to other pelvic tissues
IIC   Tumor of stage IIa or IIb also with malignant ascites or peritoneal washings; or with tumor on external surface; or with ruptured capsule(s)

Box 8-2. Definitions of Low-Risk and High-Risk Early-Stage Ovarian Carcinoma

Low Risk

Stage IA or IB, grade 1–2

High-Risk

Stage IA or IB, grade 3 or clear cell
Stage IC (rupture, positive cytology, positive capsule)
Stage II with no residual disease (pelvic disease)

Box 8-3. NIH Consensus Development Conference (1994) Recommendations for Stage I Management

Patents with stage IA grade 1 and most IB grade 1 tumors do not require adjuvant therapy

All patients with grade 3 tumors require adjuvant therapy

Patients with clear cell carcinoma require adjuvant therapy

Many but not all women with stage IC disease require adjuvant therapy

---

box, and they concluded that the most effective adjuvant therapy had not been established. The panel also recommended that patients with high-risk stage I cancers should be enrolled in clinical trials to identify adjuvant therapy that will improve survival.

These NIH recommendations point out the importance of histologic grade in the prognosis of early-stage disease. Despite numerous studies indicating the association between grade and outcome,[2-4] FIGO staging does not incorporate grade. Nevertheless, grade influences decisions on both clinical management and trial design.

Natural History of Untreated Early Ovarian Carcinoma

Knowing the natural history of untreated early ovarian cancer should identify the need for adjuvant chemotherapy. Assessing an observation arm in randomized controlled trials (RCTs) should be an accurate means of determining the true rate of recurrent cancer after surgical resection. Table 8-1 lists five prominent randomized controlled trials comparing observation with a treatment arm. The rate of cancer recurrence in the observation arm varies from 9% to 35% owing to differences in substages and grades among the trials. Once again, these trials point out the

Table 8-1. Recurrence Rate of Early Stage Ovarian Cancer in the No-Treatment Control Arms of Randomized Controlled Trials

Trial	Stage and Grade	N	5-Year Recurrence Rate
Hreshchyshyn et al (1980)[5*]	Stages IA, B, C Grades 1, 2, 3	86	17%
Young et al (1990)[6†]	Stages IA, B Grades 1, 2	81	9%
Bolis et al (GICOG, 1995)[7†]	Stages IA, B Grades 1, 2, 3	83	35%
Trope et al (2000)[8*]	Stages IA, B, C Grade 1 aneu Grades 2, 3	162	29%
Trimbos et al (ACTION, 2003)[9*]	Stages IA, B, Grade 2–3 Stage IC, all grades Stage IIA, all grades	448	32%

ACTION, Adjuvant Chemotherapy in Ovarian Neoplasm; aneu, aneuploidy; GICOG, Gruppo Italiano Collaborativo in Oncologia Ginecologica.
*Incomplete surgical staging in the majority of patients, or extent of staging unreported.
†Complete surgical staging.

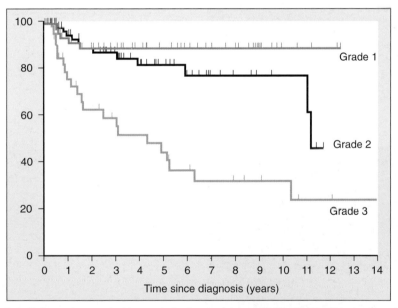

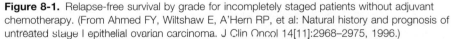

Figure 8-1. Relapse-free survival by grade for incompletely staged patients without adjuvant chemotherapy. (From Ahmed FY, Wiltshaw E, A'Hern RP, et al: Natural history and prognosis of untreated stage I epithelial ovarian carcinoma. J Clin Oncol 14[11]:2968–2975, 1996.)

importance of grade in the prognosis of early ovarian cancers. The randomized controlled trials indicate that well-differentiated tumors have less than a 10% chance of recurring after surgery only, whereas the more poorly differentiated cancers may recur in 30% to 35% of patients treated by surgery only. Figure 8-1 also demonstrates the impact of grade on survival in patients treated by surgery only.[10]

Evidence that dividing stage I disease into substages reflects differences in prognosis is seen in Table 8-2. Figures 8-2 and 8-3 show patients with stages IA and IB ovarian cancer, respectively.

Table 8-2. Five-Year Recurrence Rates for Stage I Cancer with Incomplete Surgical Staging and Without Adjuvant Chemotherapy

Stage	5-Year Recurrence Rate
IA	13% (95% CI 7.24)
IB	35% (95% CI 16.65)
IC	38% (95% CI 28.51)

Data from Ahmed FY, Wiltshaw E, A'Hern RP, et al: Natural history and prognosis of untreated stage I epithelial ovarian carcinoma. J Clin Oncol 14(11):2968–2975,1996.

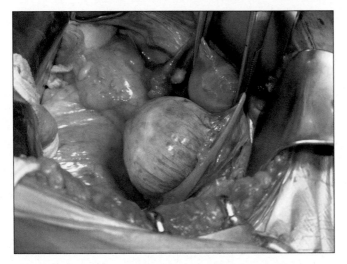

Figure 8-2. Photograph of gross stage IA ovarian cancer. The right ovarian mass is free of adhesions and visible adjacent to a normal fallopian tube and uterine corpus.

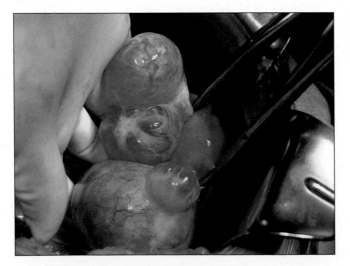

Figure 8-3. Photograph of gross stage IB ovarian cancer. Clamps have been placed across the uterine cornua. Both ovaries have cystic masses.

Importance of Surgical Staging

A major flaw in most studies of early ovarian cancer is the inconsistency in requirements for surgical staging. The Gynecologic Oncology Group's (GOG) definition of complete surgical staging is listed in Box 8-4. Obviously, gross inspection and palpation of the peritoneal cavity may miss occult or microscopic disease that would

---

Box 8-4. GOG Requirements for Surgical Staging of Ovarian Carcinoma

Staging Operative Procedures
1. Total hysterectomy with bilateral salpingo-oophorectomy
2. Infracolic omentectomy
3. Aspiration of free peritoneal fluid
4. Peritoneal washings for cytology (abdomen and pelvis)
5. Inspection of all abdominal peritoneal surfaces
6. Peritoneal biopsies from four pelvic locations and bilateral paracolic areas
7. Diaphragm scraping or biopsy
8. Bilateral selective pelvic and aortic lymph node dissections

GOG, Gynecologic Oncology Group.

---

change the stage of disease from early (stage I or II) to advanced (stage III). Thorough surgical staging procedures upstage the diagnosis in 10% to 30% of cases.[11-13] Thus, trials claiming to investigate or treat stages I and II disease without complete surgical staging may be including patients who actually have more advanced disease. Evidence for this is found in an analysis of the observation group in the ACTION trial.[9] Of the 222 patients in the observation arm, 75 had undergone optimal surgical staging, 147 nonoptimal staging. The recurrence-free survival following optimal surgical staging was significantly better than following nonoptimal staging (hazard ratio [HR] = 1.82, $P = .04$). This difference implies that more advanced, occult disease is present in cohorts not having complete surgical staging. Thus, surgical staging could affect outcomes in trials of adjuvant chemotherapy.

The inconsistent surgical staging procedures among trials of early ovarian cancer may be another reason for the range of cancer recurrence rates. The natural recurrence rates for stage I cancer treated by surgery only, depicted in Table 8-1, are mostly from trials that did not include complete surgical staging during the initial operation for most patients. The one trial that required complete surgical staging reported similar low recurrence rates for observation and treatment of low-grade cancers.[6]

Does Adjuvant Chemotherapy Improve Outcome?

Because of a relatively low rate of cancer recurrence in early ovarian cancer, the challenge of clinical trials has been to accrue enough patients to have the power to detect a clinically meaningful impact of adjuvant chemotherapy on either cancer recurrence or survival. The most notable studies indicating significant effects of adjuvant chemotherapy compared with observation are listed in Table 8-3.

In 1980, the GOG reported that an 18-month course of melphalan significantly reduced the recurrence rate compared with either observation or pelvic radiation therapy.[5] This result is surprising owing to the fact that the trial design was three arms and included only 86 patients with a large proportion of stage Ia grade 1 cancers, a group of patients who benefit the least from adjuvant chemotherapy.

All four trials found that adjuvant chemotherapy significantly reduced the risk of cancer recurrence by an absolute value of 8% to 18%. Only one study, however, also demonstrated a significant benefit on overall survival; the ICON (International Collaborative Ovarian Neoplasm)-1 trial reported an absolute improvement of 9%. The GOG trial did not report overall survival, and the GICOG trial was likely underpowered to detect a significant difference. ACTION found an absolute improvement in overall survival of 7%, very similar to ICON-1, but not reaching statistical significance despite comparable sample size.

Table 8-3. Randomized Controlled Trials Showing Benefit of Adjuvant Chemotherapy in Early-Stage Ovarian Cancer

Trial	N	Stage and Grade	Treatment	RFS % Drug vs. No Drug	OS % Drug vs. No Drug
GOG (Hreshchyshyn et al, 1980)[5]	86	Stages IA, B, C Grades 1, 2, 3	Melphalan 18 mo.	94 vs 83 $P < .05$	Not reported
GICOG (Bolis et al, 1995)[7]	83	Stages IA, B Grades 1, 2, 3	Cisplatin 6 cycles	83 vs 65 $P = .028$	88 vs 82 $P = .77$
ICON-1 (Colombo et al, 2003)[14]	477	Stages IA, B, C; ?II Grades 1, 2, 3	Carboplatin 6 cycles	73 vs 62 $P = .01$	79 vs 70 $P = .03$
ACTION (Trimbos et al, 2003)[9]	448	Stages IA, B Grades 2, 3 Stages IC and IIA All clear cell	Platinum minimum 4 cycles	76 vs 68 $P = .02$	85 vs 78 $P = .1$

OS, overall survival; RFS, recurrence-free survival.

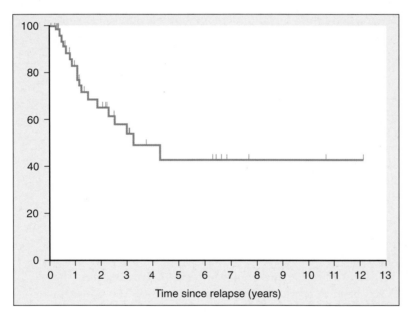

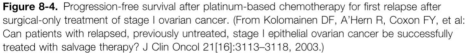

Figure 8-4. Progression-free survival after platinum-based chemotherapy for first relapse after surgical-only treatment of stage I ovarian cancer. (From Kolomainen DF, A'Hern R, Coxon FY, et al: Can patients with relapsed, previously untreated, stage I epithelial ovarian cancer be successfully treated with salvage therapy? J Clin Oncol 21[16]:3113–3118, 2003.)

Other than sample size, two other reasons might explain the fact that a reduction in the rate of cancer recurrence does not translate into improvement in overall survival. "Salvage" chemotherapy for cancer recurrence in the observation arms of these trials most likely impacted the survival for those patients, thus dampening the survival difference between the two arms. In fact, platinum-based chemotherapy for first recurrences in stage I observation groups provides 5-year progression-free survivals of 24% to 42%[10,15] (Fig. 8-4). In our opinion, the primary end point of trials in early ovarian cancer should be recurrence-free survival, since this outcome most closely approximates a true cure of the disease. Although treatment of first relapse may affect overall survival, most of these patients whose cancers recur will die of their disease.

Table 8-4. Survival After Adjuvant Chemotherapy or Observation by Completeness of Surgical Staging: The ACTION Trial

	N	RFS	P Value	OS	P Value
Complete Surgical Staging					
Observation	75	80%	.7 (HR, 95% CI 0.5–2.4)	89%	.7
Chemotherapy	76	83%		87%	
Incomplete Surgical Staging					
Observation	147	65%	.009	75%	.03
Chemotherapy	148	78%		84%	

CI, confidence interval; HR, hazard ratio; OS, 5-year overall survival; RFS, 5-year recurrence-free survival.
Data from Trimbos JB, Vergote I, Bolis G, et al: Impact of adjuvant chemotherapy and surgical staging in early-stage ovarian carcinoma: European Organisation for Research and Treatment of Cancer-Adjuvant ChemoTherapy in Ovarian Neoplasm trial. J Natl Cancer Inst 95(2):113–125, 2003.

A further explanation for trials not finding significant differences in overall survival could be the inconsistency in the degree of surgical staging. ICON-1,[14] which did report an overall survival difference between treatment and observation, did not require surgical staging as defined by GOG. Thus, the cohort undoubtedly included microscopic or occult advanced disease. Adjuvant chemotherapy is more likely to impact occult advanced disease than true pathologic stage I disease. The ACTION trial data may support this theory.[9] That trial encouraged complete surgical staging, and approximately one third of the patients underwent "optimal" surgical staging. A subanalysis of the optimally staged patients found no difference in either recurrence-free survival (83% versus 80%) or overall survival (87% versus 89%) between treatment and observation arms. On the other hand, for the group of nonoptimally staged patients, both recurrence-free and overall survivals were significantly better for the treated patients (78% versus 65%, P = .009; 84% versus 75%, P = .03, respectively) (Table 8-4). The caveat on the data from ACTION is that the number of patients in the optimally staged analysis was 151, perhaps too small to detect a significant difference. The precision of the estimated difference in recurrence rates between observation and chemotherapy in this optimal subset is wide, 0.5 to 2.4. However, a meta-analysis of randomized controlled trials that reported at least a modified surgical staging operation also did not detect a significant overall survival difference between adjuvant chemotherapy and no treatment with a more narrow precision (HR 0.81; 95% CI, 0.58–1.21).[16] These data suggest that adjuvant chemotherapy benefits nonoptimally staged patients but may not benefit optimally staged patients. Once again, this is likely due to the inclusion of occult stage III patients in cohorts not undergoing complete surgical staging.

Further evidence of the importance of thorough surgical staging on the decision for adjuvant chemotherapy comes from a non-randomized Canadian study.[17] Among 94 patients who underwent staging operations by gynecologic oncologists following a fixed protocol, 60 patients had surgical-pathologic stage I. During expectant management, only 10% of these 60 patients had recurrence—all being serous or clear cell histology. On the other hand, the recurrence rate was 25% among 25 unstaged patients managed expectantly owing to lack of risk factors. Attaining this type of thorough and regimented staging operation in a multi-institutional, randomized trial would be ideal and rewarding, but probably not feasible.

Choice of Chemotherapy and Duration of Treatment

Generally, choice of adjuvant chemotherapeutic agents for early-stage disease has been extrapolated from management of advanced-stage ovarian cancer. See the section on Advanced Ovarian Carcinoma, later in this chapter. Many of the investigational trials in early-stage ovarian cancer compared cisplatin-based combination chemotherapy to radiation therapy [18–20] (Table 8-5). Meta-analyses of these types of trials have shown no significant difference between chemotherapy and radiation therapy for disease-free and overall survival.[21]

Carboplatin replaced cisplatin as the standard platinum in treating ovarian cancer after several studies concluded that carboplatin and cisplatin had equivalent efficacy in treating advanced disease.[22] ICON-2 demonstrated that single-agent carboplatin effected the same median survival and 2-year survival (33 months and 60%) as the combination of cyclophosphamide-doxorubicin-cisplatin in advanced disease.[23] As in advanced disease, platinum-based chemotherapy can be considered standard treatment for early ovarian cancer; however, a universally accepted regimen is not evident. Two international multicenter trials of adjuvant therapy in early ovarian cancer, ACTION[9] and ICON-1,[14] allowed either single-agent carboplatin or cisplatin combination regimens for eligibility.

Since 1995, most research in chemotherapy for advanced disease has focused on incorporating paclitaxel into front-line treatment, and the combination of carboplatin and paclitaxel is currently the preferred treatment for advanced disease.[24] However, the number of trials with paclitaxel regimens in early ovarian cancer are limited.[25,26] No trials have compared combination platinum-paclitaxel with nonpaclitaxel regimens in early ovarian cancer. Without such direct comparisons, regimens other than carboplatin-paclitaxel would seem acceptable (Fig. 8-5).

The optimal duration of adjuvant therapy in early ovarian cancer is unknown. Table 8-6 shows the outcomes of trials using various regimens from three to six cycles. The GOG has conducted the only randomized trial comparing two different durations.[29] This study compared three to six cycles of adjuvant carboplatin-paclitaxel in high-risk early ovarian cancer patients who had been completely staged. It found no significant difference in the risk of cancer recurrence or 5-year survival (25% versus 20% and 81% versus 83%, respectively). Of note was the significantly greater toxicity in the six-cycle arm. The authors concluded that following complete surgical staging, three cycles of carboplatin and paclitaxel constitute a reasonable treatment option

Table 8-5. Trials Comparing Adjuvant Cisplatin with Radiation Therapy in Early-Stage Ovarian Cancer

Trial	N	Stage	Treatment	Survival
Vergote et al (1992)[18]	340	I, II, III	Cisplatin vs ^{32}P	75% DFS for cisplatin 81% DFS for ^{32}P
Chiara et al (1994)[19]	70	IA grade 3–IIC	CP vs WAR	74% DFS for chemo 50% DFS for WAR
Bolis et al (1995)[7]	161	IC	Cisplatin vs ^{32}P	81% OS for cisplatin 79% OS for ^{32}P
Kojs et al (2001)[20]	150	IA grade 2–IIC	CAP vs WAR	81% 5-year DFS for both

CAP, cyclophosphamide/doxorubicin/cisplatin; CP, cyclophosphamide and cisplatin; DFS, disease-free survival; OS, overall survival; WAR, whole abdomen radiation therapy.
Modified from Winter-Roach B, Hooper L, Kitchener H: Systematic review of adjuvant therapy for early stage (epithelial) ovarian cancer. Int J Gynecol Cancer 13(4):395–404, 2003.

Table 8-6. Duration of Adjuvant Chemotherapy in Early-Stage Ovarian Cancer

Trial	N	Stage and Grade	Treatment	No. Cycles	Survival
Rubin (1993)[27]	62	Stages IA, B, grades 2–3, IC	CP, CAP	6	73% 5-year DFS
Shimada (2005)[28]	100	Stages I, II, all grades	CAP or CT	3	100% 5-year OS for low risk 89% for high risk
Bamias (2006)[25]	69	Stages IA, B, grades 2, 3 Stages IC, II, any grade	Carboplatin Paclitaxel	4	79% 5-year DFS 87% 5-year OS
Bell (2006)[29]	427	Stages IA, B, grade 3 Stages IC, II, any grade	Carboplatin Paclitaxel	3 6	75% 5-year DFS 80% 5-year DFS

CAP, cyclophosphamide-doxorubicin-cisplatin; CP, cyclophosphamide and cisplatin; CT, carboplatin-paclitaxel.

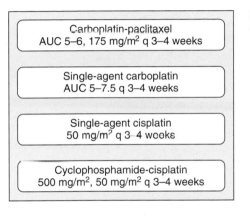

Figure 8-5. Acceptable chemotherapy regimens for non–clear cell early stage ovarian cancer.

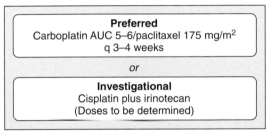

Figure 8-6. Options for treating clear cell carcinoma of the ovary.

for women with high-risk, early-stage epithelial ovarian cancer. Three additional cycles of carboplatin-paclitaxel chemotherapy are, at best, likely to provide only a modest reduction in the absolute risk of recurrence, yet are associated with increased toxicity.

Clear cell histology is generally considered an aggressive epithelial carcinoma with a worse prognosis, stage for stage,[17,30,31] or at least in stage I.[32,33] Other data do not support these opinions.[34,35] In advanced disease, the overall response rate (RR) to platinum-based chemotherapy is 11% compared with 72% for serous histology.[31] The addition of paclitaxel to platinum appears to improve the RR: 56% compared with 27% for platinum without paclitaxel.[36] More recently, a retrospective review reported that platinum with irinotecan resulted in a higher RR than paclitaxel/platinum (43% versus 32%) and also resulted in a significantly improved progression-free survival in optimally debulked patients.[37] In keeping with the general pattern of extrapolating from advanced disease, the current recommended option for adjuvant treatment of early-stage clear cell carcinoma would be combination paclitaxel-carboplatin. Although combination cisplatin-irinotecan appears promising, at this point it should be considered investigational (Fig. 8-6).

Future Directions

As intraperitoneal (IP) chemotherapy has become a recommended option for advanced ovarian cancer, trials have also assessed the benefit of intraperitoneal therapy in early stages. Several of these trials have reported similar outcomes, that is, approximately a 15% to 20% cancer recurrence rate[38-40] (Table 8-7). Since adjuvant regimens for early ovarian cancer essentially have been extrapolated from treatment of advanced disease, intraperitoneal therapy should be considered an alternative to intravenous chemotherapy for some subsets of early ovarian cancer. The National Comprehensive Cancer Network (NCCN) lists the following intraperitoneal regimen as an alternative for stage II: paclitaxel 135 mg/m^2, IV 24-hour infusion on day 1; cisplatin 100 mg/m^2, IP on day 2 after paclitaxel; paclitaxel 60 mg/m^2, IP on day 8. Cycles are repeated every 3 weeks. Use of a venous catheter with a subcutaneous access port is shown in Figure 8-7.

A review of the various adjuvant treatments for early-stage epithelial ovarian cancer over the last two to three decades reveals surprisingly similar outcomes for radiation therapy techniques and chemotherapy agents of differing classes (Fig. 8-8). The risk of recurrent cancer in this patient population seems to have remained relatively unchanged over the years. Seemingly, some proportion of patients, perhaps 20% to 25%, has cancer that is resistant to various forms of adjuvant cytotoxic therapy. The door remains open for innovative research using combination chemotherapy, biologic modifiers, and molecular targeting agents.

The two major obstacles to finding a future therapy of greater benefit in early-stage disease are (1) defining true stage I cancers by accurate surgical staging and (2) the statistical design of the trials. The potential problem of including occult stage III patients in cohorts of nonoptimally staged patients has been previously discussed. In addition, the statistical design of these trials remains a challenge because the relatively small number of recurrent events or deaths occurring over fairly long intervals after treatment requires enormous sample sizes to detect clinically reasonable differences in outcomes.

Some researchers have suggested that biologic and molecular markers can either complement or replace surgical staging in apparent early-stage disease by predicting the outcome of treatment. The magnitude of research in molecular prognostic markers for ovarian cancer is beyond the scope of this chapter, but the future of adjuvant therapy in early disease could be defined by the identification of accurate prognostic markers. Table 8-8 gives a brief summary of some of the prognostic factors other than FIGO staging.[41] Some investigators have developed models of prognostic markers. One such model in early ovarian cancer incorporated grade, p53, and EGFR.[42] The model was applied to 226 patients with stage IA-IIC who had undergone a modified surgical staging operation followed by pelvic radiation, whole-abdomen

Table 8-7. Results of Intraperitoneal Chemotherapy in Early-Stage Ovarian Cancer

Trial	Stage	N	IP Chemotherapy	Outcome
Malmstrom (1994)[38]	I, II	47	Carboplatin × 4 cycles	23% relapse
Topuz (2001)[39]	IC	13	Cisplatin and mitoxantrone median 5 cycles	84% 5-year DFS
Fujiwara (2003)[40]	I	54	Carboplatin alone or with IV cyclophosphamide or paclitaxel	81% 5-year DFS

DFS, disease-free survival; IP, intraperitoneal.

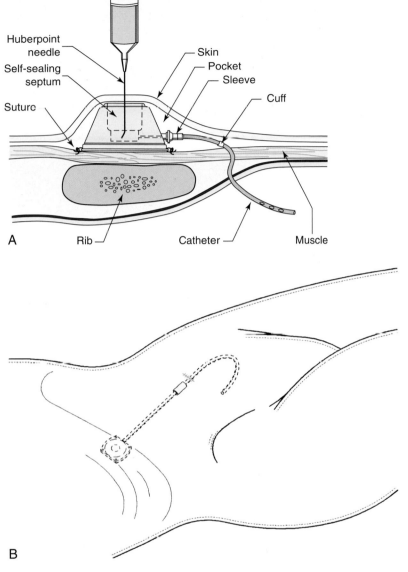

Huberpoint needle

Self-sealing septum

Suture

Skin

Pocket

Sleeve

Cuff

Rib

Catheter

Muscle

A

B

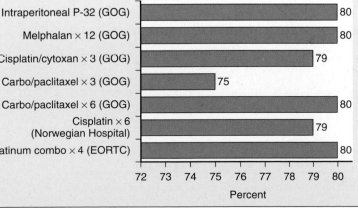

Figure 8-7. A, Implanted peritoneal access catheter with subcutaneous self-sealing port providing a path for intraperitoneal therapy. **B,** Intraperitoneal chemotherapy. (From DiSaia PJ, Creasman WT (eds): Clinical Gynecologic Oncology, 7th ed. Philadelphia: Mosby, 2007, Fig. 11–25.)

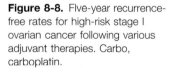

	Percent
Intraperitoneal P-32 (GOG)	80
Melphalan × 12 (GOG)	80
Cisplatin/cytoxan × 3 (GOG)	79
Carbo/paclitaxel × 3 (GOG)	75
Carbo/paclitaxel × 6 (GOG)	80
Cisplatin × 6 (Norwegian Hospital)	79
Platinum combo × 4 (EORTC)	80

Figure 8-8. Five-year recurrence-free rates for high-risk stage I ovarian cancer following various adjuvant therapies. Carbo, carboplatin.

Table 8-8. Nonstaging Factors That May Predict Outcome in Early-Stage Ovarian Cancer

Prognostic Factor	Decreased Recurrence	Increased Recurrence
Histology		Clear cell
Grade	Grade 1	Grade 3
DNA ploidy	Diploid	Aneuploid
HER2/neu	Normal expression	Overexpressed
Morphometry	Low volume	High volume
p53 mutation	Absent	Overexpressed
Bcl-2	Present	Absent
PDGF	Absent	Overexpressed
EGFR	Absent	Present

EGFR, epidermal growth factor receptor; PDGR, platelet-derived growth factor. Adapted from McGuire WP: Current aspects of adjuvant therapy of early stage ovarian cancer. Zentralbl Gynakol 120(3):93–97, 1998.

radiation, or four cycles of platinum-based chemotherapy. Patients with grade 1–2 tumors whose results were negative for *p53* and EGFR had a 5-year disease-free survival of 89% compared with 39% for patients with grade 3 tumors that were also positive for *p53* and EGFR ($P = .00008$). An intermediate risk model with any other combination of the three factors was associated with a 66% disease-free survival ($P = .0006$). In a regression analysis, FIGO substage was not significantly associated with disease-free survival, whereas grade, *p53*, and EGFR were. Since this study did not report what percentage of patients underwent the modified surgical staging operation and because lymph node dissection was not part of the operation, the model may apply only to incompletely staged patients.

Another confounding factor is the use of various adjuvant therapies. Nevertheless, it does show the potential value of combining molecular markers to better define prognosis, for example, as applied to the intermediate-risk group with grade 1 histology, positive *p53*, and positive EGFR. Such models may prove very useful in future trials whereby adjuvant therapy could be modified or tailored based on stratification into high- and low-risk groups. Such trials may also test molecular targeting for the high-risk groups as defined in Box 8-2. In addition, future strategy should include studies of prognostic factors applied to patients who are completely staged and receive no adjuvant therapy. This type of study could identify markers that are significantly associated with recurrence in true stage I disease.

Even if molecular markers were able to replace optimal surgical staging in gross stage I disease, until this happens future trials in early ovarian cancer are likely to require staging operations at least sufficient to separate stage I from stage II disease because of clinically significant different relapse rates between the two. In a recent GOG trial in which all patients received adjuvant chemotherapy, the recurrence rate for stage II was nearly twice that for stage I (33% versus 18%).[29] This inferior prognosis of stage II patients has prompted the GOG to shift stage II patients to future protocols of advanced-stage disease. In addition, the NCCN recommendations for treatment of stage II are the same as for stages III and IV (Box 8-5 and Fig. 8-9).

Summary

The benefit of adjuvant chemotherapy in most cases of true stage I ovarian cancer remains uncertain because of the lack of complete surgical staging in randomized

---

Box 8-5. Summary of Early-Stage Ovarian Cancer Treatment

All patients should have thorough surgical staging at the initial operation.

Patients with Complete Surgical Staging

1. Low-risk Stage I (see Box 8-2): No adjuvant therapy
2. High-risk Stage I (see Box 8-2):
   a. Three cycles IV carboplatin-paclitaxel (3–6 cycles = NCCN option); *or*
   b. Consider observation if not clear cell (not an NCCN guideline)
3. Stage II:
   a. Six cycles IV carboplatin-paclitaxel; *or*
   b. IP chemotherapy if <1 cm residual disease (see Fig. 8-8); *or*

Patients without Complete Surgical Staging

1. Low-risk patients:
   a. Re-operate for staging if patient accepts, or suspect residual disease; *or*
   b. Six cycles IV carboplatin/paclitaxel
2. High-risk patients:
   a. Six cycles IV carboplatin-paclitaxel if no suspicion of resectable disease; otherwise, re-operate;
      or
   b. Re-operate for staging if considering observation (not an NCCN guideline)
3. Stage II: Same as completely staged patients

IP, intraperitoneal; NCCN, National Comprehensive Care Network practice guidelines, v.1, 2007.

Preferred
Paclitaxel 175 mg/m^2 IV over 3 hours and
carboplatin AUC 5.0–7.5 q 3 weeks × 6 cycles

Alternatives
Intravenous management: Docetaxel 60–75 mg/m^2 IV over 1 hour and
carboplatin AUC 5–6 q 3 weeks × 6 cycles

Intraperitoneal (IP) management: Paclitaxel 135 mg/m^2 IV 24-hour
infusion on day 1; cisplatin 100 mg/m^2 IP on day 2; paclitaxel 60 mg/m^2
IP on day 8 (max. BSA 2.0 m^2). Repeat q 3 weeks × 6 cycles

Figure 8-9. The National Comprehensive Cancer Network (NCCN) guidelines for chemotherapy of advanced ovarian cancer. BSA, body surface area. (From NCCN practice guidelines, v. 1, 2007.)

controlled trials that used no-treatment control arms. The largest European trials (ICON-1 and ACTION) have demonstrated that adjuvant chemotherapy definitely benefits patients who have "apparent," or grossly visible, stage I disease. Data suggest that treatment of completely staged patients may not significantly reduce the cancer recurrence rate.[9,16] A randomized controlled trial to prove this concept may not be feasible because of both the sample size necessary for adequate power and the challenge of multiple institutions performing standardized complete surgical staging operations.

Observation rather than adjuvant chemotherapy in patients who have had complete surgical staging is appropriate for low-risk stage I disease and may be an option for high-risk stage I disease if the patient is fully counseled (see Box 8-5).

Complete surgical staging should be performed at the original operation if possible, and should be offered as a re-operation under certain circumstances to patients who have had incomplete staging.

When adjuvant chemotherapy is indicated, carboplatin and paclitaxel constitute the most commonly used regimen, but alternatives exist. Three to six cycles are recommended for those with completely staged high-risk stage I disease, and six cycles are recommended for incompletely staged patients with apparent stage I disease and for all those with stage II disease (see Box 8-5).

ADVANCED OVARIAN CARCINOMA (STAGES III AND IV)

Evolution of Platinum and Taxane Agents

Epithelial ovarian cancer is a chemosensitive disease, and cytotoxic chemotherapy plays a pivotal role in its management. Chemotherapy following optimal surgical cytoreduction (all tumor residual nodules less than 1 cm) achieves a complete remission for most patients with advanced epithelial ovarian cancer, which we will define as stages III and IV. In spite of this, most patients experience a relapse and ultimately develop progressive disease with their tumors becoming increasingly chemoresistant. Overall, only about 15% of women with advanced disease survive beyond 5 years. Survival rates are less than 10% for women with stage IV disease, but they may approach 35% for women with optimally debulked stage III disease.[43]

Chemotherapy for epithelial ovarian cancer has evolved dramatically over the last 25 years. In the early 1980s, the standard regimen for advanced epithelial ovarian cancer was cyclophosphamide and doxorubicin, a combination derived through studies conducted by the GOG.[44] During the 1980s and 1990s, two new classes of agents were discovered: platinums and taxanes. These agents have had a dramatic impact on outcomes for patients with advanced epithelial ovarian cancer. Platinum agents work by damaging DNA.[45] Cisplatin and carboplatin undergo hydrolysis after administration and then produce intrastrand and interstrand adducts in DNA that limit cell division, ultimately inducing apoptosis.[46] Taxanes bind to tubulin polymers (microtubules), disrupting normal microtubule activity and halting mitosis that leads to apoptosis.

Many clinical trials have shown the value of platinum in epithelial ovarian cancer. An early GOG study randomized women with large-volume advanced epithelial ovarian cancer to cyclophosphamide plus doxorubicin with or without cisplatin.[47] The addition of cisplatin resulted in significant improvements in complete response rate (51% versus 26%) and progression-free survival (13 versus 8 months). Other studies noted similar findings in which the addition of platinum to an alkylating agent improved progression-free survival in advanced epithelial ovarian cancer.[48] This clinical evidence led to the regimen of cyclophosphamide, doxorubicin, and cisplatin becoming the treatment of choice for advanced epithelial ovarian cancer during the 1980s. Doxorubicin was later removed from this standard regimen because randomized trials failed to demonstrate a survival advantage by including it in platinum-based combinations.[49] A meta-analysis demonstrated a slight survival benefit with the three-drug regimen; however, the authors concluded that the small survival advantage did not justify the added toxicity from doxorubicin.[50]

Although the addition of cisplatin to alkylating agents did appear to improve response rate and progression-free intervals in advanced disease, demonstration of a distinct survival advantage in randomized clinical trials has been elusive. In 2000, a Cochrane Database meta-analysis of over 8700 women treated on 49 different trials reported that the survival hazard ratio was 0.88 (95% CI 0.79–0.98) in favor of platinum combination chemotherapy.[51]

Equivalency of Carboplatin and Cisplatin

Several European and GOG trials over the last decade have demonstrated that carboplatin and cisplatin have equivalent efficacy in advanced epithelial ovarian cancer.[52–54] In each of these trials, carboplatin not only demonstrated activity equivalent to cisplatin, but was associated with reduced gastrointestinal toxicity, renal toxicity, and neurotoxicity. Carboplatin does cause more myelosuppression than cisplatin, but in general, quality-of-life scores are better with carboplatin than with cisplatin.[55]

Taxanes

In the late 1980s and early 1990s, paclitaxel became the next major advance in treating advanced epithelial ovarian cancer. Several phase II trials demonstrated significant activity in patients with platinum-refractory disease.[56-58] In 1990, the GOG initiated the first phase III trial, comparing six cycles of cisplatin plus paclitaxel with the control regimen of cisplatin plus cyclophosphamide in suboptimally debulked disease.[59] The paclitaxel regimen demonstrated significant improvements in overall response, clinical complete remission, median progression-free survival, and overall survival. Beyond 5 years, treatment with paclitaxel was still associated with a 34% reduction in the risk of death. The OV-10 trial, initiated by a collaborative group of European and Canadian investigators, substantiated the GOG findings.[60] A subsequent GOG trial, which randomized patients to paclitaxel only, or cisplatin only, or cisplatin/paclitaxel, somewhat challenged the superiority of cisplatin/paclitaxel by reporting similar median overall survivals (26 to 30 months) among the three groups, and no difference in first progression or death between cisplatin and cisplatin-paclitaxel.[61] However, nearly 50% of patients in each arm of the study were treated with crossover salvage therapy before radiographic disease progression. This crossover treatment may have clouded survival differences among the three arms. Additional contradictory data come from the ICON-3 trial. The authors of ICON-3 concluded that combination paclitaxel-carboplatin demonstrated no advantage over single-agent carboplatin or combined cytoxan-adriamycin-cisplatin.[62] This trial has been widely criticized for its design and methodology, and in North America the taxane-platinum combination remains the standard chemotherapy for advanced epithelial ovarian cancer.

Initially, paclitaxel infusions were given over 24 hours because of the concern for severe allergic reactions. Dose ranges for paclitaxel are 135 to 175 mg/m^2 when the drug is given every 3 to 4 weeks. Eisenhauer and colleagues[63] demonstrated that response rates were similar for 3-hour and 24-hour infusions; however, 3-hour paclitaxel infusions appear to be associated with more neurotoxicity and less myelosuppression than 24-hour infusions. Currently, in the United States the most common administration is 3-hour infusions followed by carboplatin in the outpatient setting. Although this administration is more convenient for patients, paclitaxel-associated neuropathy can be a significant chronic problem for some patients.

A newer taxane, docetaxel, may offer less toxicity than paclitaxel. In the SCOTROC study, 1077 women were randomized to docetaxel-carboplatin versus paclitaxel-carboplatin.[64] Patients in the docetaxel arm reported less neurotoxicity, less muscle and joint pain, and less musculoskeletal weakness. However, docetaxel was associated with more gastrointestinal toxicity and neutropenia. Docetaxel is currently being studied in advanced epithelial ovarian cancer at several U.S. centers, and the results of these trials are pending.

NCCN guidelines list carboplatin-paclitaxel as the preferred regimen in advanced disease, but carboplatin-docetaxel is an alternative (see Fig. 8-8).

New Combinations and Dose Schedules

GOG 182/ICON-5 is a large multicenter randomized trial, which closed to accrual in 2005 (Fig. 8-10). The aim of this study was to determine whether adding a third drug (topotecan, liposomal doxorubicin, or gemcitabine) and adjusting schedules

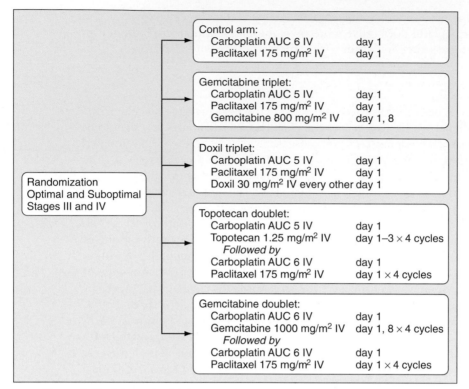

Figure 8-10. Schema for GOG 182: triplet and sequential doublet chemotherapy.

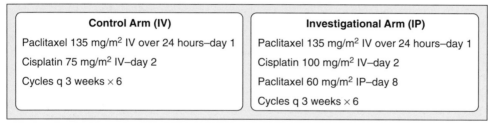

Figure 8-11. Schema for GOG 172 trial of intraperitoneal (IP) chemotherapy.

(i.e., using sequential doublets) could improve outcomes of patients with advanced epithelial ovarian cancer. Carboplatin and paclitaxel served as the control arm in this five-arm trial. These data are maturing and results are pending.[65]

Intraperitoneal Chemotherapy

The concept of treating optimally debulked patients with intraperitoneal chemotherapy has appealed to clinicians for over two decades. In early 2006, a GOG study concluded that intraperitoneal treatment appeared superior in this subset of patients.[66] This trial randomized 429 patients to either standard intravenous cisplatin plus paclitaxel or intraperitoneal/intravenous cisplatin plus paclitaxel (Fig. 8-11). The patients receiving intraperitoneal chemotherapy had a significant improvement in overall survival (median survival 65.6 versus 49.7 months). Toxicity, particularly neurotoxicity, was greater and quality-of-life scores were initially lower in patients treated with intraperitoneal chemotherapy. An earlier GOG randomized trial also provided strong evidence for the utility of intraperitoneal chemotherapy in optimally debulked patients.[67] The NCCN has listed intraperitoneal therapy as an alternative management for patients with optimal residual disease after primary cytoreduction, using the GOG regimen (see Fig. 8-8). Physicians may choose to prescribe this regimen or a modification of it to reduce the associated toxicity. The GOG is currently conducting phase I studies of intraperitoneal paclitaxel and intraperitoneal carboplatin to derive regimens with reduced toxicity.

Maintenance Therapy

Another concept, maintenance therapy, has been studied and debated among investigators over the last 5 years. Maintenance therapies focus on extending the duration of frontline treatment. There have been several reports concerning cytotoxic chemotherapy, hormonal therapy, and immunotherapy used in this manner.[68-70] In 2003, a GOG trial demonstrated that maintenance paclitaxel given every 4 weeks for 12 months to patients in complete remission following standard intravenous paclitaxel-carboplatin significantly increased the progression-free survival by 7 months compared with maintenance therapy for 3 months.[71] This study's value has been controversial owing to lack of overall survival data following early closure by the data monitoring committee. Nonetheless, this was a significant improvement for these patients, some of whom began therapy with bulky, suboptimal disease; therefore, maintenance therapy should be a discussion point with patients with advanced epithelial ovarian cancer. Currently, GOG 212 is further investigating this concept in a randomized three-arm study comparing 12 months of paclitaxel versus xyotax versus observation following complete clinical response to frontline platinum/taxane treatment.

Neoadjuvant Therapy

Neoadjuvant chemotherapy in advanced epithelial ovarian cancer is the final concept that merits discussion for treatment of advanced disease. Neoadjuvant implies delivering chemotherapy before a cytoreductive operation. Maximal operative effort with the goal of optimal (less than 1 cm disease) cytoreduction or "debulking" is the current cornerstone of surgical management in advanced epithelial ovarian cancer. Some series indicate that approximately 50% of patients can be primarily optimally debulked. The reasons for surgeons not being able to complete optimal cytoreductions are many, but clearly biologic tumor heterogeneity is an important factor.[72] Furthermore, for patients with poor performance status and severe debilitation from their disease, or comorbidities, aggressive surgical cytoreduction can be extremely hazardous. Given these concepts, there has been increasing enthusiasm in recent years for using neoadjuvant chemotherapy to reduce tumor burden and improve patient performance status before an aggressive attempt at cytoreduction. Currently, a randomized trial is underway to evaluate the role of neoadjuvant chemotherapy in advanced epithelial ovarian cancer.[73] To date, several investigators have reported data on this therapy, but no distinct standard protocol for the use of neoadjuvant chemotherapy has been defined or accepted by clinicians.[74-76]

References

1. National Institutes of Health consensus development conference statement. Gynecol Oncol 55:S4–S14, 1994.
2. Vergote I, De Brabanter J, Fyles A, et al: Prognostic importance of degree of differentiation and cyst rupture in stage I invasive epithelial ovarian carcinoma. Lancet 357(9251):176–182, 2001.
3. Winter-Roach B, Hooper L, Kitchener H: Systematic review of adjuvant therapy for early stage (epithelial) ovarian cancer. Int J Gynecol Cancer 13(4):395–404, 2003.
4. Bertelsen K, Holund B, Andersen JE, et al: Prognostic factors and adjuvant treatment in early epithelial ovarian cancer. Int J Gynecol Cancer 3(4):211–218, 1993.
5. Hreshchyshyn MM, Park RC, Blessing JA, et al: The role of adjuvant therapy in Stage I ovarian cancer. Am J Obstet Gynecol 138(2):139–145, 1980.
6. Young RC, Walton LA, Ellenberg SS, et al: Adjuvant therapy in stage I and stage II epithelial ovarian cancer. Results of two prospective randomized trials. N Engl J Med 322(15):1021–1027, 1990.

7. Bolis G, Colombo N, Pecorelli S, et al; (GICOG: Gruppo Interregionale Collaborativo in Ginecologia): Adjuvant treatment for early epithelial ovarian cancer: results of two randomised clinical trials comparing cisplatin to no further treatment or chromic phosphate (^{32}P). Ann Oncol 6(9):887–893, 1995.

8. Trope C, Kaern J, Hogberg T, et al: Randomized study on adjuvant chemotherapy in stage I high-risk ovarian cancer with evaluation of DNA-ploidy as prognostic instrument. Ann Oncol 11(3):281–288, 2000.

9. Trimbos JB, Vergote I, Bolis G, et al: Impact of adjuvant chemotherapy and surgical staging in early-stage ovarian carcinoma: European Organisation for Research and Treatment of Cancer-Adjuvant ChemoTherapy in Ovarian Neoplasm trial. J Natl Cancer Inst 95(2):113–125, 2003.

10. Ahmed FY, Wiltshaw E, A'Hern RP, et al: Natural history and prognosis of untreated stage I epithelial ovarian carcinoma. J Clin Oncol 14(11):2968–2975, 1996.

11. Buchsbaum HJ, Brady MF, Delgado G, et al: Surgical staging of carcinoma of the ovaries. Surg Gynecol Obstet 169(3):226–232, 1989.

12. Young RC, Decker DG, Wharton JT, et al: Staging laparotomy in early ovarian cancer. JAMA 250(22):3072–3076, 1983.

13. Leblanc E, Querleu D, Narducci F, et al: Laparoscopic restaging of early stage invasive adnexal tumors: a 10-year experience. Gynecol Oncol 94(3):624–649, 2004.

14. Colombo N, Guthrie D, Chiari S, et al: International Collaborative Ovarian Neoplasm trial 1: a randomized trial of adjuvant chemotherapy in women with early-stage ovarian cancer. J Natl Cancer Inst 95(2):125–132, 2003.

15. Kolomainen DF, A'Hern R, Coxon FY, et al: Can patients with relapsed, previously untreated, stage I epithelial ovarian cancer be successfully treated with salvage therapy? J Clin Oncol 21(16):3113–3118, 2003.

16. Elit L, Chambers A, Fyles A, et al: Systematic review of adjuvant care for women with Stage I ovarian carcinoma. Cancer 101(9):1926–1935, 2004.

17. Le T, Adolph A, Krepart GV, et al: The benefits of comprehensive surgical staging in the management of early-stage epithelial ovarian carcinoma. Gynecol Oncol 85(2):351–355, 2002.

18. Vergote IB, Vergote-De Vos LN, Abeler VM, et al: Randomized trial comparing cisplatin with radioactive phosphorus or whole-abdomen irradiation as adjuvant treatment of ovarian cancer. Cancer 69(3):741–749, 1992.

19. Chiara S, Conte P, Franzone P, et al: High-risk early-stage ovarian cancer. Randomized clinical trial comparing cisplatin plus cyclophosphamide versus whole abdominal radiotherapy. Am J Clin Oncol 17(1):72–76, 1994.

20. Kojs Z, Glinski B, Reinfuss M, et al: Results of a randomized prospective trial comparing postoperative abdominopelvic radiotherapy with postoperative chemotherapy in early ovarian cancer [in French]. Cancer Radiother 5(1):5–11, 2001.

21. Winter-Roach B, Hooper L, Kitchener H: Systematic review of adjuvant therapy for early stage (epithelial) ovarian cancer. Int J Gynecol Cancer 13(4):395–404, 2003.

22. Ozols RF, Bundy BN, Greer BE, et al: Phase III trial of carboplatin and paclitaxel compared with cisplatin and paclitaxel in patients with optimally resected stage III ovarian cancer: a Gynecologic Oncology Group study. J Clin Oncol 21(17):3194–3200, 2003.

23. ICON Collaborators. International Collaborative Ovarian Neoplasm Study: ICON2: randomized trial of single-agent carboplatin against three-drug combination of CAP (cyclophosphamide, doxorubicin, and cisplatin) in women with ovarian cancer. Lancet 352(9140):1571–1576, 1998.

24. Ozols RF: Paclitaxel plus carboplatin in the treatment of ovarian cancer. Semin Oncol 26(1 Suppl 2):84–89, 1999.

25. Bamias A, Papadimitriou C, Efstathiou E, et al: Four cycles of paclitaxel and carboplatin as adjuvant treatment in early-stage ovarian cancer: a six-year experience of the Hellenic Cooperative Oncology Group. BMC Cancer 6:228, 2006.

26. Chi DS, Waltzman RJ, Barakat RR, et al: Primary intravenous paclitaxel and platinum chemotherapy for high-risk Stage I epithelial ovarian carcinoma. Eur J Gynaecol Oncol 20(4):277–280, 1999.

27. Rubin SC, Wong GY, Curtin JP, et al: Platinum-based chemotherapy of high-risk stage I epithelial ovarian cancer following comprehensive surgical staging. Obstet Gynecol 82(1):143–147, 1993.

28. Shimada M, Kigawa J, Kanamori Y, et al: Outcome of patients with early ovarian cancer undergoing three courses of adjuvant chemotherapy following complete surgical staging. Int J Gynecol Cancer 15(4):601–605, 2005.

29. Bell J, Brady MF, Young RC, et al; Gynecologic Oncology Group: Randomized phase III trial of three versus six cycles of adjuvant carboplatin and paclitaxel in early stage epithelial ovarian carcinoma: a Gynecologic Oncology Group study. Gynecol Oncol 102(3):432–439, 2006.

30. Tumors of the ovary: neoplasms derived from celomic epithelium. In Morrow CP, Curtin JP (eds): Synopsis of Gynecologic Oncology. Philadelphia: Churchill Livingstone, 1975, p 249.

31. Sugiyama T, Kamura T, Kigawa J, et al: Clinical characteristics of clear cell carcinoma of the ovary: a distinct histologic type with poor prognosis and resistance to platinum-based chemotherapy. Cancer 88(11):2584–2589, 2000.

32. O'Brien ME, Schofield JB, Tan S, et al: Clear cell epithelial ovarian cancer (mesonephroid): bad prognosis only in early stages. Gynecol Oncol 49(2):250–254, 1993.

33. Kennedy AW, Biscotti CV, Hart WR, et al: Ovarian clear cell adenocarcinoma. Gynecol Oncol 32(3):342–349, 1989.

34. Crozier MA, Copeland LJ, Silva EG, et al: Clear cell carcinoma of the ovary: a study of 59 cases. Gynecol Oncol 35(2):199–203, 1989.

35. Mizuno M, Kikkawa F, Shibata K, et al: Long-term follow-up and prognostic factor analysis in clear cell adenocarcinoma of the ovary. J Surg Oncol 94(2):138–143, 1993.

36. Ho CM, Huang YJ, Chen TC, et al: Pure-type clear cell carcinoma of the ovary as a distinct histological type and improved survival in patients treated with paclitaxel-platinum-based chemotherapy in pure-type advanced disease. Gynecol Oncol 94(1):197–203, 2004.

37. Takano M, Kikuchi Y, Yaegashi N, et al: Adjuvant chemotherapy with irinotecan hydrochloride and cisplatin for clear cell carcinoma of the ovary. Oncol Rep 16(6):1301–1306, 2006.

38. Malmstrom H, Simonsen E, Westberg R: A phase II study of intraperitoneal carboplatin as adjuvant treatment in early-stage ovarian cancer patients. Gynecol Oncol 52(1):20–25, 1994.

39. Topuz E, Eralp Y, Saip P, et al: The efficacy of combination chemotherapy including intraperitoneal cisplatinum and mitoxantrone with intravenous ifosfamide in patients with FIGO stage IC ovarian carcinoma. Eur J Gynaecol Oncol 22(1):70–73, 2001.

40. Fujiwara K, Sakuragi N, Suzuki S, et al: First-line intraperitoneal carboplatin-based chemotherapy for 165 patients with epithelial ovarian carcinoma: results of long-term follow-up. Gynecol Oncol 90(3):637–643, 2003.

41. McGuire WP: Current aspects of adjuvant therapy of early stage ovarian cancer. Zentralbl Gynakol 120(3):93–97, 1998.

42. Skirnisdottir I, Seidal T, Sorbe B: A new prognostic model comprising p53, EGFR, and tumor grade in early stage epithelial ovarian carcinoma and avoiding the problem of inaccurate surgical staging. Int J Gynecol Cancer 14(2):259–270, 2004.

43. Heintz AP, Odicino F, Maisonneuve P, et al: Carcinoma of the ovary. J Epidemiol Biostat 6:107–138, 2001.

44. Omura GA, Morrow CP, Blessing JA, et al: A randomized comparison of melphalan versus melphalan plus hexamethylmelamine versus adriamycin plus cyclophosphamide in ovarian carcinoma. Cancer 51:783, 1983.

45. Dumontet C, Sikic BI: Mechanisms of action of and resistance to antitubulin agents: microtubule dynamics, drug transport, and cell death. J Clin Oncol 17:1061–1070, 1999.

46. Go RS, Adjei AA: Review of the comparative pharmacology and clinical activity of cisplatin and carboplatin. J Clin Oncol 17:409–422, 1999.

47. Omura G, Blessing JA, Ehrlich CE, et al: A randomized trial of cyclophosphamide and doxorubicin with or without cisplatin in advanced ovarian carcinoma. A Gynecologic Oncology Group study. Cancer 57:1725, 1986.

48. McGuire W, Ozols RF: Chemotherapy of advanced ovarian cancer [published erratum appears in Semin Oncol 25(6):707]. Semin Oncol 25:340, 1998.

49. Omura GA, Bundy BN, Berek JS, et al: Randomized trial of cyclophosphamide plus cisplatin with or without doxorubicin in ovarian cancer: a Gynecologic Oncology Group study. J Clin Oncol 7:457, 1989.

50. Fanning J, Bennett TZ, Hilgers RD: Meta-analysis of cisplatin, doxorubicin and cyclophosphamide versus cisplatin and cyclo-

phosphamide chemotherapy of ovarian carcinoma. Obstet Gynecol 80:954, 1992.

51. Chemotherapy for advanced ovarian cancer. Advanced Ovarian Cancer Trialists Group. Cochrane Database Syst CD001418, Rev 2000.

52. Aabo K, Adams M, Adnitt P, et al: Chemotherapy in advanced ovarian cancer: four systematic metastatic disease-analyses of individual patient data from 37 randomized trials. Advanced Ovarian Cancer Trialists Group. Br J Cancer 78:1479, 1998.

53. Neijt JP, Engelholm SA, Tuxen MK, et al: Exploratory phase III study of paclitaxel and cisplatin versus paclitaxel and carboplatin in advanced ovarian cancer. J Clin Oncol 18:3084, 2000.

54. Ozols RF, Bundy BN, Greer BE, et al: Phase III trial of carboplatin and paclitaxel compared with cisplatin and paclitaxel in patients with optimally resected stage III ovarian cancer: a Gynecologic Oncology Group study. J Clin Oncol 21:3194, 2003.

55. Du Bois A, Luck HJ, Meier W, et al: A randomized clinical trial of cisplatin/paclitaxel versus carboplatin/paclitaxel as first-line treatment of ovarian cancer. J Natl Cancer Inst 95:1320, 2003.

56. Einzig AI, Wiernik PH, Sasloff J, et al: Phase II study and long-term follow-up of patients treated with Taxol for advanced ovarian adenocarcinoma. J Clin Oncol 10:1748, 1992.

57. Kohn EC, Sarosy G, Bicher A, et al: Dose-intense Taxol: high response rate in patients with platinum-resistant recurrent ovarian cancer. J Natl Cancer Inst 86:18, 1994.

58. Thigpen JT, Blessing JA, Ball H, et al: Phase II trial of paclitaxel in patients with progressive ovarian carcinoma after platinum-based chemotherapy: a Gynecologic Oncology Group Study. J Clin Oncol 12:1748, 1994.

59. McGuire WP, Hoskins WJ, Brady MF, et al: Cyclophosphamide and cisplatin compared with paclitaxel and cisplatin in patients with stage III and stage IV ovarian cancer. N Engl J Med 334:1, 1996.

60. Piccart MJ, Bertelsen K, James K, et al: Randomized intergroup trial of cisplatin-paclitaxel versus cisplatin-cyclophosphamide in women with advanced epithelial ovarian cancer: three-year results. J Natl Cancer Inst 92:699, 2000.

61. Muggia FM, Braly PS, Brady MF, et al. Phase III randomized study of cisplatin versus paclitaxel versus cisplatin and paclitaxel in patients with suboptimal stage III or IV ovarian cancer: a Gynecologic Oncology Group study. J Clin Oncol 18:106, 2000.

62. International Collaborative Ovarian Neoplasm (ICON) group: Paclitaxel plus carboplatin versus standard chemotherapy with either single agent carboplatin or cyclophosphamide, doxorubicin, and cisplatin in women with ovarian cancer: the ICON3 randomised trial. Lancet 360:505, 2002.

63. Eisenhauer EA, ten Bokkel Huinink WW, Swenerton KD, et al: European-Canadian randomized trial of paclitaxel in relapsed ovarian cancer: high-dose versus low-dose and long versus short infusion. J Clin Oncol 12:2654, 1994.

64. Vasey PA, Jayson GC, Gordon A, et al: Phase III randomized trial of docetaxel-carboplatin versus paclitaxel-carboplatin as first-line chemotherapy for ovarian carcinoma. J Natl Cancer Inst 96:1682, 2004.

65. Bookman MA, Alberts DS, Brady MF, et al: GOG182-ICON5: 5-arm phase III randomized trial of paclitaxel and carboplatin versus combinations with gemcitabine, PEG-liposomal doxorubicin, or Topotecan in patients with advanced-stage epithelial ovarian or primary peritoneal carcinoma. 2006 ASCO Annual Meeting Proceedings, J Clin Oncol 24(18S):5002, 2006.

66. Armstrong DK, Bundy B, Wenzel L, et al: Intraperitoneal cisplatin and paclitaxel in ovarian cancer. N Engl J Med 354:34, 2006.

67. Markman M, Bundy BN, Alberts DS, et al: Phase III trial of standard-dose intravenous cisplatin plus paclitaxel versus moderately high-dose carboplatin followed by intravenous paclitaxel and intraperitoneal cisplatin in small-volume stage III ovarian carcinoma: an intergroup study of the Gynecologic Oncology Group, Southwestern Oncology Group, and Eastern Cooperative Oncology Group. J Clin Oncol 19:1001, 2001.

68. Pfisterer J, Weber B, Reuss A, et al: Randomized phase III trial of Topotecan following carboplatin and paclitaxel in first-line treatment of advanced ovarian cancer: a gynecologic cancer intergroup trial of the AGO-OVAR and GINECO. J Natl Cancer Inst 98:1036, 2006.

69. Hall GD, Brown JM, Coleman RE, et al: Maintenance treatment with interferon for advanced ovarian cancer: results of the Northern and Yorkshire gynecology group randomized phase III study. Br J Cancer 91:621, 2004.

70. Perez-Gracia JL, Carrasco EM: Tamoxifen therapy for ovarian cancer in the adjuvant and advanced settings: systematic review of the literature and implications for future research. Gynecol Oncol 84:201, 2002.

71. Markman M, Liu PY, Wilczynski S, et al: Phase III randomized trial of 12 versus 3 months of maintenance paclitaxel in patients with advanced ovarian cancer after complete response to platinum and paclitaxel-based chemotherapy: a Southwest Oncology Group and Gynecologic Oncology Group trial. J Clin Oncol 21:2460, 2003.

72. Ansquer Y, Leblanc E, Clough K, et al: Neoadjuvant chemotherapy for resectable ovarian carcinoma. Cancer 91:2329–2334, 2001.

73. Vergote IB, De Wever I, Decloedt J, et al: Neoadjuvant chemotherapy versus primary debulking surgery in advanced ovarian cancer. Semin Oncol 27:31, 2000.

74. Schwartz PE, Rutherford TJ, Chambers JT, et al: Neoadjuvant chemotherapy for advanced ovarian cancer: long-term survival. Gynecol Oncol; 72:93, 1999.

75. Kuhn W, Rutke S, Spathe K, et al: Neoadjuvant chemotherapy followed by tumor debulking prolongs survival for patients with poor prognosis in International Federation of Gynecology and Obstetrics Stage IIIC ovarian carcinoma. Cancer 92:2585, 2001.

76. Mazzeo F, Berliere M, Kerger J, et al: Neoadjuvant chemotherapy followed by surgery and adjuvant chemotherapy in patients with primarily unresectable, advanced-stage ovarian cancer. Gynecol Oncol 90:163, 2003.

9 Management of Recurrent Ovarian Cancer: Chemotherapy and Clinical Trials

Maurie Markman

> **KEY POINTS**
>
> - Although there is no evidence for the curative potential of chemotherapy in recurrent or resistant ovarian cancer, improved survival associated with the delivery of several cytotoxic regimens has been documented.
> - Treatment in the second-line setting must attempt to carefully balance the desired effects (e.g., improvement in symptoms, delay in subsequent progression) with potential serious adverse effects.
> - Existing evidence supports the superiority of combination platinum-based chemotherapy, compared with single-agent platinum when used as second-line treatment of recurrent (potentially platinum-sensitive) ovarian cancer.

Background

Ovarian cancer is one of the most chemotherapy-sensitive malignancies, with 60% to 80% of women with newly diagnosed advanced disease anticipated to achieve both substantial objective and subjective responses to primary therapy.[1] Despite this fact, most women who respond to this treatment ultimately experience a relapse of the disease process.[2] Thus, the need to ultimately consider a second-line treatment strategy in ovarian cancer is the rule, rather than the exception. This chapter reviews the status of chemotherapeutic management options in the ovarian cancer patient who fails to respond to primary treatment or whose disease progresses after a response to initial therapy.

Definition of Recurrent versus Platinum-Resistant Ovarian Cancer

It has long been recognized that ovarian cancer patients whose tumors exhibit objective evidence of a response to chemotherapy may respond a second time to the same (or a similar) treatment program.[3,4] In fact, this observation is not unique to ovarian cancer, having been demonstrated relatively early in the development of modern chemotherapy in the management of hematologic malignancies.[5]

Because of the central role of the platinum agents in ovarian cancer,[6] it should come as no surprise that the greatest experience with re-treatment in this malignancy has been with platinum-based strategies, delivered either as single agents or as a component of a combination chemotherapy program.[7-11] As a result of its more favorable toxicity profile, carboplatin is generally the platinum of choice in the second-line setting.[2]

It has also been demonstrated that the opportunity that a particular individual's ovarian cancer will respond a second (or third, etc.) time to a platinum-based chemotherapy is a *continuum*, with the longer the duration of the platinum- or treatment-free interval, the greater the statistical likelihood that the patient will again experience objective and subjective benefit from this approach[7-9] (Table 9-1; Fig. 9-1).

Thus, for a woman who develops recurrent disease approximately 8 to 10 months after completing primary treatment, the probability of a second response ranges from 20% to 30%. However, for the patient experiencing disease recurrence with a treatment-free interval of 2 years, the chances of her experiencing a response to re-treatment is greater than 50%.

For the purpose of designing relatively homogeneous prospective clinical trials, "platinum-resistant" and "recurrent" (potentially platinum-sensitive) disease has been defined[12,13] (Box 9-1). Again, it is critical to remember that although these defi-

Table 9-1. Relationship Between Response Rates to Second-Line Platinum-Based Chemotherapy and the Platinum or Treatment-Free Interval

Platinum-Free Interval	Percentage
0–6 months	10
7–12 months	20–30
13–18 months	30–40
19–24 months	40–50
>24 months	>50

Data from references 7, 8, and 9.

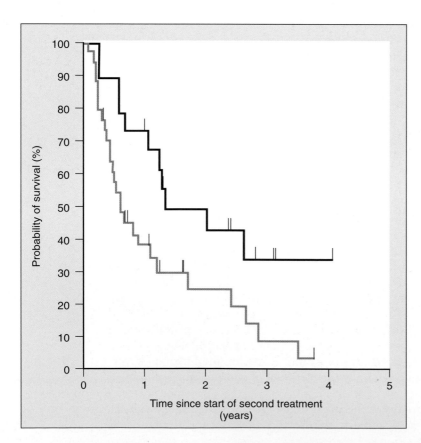

Figure 9-1. Survival from the start of treatment for relapse (second treatment). The time lapsed since the end of treatment to relapse has a tremendous bearing on probability of survival. *Lighter red*, relapse or progression within 18 months of completing initial treatment; *darker red*, relapse or progression after 18 months of completing initial treatment. (From Gore ME, Fryatt I, Wiltshaw E, et al: Treatment of relapsed carcinoma of the ovary with cisplatin or carboplatin following initial treatment with these compounds. Gynecol Oncol 36:207–211, 1990, Fig. 3.)

Box 9-1. Definition of Recurrent and Platinum-Resistant Ovarian Cancer

Recurrent ovarian cancer:
Prior response to a platinum-based chemotherapy regimen *and* a treatment-free interval of ≥6 months

Platinum-resistant ovarian cancer:
No response to prior platinum-based chemotherapy (e.g., "best response" stable disease or actual disease progression) *or* response to platinum-based therapy with a treatment-free interval of <6 months

---

Box 9-2. Considerations in the Selection of Second-Line Therapy in Ovarian Cancer

- Prior response to treatment (including treatment-free interval)
- Toxicity from prior therapy (including any residual effects)
- Evidence-based phase III trial data supporting strategies in the particular setting (e.g., recurrent disease)
- Non–evidence-based (phase II studies) supporting potential treatment programs
- Availability of, and interest in, clinical trials
- Patient choice

Box 9-3. Reasonable Objectives of Second-Line Therapy of Ovarian Cancer

1. Extend survival
2. Improve cancer-related symptoms
3. Prolong the time to the development or worsening of symptoms
4. Prolong the time to the documentation of progressive disease
5. Improve or maintain overall quality of life

---

nitions are useful (particularly in the context of eligibility criteria for clinical studies), no single duration of a platinum- or treatment-free interval can specifically differentiate the individual patient who will, or will not, achieve benefit from re-treatment with a platinum drug. Selection of optimal therapy in this setting must include consideration of available trial data (especially evidence-based randomized phase III studies), the toxicity previously experienced by the patient during prior treatment regimens, and patient choice (Box 9-2).

Goals of Second-Line Chemotherapy in Ovarian Cancer

Unfortunately, available data fail to provide evidence for the legitimate curative potential of any existing second-line chemotherapeutic strategy in ovarian cancer.[2,7–11] This is an important point and clearly distinguishes secondary from primary treatment, where it is rational to suggest that such treatment *is being delivered to many patients with curative intent*, even if only a limited percentage of individuals ultimately achieve this goal.[1,2]

In the absence of "cure" as an aim of treatment, what are the overall goals of second-line treatments in ovarian cancer? There are a number of highly clinically relevant objectives of such therapy, as outlined in Box 9-3. A critically important aspect of anticancer management in this setting is to carefully balance the meaningful goals of therapy with the potential adverse effects of treatment, particularly when certain toxicities may be cumulative and persistent in their impact on an individual's quality of life (e.g., neuropathy).

Chemotherapy of Recurrent (Potentially Platinum-Sensitive) Ovarian Cancer

As previously noted, there is very strong evidence to support delivery of a platinum-based chemotherapy regimen in the second-line setting in women who have previously experienced an objective response to therapy with this class of drugs.[7–11] Unfortunately, there has been a rather profound absence of evidence-based studies that have directly compared a platinum-based regimen with a non-platinum program in the setting of recurrent ovarian cancer. However, the limited randomized experience does suggest superiority of a platinum-containing program in this clinical setting[14] (Table 9-2; Fig. 9-2).Despite this fact, there are a number of reasons why an individual physician and patient may decide to avoid platinum in the second-line setting, despite a prior response to the drug (Box 9-4).

The risk for the development of a platinum-associated hypersensitivity reaction is increasingly recognized as an important concern in this patient population. Up to 15% to 20% of women receiving a second-line platinum-based chemotherapy program experience this toxic reaction, with signs and symptoms ranging from a mild rash to cardiovascular and respiratory arrest[15,16] (Fig. 9-3). Fatal episodes related to re-treatment with a platinum agent following the demonstration of a platinum allergy have been reported.[17]

Several desensitization programs have been developed to permit the continuation of therapy with platinum in this patient population, with a variable degree of reported success.[18–20] These programs are patterned after strategies used in individuals documented to have hypersensitivity to antibiotics (e.g., penicillin), in which initiation or continuation of treatment with the agents is highly relevant, despite the potential risk.

The decision to continue a patient with a platinum drug in this setting should reasonably be based on several factors, including: (a) severity of the reaction; (b) objective evidence for the activity of the second-line program that contains the platinum (e.g., major reduction in abdominal pain or disappearance of symptomatic

Table 9-2. Combination Platinum-Based Chemotherapy versus a Non-Platinum Regimen in Recurrent Ovarian Cancer

	Complete Response	Progression-free Survival (Median)	Overall Survival (Median)
Paclitaxel	17%	9 months	25.8 months
CAP	30%	15.7 months ($P = .038$)	34.7 months ($P = .043$)

CAP, cyclophosphamide, doxorubicin, cisplatin.
Data from Cantu MG, Buda A, Parma G, et al: Randomized controlled trial of single-agent paclitaxel versus cyclophosphamide, doxorubicin, and cisplatin in patients with recurrent ovarian cancer who responded to first-line platinum-based regimens. J Clin Oncol 20:1232–1237, 2002.

Box 9-4. Reasons for Not Using Platinum-Based Therapy in Recurrent Ovarian Cancer

- Prior serious acute toxicity (e.g., severe emesis; grade 3 neuropathy; grade 3–4 thrombocytopenia)
- Persistent toxicity, even if not severe (e.g., grade 1 neuropathy)
- Highly unpleasant adverse effects of prior platinum therapy (e.g., grade 1–2 emesis lasting 5–7 days after each treatment)
- Development of a clinically relevant platinum hypersensitivity reaction
- Modest activity of prior platinum therapy (e.g., treatment-free interval of only 6–8 months)

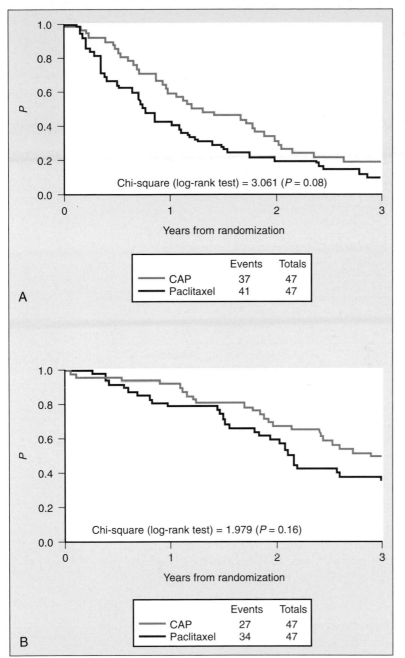

Figure 9-2. Comparison of single-agent versus multiagent therapy. A, Kaplan-Meier plot of progression-free intervals by treatment. **B,** Kaplan-Meier plot of overall survival by treatment. Few evidence-based studies directly compare a platinum-based regimen with a non-platinum program in the setting of recurrent ovarian cancer. However, the limited randomized experience does suggest superiority of a platinum-containing program. CAP, cyclophosphamide, doxorubicin (Adriamycin), and cisplatin. (Data from Cantu MG, Buda A, Parma G, et al: Randomized controlled trial of single-agent paclitaxel versus cyclophosphamide, doxorubicin, and cisplatin in patients with recurrent ovarian cancer who responded to first-line platinum-based regimens. J Clin Oncol 20:1232–1237, 2002, Figs. 2 and 3.)

ascites versus a minimal fall in the CA-125 level after the initial course of second-line platinum); (c) available alternative options; and (d) patient choice.[21] Patients and their families need to be included in the discussion regarding re-treatment with a platinum agent after the development of platinum hypersensitivity, since the risk of a severe, even fatal, reaction is more than a theoretical possibility.[17]

Combination Platinum-Based Chemotherapy versus Single-Agent Platinum

If a patient is to receive a platinum agent, the next question is: Should the platinum drug be administered alone or in combination with a second non-platinum drug?

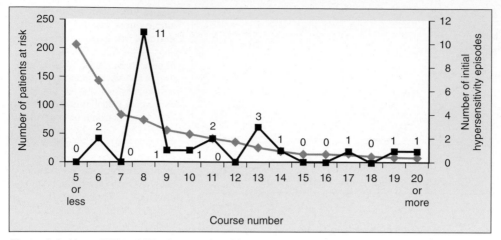

Figure 9-3. Up to 15% to 20% of women receiving a second-line platinum-based chemotherapy program will experience a toxic reaction. (Data from Markman M, Kennedy A, Webster K, et al: Clinical features of hypersensitivity reactions to carboplatin. J Clin Oncol 17:1141, 1999, Table 1.)

Table 9-3. Phase III Randomized Trials of Combination Platinum-Based Therapy versus Single-Agent Platinum in Recurrent Ovarian Cancer

	Response Rate	Progression-Free Survival (Median)	Overall Survival (Median)
Carboplatin + paclitaxel versus carboplatin (ICON-4)[10]	66% vs 54% (P = .06)	12 vs 9 months (HR 0.76, P = .0004)	29 vs 24 months (HR 0.82, P = .02)
Carboplatin + gemcitabine versus carboplatin (AGO)[11]	47.2% vs 30.9% (P = .016)	8.6 vs 5.8 months (HR 0.72, P = .003)	18 vs 17.3 months (HR 0.96, P = .74)

Data from The ICON and AGO Collaborators. Paclitaxel plus platinum-based chemotherapy versus conventional platinum-based chemotherapy in women with relapsed ovarian cancer: the ICON4/AGO-OVAR-2.2 trial. Lancet 361:2099–2106, 2003; Pfisterer J, Plante M, Vergote I, et al: Gemcitabine plus carboplatin compared with carboplatin in patients with platinum-sensitive recurrent ovarian cancer: an intergroup trial of the AGO-OVAR, the NCIC CTG, and the EORTC GCG. J Clin Oncol 24:4699–4707, 2006.

The results of two phase III randomized trials have provided important support for the conclusion that combination platinum-based chemotherapy is therapeutically superior to single-agent platinum when used in recurrent ovarian cancer[10,11] (Table 9-3).

The first reported trial (International Collaborative Ovarian Neoplasm [ICON]-4) was rather complex in its design, but it is reasonable to conclude that the study essentially compared a regimen of single-agent carboplatin with the combination of carboplatin plus paclitaxel.[10] This trial revealed an improvement in both progression-free and overall survival in favor of the combination program. At 2 years' follow-up, a 7% absolute improvement (57% versus 50%) was seen in overall survival in favor of the carboplatin plus paclitaxel regimen.

Unfortunately, this clear survival benefit must be viewed in the context of the documented substantial increase in neurotoxicity observed in the population randomized to the combination regimen, compared with single-agent carboplatin (grades 2–3: 20% versus 1%)[10] (Fig. 9-4).

The second reported randomized study in recurrent ovarian cancer directly compared single-agent carboplatin with the combination of carboplatin plus gemcitabine.[11] This trial also demonstrated an improvement in progression-free survival associated with the combination program, but surprisingly (in view of the previously known results from ICON-4), no improvement in overall survival.

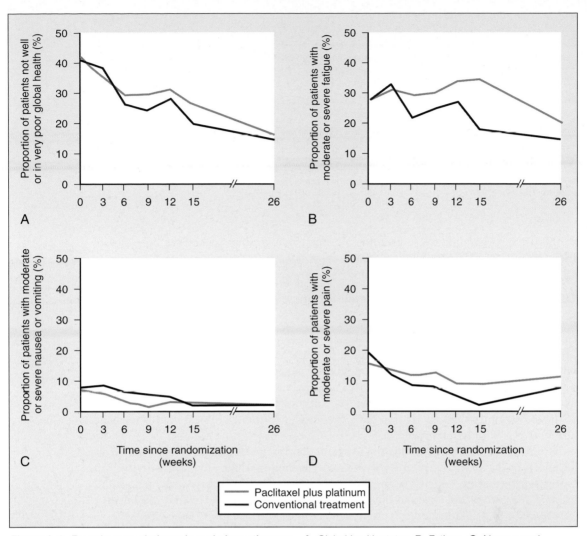

Figure 9-4. Reactions to platinum-based chemotherapy. A, Global health status. **B,** Fatigue. **C,** Nausea and vomiting. **D,** Pain over time. The same patients do not contribute to each point. (From The ICON and AGO Collaborators. Paclitaxel plus platinum-based chemotherapy versus conventional platinum-based chemotherapy in women with relapsed ovarian cancer: the ICON4/AGO-OVAR-2.2 trial. Lancet 361:2099–2106, 2003, Fig. 6.)

Although several hypotheses may be proposed to explain the lack of overall survival benefits observed in this trial, perhaps the most likely is the fact that a larger percentage of patients in the carboplatin versus carboplatin plus gemcitabine trial received further chemotherapy *after progression* compared with the number of individuals receiving additional treatment when therapy on ICON-4 was completed. Though only a theory, it has recently been documented that active chemotherapy in the third-line setting can exert a statistically significant impact on survival *independent of prior therapy* the patient may have received[22] (Table 9-4).

As might have been anticipated, no difference was seen in the risk of serious neuropathy between the two treatment regimens (carboplatin plus gemcitabine versus carboplatin), since gemcitabine is itself not considered neurotoxic.[11]

A randomized phase III trial that compared the combination of carboplatin plus liposomal doxorubicin with carboplatin plus paclitaxel is currently nearing completion, with the results hoped to be available in the near future.[23] It is possible that the outcome of this study will permit the addition of another combination regimen

Table 9-4. Evidence for the Impact of Third-Line Therapy on Survival in Ovarian Cancer

Randomized Phase III Trial Comparison	Canfosfamide (TLK 286) (Experimental Arm)	Liposomal Doxorubicin or Topotecan (Control Arm)
Objective response rate	4.3%	10.9%
Progression-free survival (median)	2.3 months	4.4 months ($P = .0001$)
Overall survival (median)	8.5 months	13.6 months ($P = .0001$)

Data from Vergote I, Finkler N, del Campo J, et al: Single agent, canfosfamide versus pegylated doxorubicin or topotecan in 3rd line treatment of platinum refractory or resistant ovarian cancer: phase 3 study results. J Clin Oncol 25 (18S) (part II):966s- (Abstract #LBA55289), 2007.

to the list of programs whose usefulness in recurrent ovarian cancer has been documented in evidence-based clinical trials.

Other Options in the Recurrent Disease Setting

Despite the important data supporting the usefulness of carboplatin-based combination chemotherapy in recurrent ovarian cancer, it is not known whether the outcome of treatment (progression-free and overall survival) would be equivalent, but perhaps with less toxicity, if the agents were delivered in sequence rather than together.[6,24] For example, patients could receive three cycles of carboplatin, followed by three cycles of paclitaxel (or gemcitabine, or liposomal doxorubicin). Unfortunately, without randomized phase III trial data, the answer to the usefulness of this rational alternative is simply unknown.

The delivery of non-platinum single-agent therapy in recurrent ovarian cancer is another option, particularly in a patient experiencing platinum hypersensitivity[21] or who has preexisting toxicity from primary platinum-based therapy (e.g., persistent grade 2–3 neuropathy). Even in the setting of prior modestly severe (but disconcerting) toxicity (e.g., grade 2 emesis after each chemotherapy regimen lasting for several days), a patient may elect to be treated with a non-platinum strategy.

In addition, for patients whose treatment- or platinum-free interval minimally satisfies the definition of recurrent disease (e.g., 6 to 9 months), a reasonable case can be made to initiate treatment with an alternative drug.[7–9] Of course, this argument is made stronger if the patient experienced difficulty tolerating the initial treatment program.

A number of cytotoxic agents have been shown to possess a sufficient level of biologic activity in phase II studies in recurrent or resistant ovarian cancer such that they may reasonably be considered to be used in this setting[25] (Box 9-5). Unfortunately, very limited randomized phase III data exist to help in the selection of the best single agent to use in this patient population (Fig. 9-5).

One phase III study should be highlighted because the results appear to indicate the superiority (both an improvement in progression-free and overall survival) of single-agent liposomal doxorubicin, compared with single-agent topotecan, in recurrent ovarian cancer[12,26] (Fig. 9-6). Although the data are of considerable interest and certainly document the clinical utility of liposomal doxorubicin in this setting, it must be noted that neither of these single agents has been compared with a platinum drug—either alone or as a component of a combination strategy.[14]

Furthermore, this trial is also notable for the fact that a rather modest improvement in progression-free survival in favor of the liposomal doxorubicin regimen (median: 5.6 weeks) translates to a substantial difference in overall survival (median:

Box 9-5. Antineoplastic Agents with Demonstated Activity in Recurrent or Platinum-Resistant Ovarian Cancer

Altretamine	Liposomal doxorubicin
Bevacizumab	Oxaliplatin
Docetaxel	Paclitaxel (q3 weeks, weekly)
Epirubicin	Pemetrexed
Etoposide (orally for 21 days)	Tamoxifen
Gemcitabine	Topotecan (q3 weeks, weekly)
Ifosfamide	Trabectedin (not FDA-approved)
Irinotecan	Vinorelbine

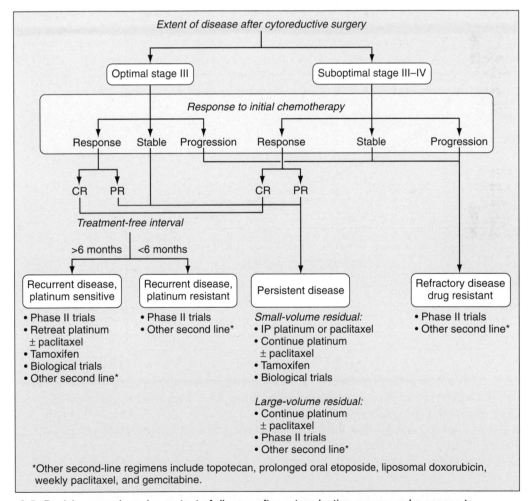

Figure 9-5. Decision map, based on extent of disease after cytoreductive surgery and response to chemotherapy. More precise definition of the treated population helps inform the use of a particular regimen in routine clinical practice. Unfortunately, limited randomized phase III data exist to help in the selection of the "best" single agent. CR, complete response; IP, intraperitoneal; PR, partial response. (From Markman M, Bookman MA: Second-line treatment of ovarian cancer. Oncologist 5:26–35, 2000, Fig. 1.)

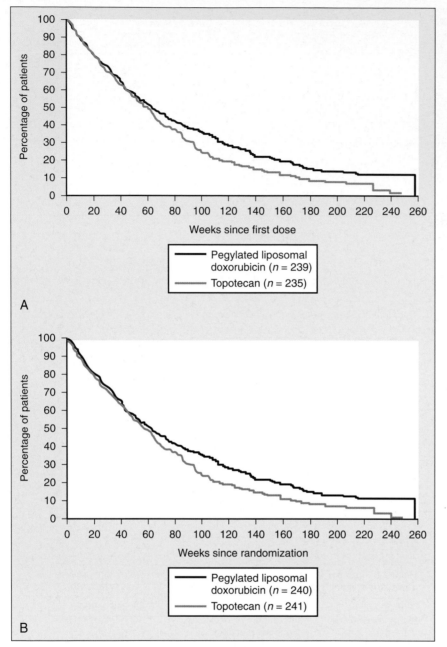

Figure 9-6. Kaplan-Meier curves of survival for patients treated with pegylated liposomal doxorubicin or topotecan. Survival was significantly prolonged for patients treated with pegylated liposomal doxorubicin compared with those treated with topotecan. Neither of these single agents has been compared in any study with a platinum drug (see Fig. 9-2). (From Gordon AN, Tonda M, Sun S, et al: Long-term survival advantage for women treated with pegylated liposomal doxorubicin compared with topotecan in a phase 3 randomized study of recurrent and refractory epithelial ovarian cancer. Gynecol Oncol 95:1–8, 2004, Figs. 1–4.)

37 weeks).[12,26] One possible explanation for this somewhat surprising finding is that much of the difference in overall survival resulted from what happened to patients *after* they completed treatment on this protocol.

It is reasonable to speculate that for the women entered into this trial oncologists would subsequently have desired to administer carboplatin *after progression*, because this was a potentially platinum-sensitive patient population (although the individuals entered into this trial initially received the study medications before re-treatment with the platinum). It is possible (although no specific data are available to prove this hypothesis) that patients who received the relatively nonmyelosuppressive liposomal doxorubicin were able to be treated with a reasonable course of carboplatin following progression, whereas it was more difficult to deliver carboplatin after treatment with topotecan, a recognized more myelotoxic antineoplastic agent.[12,26]

Figure 9-6, cont'd.

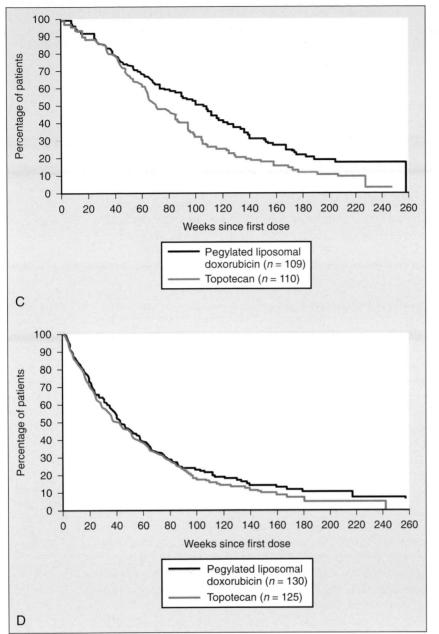

Note that it has been theorized that by treating recurrent ovarian cancer patients with a non-platinum agent before a platinum drug in the recurrent disease setting (so-called "artificially extending the platinum-free interval"), it may be possible to increase the percentage of individuals who respond to the platinum drug when it is subsequently administered. Although this is a provocative concept, unfortunately no prospectively obtained randomized clinical data are available to support this proposal. Moreover, it is at least equally possible that by delaying the administration of platinum until the third-line setting, the effectiveness of the platinum agent may be reduced.[27] Furthermore, as previously noted, the toxicity produced by the second-line nonplatinum strategy may even make it more difficult to deliver an optimal subsequent course of a platinum drug.[12,26]

It is also relevant to note that currently no evidence exists for the superiority of any combination non–platinum-containing regimen in recurrent ovarian cancer compared with the administration of a single agent. Therefore, with the exception of individuals participating in clinical trials, single-agent therapy is the preferred choice in this clinical setting.

Finally, the potential role of surgery in recurrent ovarian cancer must be considered in the context of the decision to deliver chemotherapy in this patient population. Although there are no evidence-based trials that have documented the usefulness of this therapeutic approach or that critically define the specific patient subgroups for whom such surgery should be carried out, considerable retrospective data suggest that patients with relatively long treatment-free intervals and potentially surgically resectable disease may benefit from this strategy *prior to* the delivery of second-line cytotoxic chemotherapy.[28] The results of ongoing phase III trials directly addressing the issue of defining a role for secondary cytoreductive surgery in the management of ovarian cancer are awaited with considerable interest.

Treatment of Platinum-Resistant Ovarian Cancer

A relatively large number of antineoplastic agents have demonstrated activity in platinum-resistant ovarian cancer[25] (see Box 9-5). To date, there is no evidence for the superiority of any specific single agent over another drug in this setting based on the results of data from phase III randomized controlled trials.

How should therapy in resistant disease be selected if data from phase III trials are not available to guide the choice of treatment? As previously noted, a number of relevant factors can be suggested that may help in the selection of treatment (see Box 9-3). In addition, it is likely that an individual ovarian cancer patient will be treated with several of these drugs during the course of her illness.[29] Thus, the question of selection may in reality be one of "when" a particular drug will be delivered rather than "if" it will be administered.

Of critical relevance to the management of the patients in this frequently chronic disease setting is the often delicate balance between improving existing (or delaying the development of) cancer-related symptoms while at the same time not producing toxic effects that may negate potentially beneficial effects of the therapeutic regimen.[30] For those who challenge the concept that treatment in this advanced setting has any impact on survival, evidence-based data now exist to refute this perspective (at least for the overall population of patients in this clinical setting).[22]

No discussion of the treatment of platinum-resistant ovarian cancer would be complete without mention of the potentially important role of radiation therapy in individual patient management. Radiation is particularly useful in patients with relatively isolated pelvic progression in whom pain is the major symptom and in whom it is possible to define radiation portals that will not require exposure of substantial volume of bowel. While it is appropriate to note that this strategy may have a negative impact on the ability to administer myelosuppressive chemotherapy in the future, in the setting of platinum-resistant disease it is unlikely that this factor will be of substantial clinical consequence.

Finally, it is important to acknowledge that at some poorly defined point in the care of almost all patients with platinum-resistant ovarian cancer, the issue of continuation of antineoplastic therapy versus a focus on symptom management or palliative/hospice care becomes a relevant discussion for the oncologist to have with the patient and her family.

Chemoresistance and Chemosensitivity Testing in the Selection of Second-Line Anti-Neoplastic Drug Delivery

A number of retrospective and fewer prospective reports have suggested the potential for in vitro testing of ovarian cancer tumor samples to select treatment, particularly in the setting of recurrent or resistant disease.[31-33] The goal of all such testing would be to provide the clinician with a tool that will permit the delivery of a treatment strategy that is more likely to be beneficial, compared with empiric decisions regarding treatment based on evidence-based (and other) clinical data, and good clinical judgment.[34,35]

Before briefly discussing the evidence supporting the clinical usefulness of these claims, it is important to appreciate the critical distinction between a prognostic and a predictive test in the oncology arena.

A *prognostic test* provides information regarding the statistical likelihood of a more or less favorable outcome. For example, women with advanced-stage or high-grade ovarian cancer are more likely to have a poorer survival outcome compared with individuals with early-stage or low-grade disease. This is an example of a prognostic test, since there is nothing in the information that permits the clinician to specifically select a treatment program that can actually improve that survival.

In contrast, a *predictive test* provides data that allow the clinician to use the information to select a particular management strategy that has been shown to enhance the opportunity for a more favorable outcome. Excellent examples of predictive tests in oncology are the estrogen receptor, which suggests the potential utility of hormonal therapy, and *Her2* overexpression, which predicts the activity of treatment containing trastuzumab.

Unfortunately, to date, the only available evidence reveals several of these chemosensitivity or chemoresistance assays to be of possible prognostic value in ovarian cancer.[34,35] For example, an ovarian cancer shown to be highly resistant to a number of chemotherapeutic agents may have a particularly poor outcome, but there is currently no prospective evidence that the active selection of a particular drug (e.g., low level of resistance or suggested high degree of sensitivity in vitro), based on an assay result, will improve the chances for a favorable outcome (again, compared with the judgment of an experienced oncologist).

It is hoped that future trials in this general area will be able to either establish the clinical utility of one (or more) of these assay systems or continue to reveal them to be solely of prognostic (and therefore quite limited) clinical value in this setting.

Ongoing Research in Recurrent and Resistant Ovarian Cancer

A relatively large number of phase II and phase III trials that are examining novel strategies in the management of recurrent and resistant ovarian cancer are currently in progress.

Of particular interest are studies exploring the role of antiangiogenesis agents, based on the provocative phase II trial experience with second-line single-agent bevacizumab in ovarian cancer (objective response rate: 15–20%).[36,37] Phase III trials examining the use of this drug in both the primary and second-line settings are ongoing.

The activity of a novel PARP (poly-ADP-ribose polymerase) inhibitor has recently been reported to exceed 20% to 30% in women with recurrent or resistant ovarian cancer who possess a *BRCA1* or *BRCA2* mutation.[38,39] Again, a phase III randomized trial examining this novel compound is in progress.

Other drugs being explored in individual phase III studies in platinum-resistant disease include trabectedin, karenitecin, phenoxodiol, and patupilone. It is hoped that the results of one or more of these ongoing studies will reveal a new management paradigm that will improve both the survival and quality of life for women with recurrent and resistant ovarian cancer.

References

1. Covens A, Carey M, Bryson P, et al: Systematic review of first-line chemotherapy for newly diagnosed postoperative patients with stage II, III, or IV epithelial ovarian cancer. Gynecol Oncol 85:71–80, 2002.
2. Ozols RF, Bundy BN, Greer BE, et al: Phase III trial of carboplatin and paclitaxel compared with cisplatin and paclitaxel in patients with optimally resected stage III ovarian cancer: a Gynecologic Oncology Group study. J Clin Oncol 21:3194–3200, 2003.
3. Gershenson DM, Kavanagh JJ, Copeland LJ, et al: Re-treatment of patients with recurrent epithelial ovarian cancer with cisplatin-based chemotherapy. Obstet Gynecol 73:798–802, 1989.
4. Seltzer V, Vogl S, Kaplan B: Recurrent ovarian carcinoma: retreatment utilizing combination chemotherapy including cis-diamminedichloroplatinum in patients previously responding to this agent. Gynecol Oncol 21:167–176, 1985.
5. Fisher RI, DeVita VT, Hubbard SP, et al: Prolonged disease-free survival in Hodgkin's disease with MOPP reinduction after first relapse. Ann Intern Med 90:761–763, 1979.
6. Muggia FM, Braly PS, Brady MF, et al: Phase III randomized study of cisplatin versus paclitaxel versus cisplatin and paclitaxel in patients with suboptimal stage III or IV ovarian cancer: a Gynecologic Oncology Group study. J Clin Oncol 18:106–115, 2000.
7. Markman M, Rothman R, Hakes T, et al: Second-line platinum therapy in patients with ovarian cancer previously treated with cisplatin. J Clin Oncol 9:389–393, 1991.
8. Hoskins PJ, O'Reilly SE, Swenerton KD: The 'failure free interval' defines the likelihood of resistance to carboplatin in patients with advanced epithelial ovarian cancer previously treated with cisplatin: relevance to therapy and new drug testing. Int J Gynecol Cancer 1:205–208, 1991.
9. Gore ME, Fryatt I, Wiltshaw E, et al: Treatment of relapsed carcinoma of the ovary with cisplatin or carboplatin following initial treatment with these compounds. Gynecol Oncol 36:207–211, 1990.
10. The ICON and AGO Collaborators. Paclitaxel plus platinum-based chemotherapy versus conventional platinum-based chemotherapy in women with relapsed ovarian cancer: the ICON4/AGO-OVAR-2.2 trial. Lancet 361:2099–2106, 2003.
11. Pfisterer J, Plante M, Vergote I, et al: Gemcitabine plus carboplatin compared with carboplatin in patients with platinum-sensitive recurrent ovarian cancer: an intergroup trial of the AGO-OVAR, the NCIC CTG, and the EORTC GCG. J Clin Oncol 24:4699–4707, 2006.
12. Gordon AN, Fleagle JT, Guthrie D, et al: Recurrent epithelial ovarian carcinoma: a randomized phase III study of pegylated liposomal doxorubicin versus topotecan. J Clin Oncol 19:3312–3322, 2001.
13. Thigpen JT, Blessing JA, Ball H, et al: Phase II trial of paclitaxel in patients with progressive ovarian carcinoma after platinum-based chemotherapy: a Gynecologic Oncology Group study. J Clin Oncol 12:1748–1753, 1994.
14. Cantu MG, Buda A, Parma G, et al: Randomized controlled trial of single-agent paclitaxel versus cyclophosphamide, doxorubicin, and cisplatin in patients with recurrent ovarian cancer who responded to first-line platinum-based regimens. J Clin Oncol 20:1232–1237, 2002.
15. Markman M, Kennedy A, Webster K, et al: Clinical features of hypersensitivity reactions to carboplatin. J Clin Oncol 17:1141, 1999.
16. Navo M, Kunthur A, Badell ML, et al: Evaluation of the incidence of carboplatin hypersensitivity reactions in cancer patients. Gynecol Oncol 103:608–613, 2006.
17. Zweizig S, Roman LD, Mudersbach LI: Death from anaphylaxis to cisplatin: a case report. Gynecol Oncol 53:121–122, 1994.
18. Robinson JB, Singh D, Bodurka-Bevers DC, et al: Hypersensitivity reactions and the utility of oral and intravenous desensitization in patients with gynecologic malignancies. Gynecol Oncol 82:550–558, 2001.
19. Rose PG, Fusco N, Smrekar M, et al: Successful administration of carboplatin in patients with clinically documented carboplatin hypersensitivity. Gynecol Oncol 89:429–433, 2003.
20. Markman M, Hsieh F, Zanotti K, et al: Initial experience with a novel desensitization strategy for carboplatin-associated hypersensitivity reactions. J Cancer Res Clin Oncol 130:25–28, 2004.
21. Markman M: The dilemma of carboplatin-associated hypersensitivity reactions in ovarian cancer management. Gynecol Oncol 107:163–165, 2007.
22. Vergote I, Finkler N, del Campo J, et al: Single agent, canfosfamide versus pegylated doxorubicin or topotecan in 3rd line treatment of platinum refractory or resistant ovarian cancer: phase 3 study results. J Clin Oncol 25 (18S) (part II):966s-(Abstract #LBA55289), 2007.
23. Avall-Lundqvist E, Wimberger P, Gladieff L, et al: Pegylated liposomal doxorubicin-carboplatin vs. paclitaxel-carboplatin in relapsing sensitive ovarian cancer: a 500-patient interim safety analysis of the CALYPSO GCIG Intergroup phase III study. J Clin Oncol 26(15S):308s, 2008.
24. The International Collaborative Ovarian Neoplasm (ICON) Group: Paclitaxel plus carboplatin versus standard chemotherapy with either single-agent carboplatin or cyclophosphamide, doxorubicin, and cisplatin in women with ovarian cancer: the ICON3 randomised trial. Lancet 360:505–515, 2002.
25. Markman M, Bookman MA: Second-line treatment of ovarian cancer. Oncologist 5:26–35, 2000.
26. Gordon AN, Tonda M, Sun S, et al: Long-term survival advantage for women treated with pegylated liposomal doxorubicin compared with topotecan in a phase 3 randomized study of recurrent and refractory epithelial ovarian cancer. Gynecol Oncol 95:1–8, 2004.
27. Pignata S, Ferrandina G, Scarfone G, et al: Extending the platinum-free interval with a non-platinum therapy in platinum-sensitive recurrent ovarian cancer. Results from the SOCRATES Retrospective Study. Oncology 71:320–326, 2006.
28. Bristow RE, Lagasse LD, Karlan BY: Secondary surgical cytoreduction for advanced epithelial ovarian cancer. Cancer 78:2049–2062, 1996.
29. Markman M: Why study third-, fourth-, fifth-line chemotherapy of ovarian cancer? Gynecol Oncol 83:449–450, 2001.
30. Markman M: Viewing ovarian cancer as a "chronic disease": what exactly does this mean? Gynecol Oncol 100:229–230, 2006.
31. Holloway RW, Mehta RS, Finkler NJ, et al: Association between in vitro platinum resistance in the EDR assay and clinical outcomes for ovarian cancer patients. Gynecol Oncol 87:8–16, 2002.
32. Sharma S, Neale MH, Di NF, et al: Outcome of ATP-based tumor chemosensitivity assay directed chemotherapy in heavily pre-treated recurrent ovarian carcinoma. BMC Cancer 3:19–28, 2003.
33. Gallion H, Christopherson WA, Coleman RL, et al: Progression-free interval in ovarian cancer and predictive value of an ex vivo chemoresponse assay. Int J Gynecol Cancer16:194–201, 2006.
34. Samson DJ, Seidenfeld J, Ziegler K, et al: Chemotherapy sensitivity and resistance assays: a systematic review. J Clin Oncol 22:3618–3630, 2004.
35. Schrag D, Garewal HS, Burstein HJ, et al: American Society of Clinical Oncology Technology Assessment: chemotherapy sensitivity and resistance assays. J Clin Oncol 22:3631–3638, 2004.

36. Burger RA, Sill M, Monk BJ, et al: Phase II trial of bevacizumab in persistent or recurrent epithelial ovarian cancer or primary peritoneal cancer: a Gynecologic Oncology Group study. J Clin Oncol 25:5165–5171, 2007.
37. Cannistra SA, Matulonis UA, Penson RT, et al: Phase II study of bevacizumab in patients with platinum-resistant ovarian cancer or peritoneal serous cancer. J Clin Oncol 25:5180–5186, 2007.
38. Fong PC, Boss DS, Carden CP, et al: AZD2281, a PARP inhibitor with single agent anticancer activity in patients with BRCA deficient ovarian cancer: results from a phase I study. J Clin Oncol 26(15S):295s, 2008.
39. Ashworth A: A synthetic lethal therapeutic approach: poly(ADP) ribose polymerase inhibitors for the treatment of cancer deficient in DNA double-strand break repair. J Clin Oncol 26:3785–3790, 2008.

Secondary Cytoreduction in the Treatment of Recurrent Ovarian Cancer

Ram Eitan and Dennis S. Chi

KEY POINTS

- Surgical cytoreduction is the cornerstone of treatment in newly diagnosed ovarian carcinoma.
- Surgery should also be considered as a treatment option for patients with recurrent ovarian carcinoma.
- Patient selection depends on several factors: (1) disease-free interval, (2) extent of disease recurrence, (3) performance status, and (4) history of response to chemotherapy.

Introduction

Surgery remains the cornerstone of treatment in primary epithelial ovarian carcinoma (EOC). Extensive cytoreduction is used in the treatment of advanced-stage disease, and thorough surgical staging procedures are used in apparent early-stage cases. Both procedures have been well established in the care of epithelial ovarian carcinoma and have been shown to influence prognosis, decisions regarding further therapy, and long-term outcome.

The treatment of recurrent epithelial ovarian carcinoma relies heavily on chemotherapy with various protocols and drug regimens used, depending on the length of time from the previous treatment, line of therapy, performance status, and pattern of disease spread on recurrent disease. Surgery also has an important role in the treatment of recurrent epithelial ovarian carcinoma and is the focus of this chapter.

Clinical and Theoretical Background of Surgical Cytoreduction

The concept of cytoreductive surgery for ovarian cancer has evolved since Meigs[1] first proposed in 1934 that as much tumor as possible should be removed to enhance the effects of postoperative radiation. Forty years after Meigs' initial proposition, Griffiths[2] published the landmark study that first clearly delineated the inverse relationship between postoperative residual tumor size and ovarian cancer patient survival. More contemporary studies published by Hoskins and the Gynecologic Oncology Group (GOG) demonstrated two important principles with respect to residual disease after primary surgery for advanced-stage ovarian cancer.[3] First, there is a threshold effect, or a maximal diameter of residual disease above which even extensive efforts at cytoreduction will not impact survival. Second, below this threshold there is also a continuum effect—such that the smaller the residuum, the better the survival outcome—with patients who are left with no gross residual disease having the most favorable prognosis.[4]

Box 10-1. Benefits of Tumor Cytoreduction

- Log-kill of tumors with chemotherapy is greater in small volume tumors
- Elimination of chemotherapy-resistant cells
- Removal of large tumor masses with poor blood flow
- Improved intestinal tract function
- Higher response rate to chemotherapy
- Prolonged disease-free survival
- Improved overall survival

Tumor cytoreduction of advanced epithelial ovarian carcinoma has both theoretical and clinical benefits (Box 10-1). A key concept in understanding the potential benefits of tumor cytoreduction is the Gompertzian cell growth curve. Tumor cell numbers tend to increase exponentially over time, and the rate of growth is faster in the earlier part of the curve when tumors are relatively small.[5] Chemotherapy works by killing rapidly growing and dividing cells. Log-kill of tumors with chemotherapy is therefore thought to be greater in tumors of smaller volume, which are made up of rapidly growing and dividing cells. Surgical cytoreduction of tumor volume from larger slow-growing tumors to smaller rapid-growing ones thereby offers patients a greater chance of response to chemotherapy.

The elimination of potentially chemotherapy-resistant cells is another benefit of surgical cytoreduction. The probability of spontaneous mutations and drug-resistant phenotypes increases as tumor size and cell numbers increase, according to the mathematical model of Goldie and Coldman.[6] Therefore, by decreasing tumor size and cell numbers, cytoreductive surgery has the ability to remove existing resistant tumor cells and to decrease the spontaneous development of additional resistant cells. In addition, surgery has the potential to remove large tumor masses with poor blood flow, allowing better distribution of intratumoral chemotherapy. These possible benefits are supported by the numerous reports on the clinical benefits of cytoreduction and theoretically hold true for both primary and secondary clinical scenarios.

Although the basic treatment paradigm of a maximum cytoreductive surgical effort before initiating platinum- and taxane-based chemotherapy is well established, the majority of patients with advanced-stage epithelial ovarian cancer ultimately experience tumor recurrence.[7,8] For this reason, the therapeutic value of repeating the initial surgical treatment plan (cytoreduction) has been widely debated. Since the publication by Berek and associates[9] in 1983, which first introduced the term "secondary cytoreduction," the clinical scenarios, indications for, and anticipated outcomes of repeat tumor-reductive operations for recurrent ovarian cancer have been better defined.[10]

By most accounts, cytoreductive surgery for recurrent ovarian cancer is defined as an operative procedure performed at some time remote (disease-free interval of more than 6 to 12 months) from the completion of primary therapy with the intended purpose of tumor reduction. Even within this narrowly defined clinical scenario, the potential usefulness of surgical cytoreduction remains controversial. Operative therapy plays only a minor role in the treatment of recurrent ovarian cancer in routine clinical practice. This might be based on the one hand on the technical complexity of secondary surgery in patients with repetitive abdominal procedures, and on the other hand on the lack of conclusive evidence and existence of several unanswered questions regarding cytoreductive surgery in this setting. The survival impact of successful tumor reduction has been difficult to quantify in relation to other relevant clinical and biologic prognostic characteristics.

> **Box 10-2.** 1998 International Ovarian Cancer Consensus Conference Criteria for Optimal Candidates for Secondary Cytoreductive Surgery
>
> - Disease-free interval >12 months
> - Response to first-line therapy
> - Potential for complete resection based on preoperative evaluation
> - Good performance status
> - Younger age

Secondary Cytoreduction

As in most clinical situations in medicine, patient selection for a chosen treatment modality is a significant factor in the success of this treatment. In the setting of recurrent ovarian cancer, in which cure is rarely a reasonable outcome to hope for, the clinician's role is to choose among several treatment schemes meant to prolong survival with good quality of life and minimal morbidity. It is not always possible to predict the patient's response to chemotherapy or how much she will benefit from surgery, but the morbidity associated with either modality should be taken into account during counseling when recurrence is diagnosed.

In 1998, the Second International Ovarian Cancer Consensus Conference suggested several criteria for optimal candidates for secondary cytoreductive surgery[11] (Box 10-2). This was an important statement that set forth long-awaited guidelines for surgery in the recurrent disease setting but that was based more on experts' opinions than on published peer-reviewed data. Several questions were still to be answered concerning secondary cytoreduction—questions regarding patient selection and goals of secondary surgery.

Patient Selection

Numerous series have been published on secondary cytoreduction, and almost all have concluded that there is a benefit to secondary surgical cytoreduction.[12–23] However, because of the nonrandomized nature of all the series on this topic, patient selection undoubtedly played a significant role in the findings and conclusions of these studies.

Disease-free Interval

In many series, an important prognostic and therefore selection factor is the disease-free interval (DFI), defined as the interval from the completion of chemotherapy to the diagnosis of recurrence. The platinum-free interval is the interval of time between the last dose of platinum-based chemotherapy and the diagnosis of recurrence. Generally, the DFI and the platinum-free interval are the same, since almost all patients receive primary platinum-based chemotherapy.

The importance of the DFI in patient selection for secondary cytoreduction was demonstrated by Morris and colleagues[24] in a retrospective series of 33 patients with advanced ovarian cancer who did not respond to first-line chemotherapy. In this cohort of patients with essentially no DFI, secondary cytoreduction was found to be of no benefit. However, numerous studies have demonstrated a survival benefit for patients whose DFI was longer than 12 months.

In 2006, the AGO (Arbeitsgemeinschaft Gynaekologische Onkologie) published a multicenter study on secondary cytoreductive surgery.[21] This was a large trial evaluating 267 patients with recurrent ovarian cancer. The Descriptive Evaluation of

Preoperative Selection Kriteria for Operability in Recurrent Ovarian Cancer (DESKTOP) trial was an exploratory study based on data from a retrospective analysis of hospital records. Regarding DFI, the authors of DESKTOP could not detect any impact of DFI on outcome in patients with DFIs when comparing 6 to 12 months with more than 12 months. Other series have reported a significant survival impact for DFIs exceeding 12 months and up to 36 months,[14,25–27] whereas other series did not detect any impact.[28–31]

In the same year as the AGO study, Chi and associates[20] applied a statistical analysis called *smoothing techniques* to analyze survival as a function of DFI in a large cohort of patients who underwent secondary cytoreduction for recurrent ovarian cancer (Fig. 10-1). The analysis identified optimal DFI cut-points of 6 to 12 months, 13 to 30 months, and more than 30 months. Survival after secondary cytoreduction was significantly improved in the longer DFI groups (Fig. 10-2).

Although DFI is one of the most frequently reported prognostic factors, it should not be the sole factor in deciding whether to offer secondary cytoreduction to women with recurrent ovarian cancer. Other factors, discussed in the following text, also carry weight in decision making. Moreover, some patients should not be offered surgery. For instance, women whose disease is persistent or progressive while they

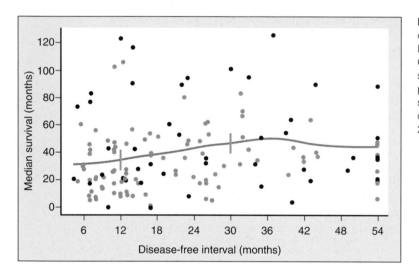

Figure 10-1. Survival as a function of disease-free interval. (From Chi DS, McCaughty K, Diaz JP, et al: Guidelines and selection criteria for secondary cytoreductive surgery in patients with recurrent, platinum-sensitive epithelial ovarian carcinoma. Cancer 106:1933–1939, 2006, Figure 4.)

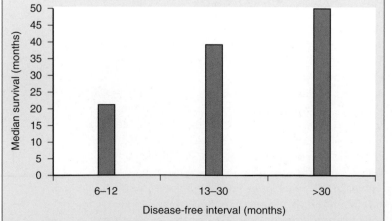

Figure 10-2. Disease-free interval and survival after secondary cytoreduction.

are receiving primary chemotherapy should not be offered surgical cytoreduction. Women with recurrent disease within 6 months of completing chemotherapy have a poor prognosis and generally gain little but morbidity from attempts at surgical cytoreduction. Women with a recurrence 6 to 12 months after completing chemotherapy can sometimes be offered surgical cytoreduction based on other variables. Patients with later recurrences and DFIs of 12 months to 30 months may be considered for secondary cytoreduction based on other factors, whereas patients with DFIs of 30 months or more should be assessed for surgical cytoreduction.

Extent of Disease and Ascites

Several factors regarding the pattern of recurrent disease should be taken into account before reaching a decision on surgical cytoreduction. These include the anatomic sites of recurrence, the number of lesions, the presence of carcinomatosis, and ascites (Box 10-3). Through imaging and physical examination, most of these factors can be assessed. Assessment of carcinomatosis is not always possible on imaging.

DESKTOP investigators evaluated the predictive value of ascites, localization of recurrence to the pelvis or other parts of the abdomen, and preoperative diagnosis of carcinomatosis.[21] These and other variables were appraised for their correlation with complete resection of tumor. On univariate analysis with respect to operability, ascites less than 500 mL, recurrent disease limited to the pelvis only, and no radiologic diagnosis of peritoneal carcinomatosis were predictors of complete resection. Regarding preoperative tumor assessment, they limited further analysis to ascites volume and when included on multivariate analysis, ascites less than 500 mL showed an independent and significant impact on the probability of achieving complete resection without macroscopically visible residual tumor. On multivariate analysis, the presence of ascites also had a negative impact on survival. Chi and associates[20] also found the presence of ascites to be a significant factor for survival on univariate but not multivariate analysis.

Localized recurrence of ovarian cancer with a small number of lesions is considered a favorable prognostic factor. It is thought that the likelihood of successful secondary cytoreduction is greater and that postrecurrence survival is superior. Most of the studies in the literature compare a solitary site with multiple sites of recurrence. Gronlund and associates[32] noted that a solitary recurrence was associated with the ability to achieve complete tumor resection and that patients who had complete cytoreduction experienced improved overall survival. Munkarah and colleagues[28] also evaluated the role of cytoreductive surgery for solitary versus multiple intra-abdominal recurrence sites of ovarian carcinoma. Survival was not evaluated on the basis of recurrent disease sites, but they were able to achieve optimal cytoreduction in a greater percentage of patients with isolated recurrence sites, which resulted in a trend toward improved survival. Zang and associates[18] noted improved ability to perform optimal cytoreduction in patients with a solitary lesion and also observed a significant 5-year survival advantage for patients who had one recurrent disease site (49.8%) compared with patients who had multiple recurrent disease sites (5.4%). Gadducci

---

Box 10-3. Patterns of Recurrence to Be Evaluated

- Anatomic sites of recurrence
- Number of lesions
- Lesion size
- Presence of carcinomatosis
- Ascites

and associates[33] reported a median survival of 40 months for patients who had an isolated, solitary recurrence versus 19 months for patients who had multiple recurrence sites. Other studies, including an evaluation of isolated lymph nodal recurrences, have also demonstrated notable survival benefits for secondary cytoreductive surgery in patients who have a single site of recurrence.[14,27,34-36]

To evaluate a wider spectrum of patients, Chi and associates[20] demonstrated that patients with a single site of recurrence had a median survival of 60 months compared with 42 months for patients with multiple sites of recurrence and 28 months for patients with carcinomatosis (Fig. 10-3).

Salani and colleagues[22] divided a cohort of patients who underwent secondary cytoreduction into two groups with up to five and with more then five sites of recurrence on preoperative imaging studies. The median survival of 48 months from the time of secondary cytoreductive surgery suggested that patients with less than five lesions on imaging studies in general have a better prognosis.

Larger tumor diameter at the time of recurrence has been shown by some investigators to adversely affect survival, although this varies from 5 to 10 cm depending on the study.[9,14,27] Others could not show an association of lesion size with either complete cytoreduction or survival.[15,19,30,33,34]

Overall, the literature consistently supports the idea that a patient with a long DFI and a solitary lesion less than 5 cm with no ascites or carcinomatosis will benefit from secondary cytoreduction. Unfortunately, the woman with a short DFI, extensive disease involving peritoneal surfaces with carcinomatosis, and ascites was in the majority and not the optimal candidate just mentioned (Fig. 10-4). There is a spectrum of recurrence patterns, and few patients fit into the optimal category slot. Logic should be used in determining the pattern of tumor spread that most likely fits surgical ability for resection. Imaging is an important tool for preoperative assessment and is discussed further.

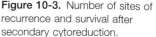

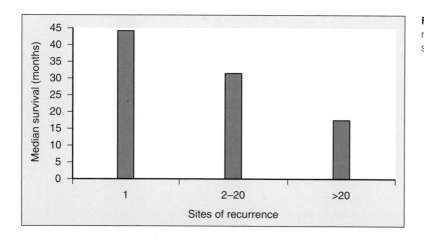

Figure 10-3. Number of sites of recurrence and survival after secondary cytoreduction.

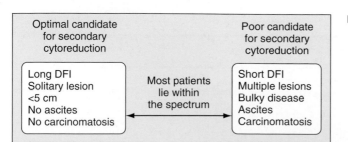

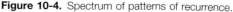

Figure 10-4. Spectrum of patterns of recurrence.

Variables Related to Adjuvant Chemotherapy and Response

Eisenkop and colleagues[14] examined the effect of the use of salvage chemotherapy before attempting surgical cytoreduction. Patients who had not received salvage chemotherapy experienced improved survival after surgery for recurrence. The investigators also evaluated the effect of previous response to chemotherapy in the course of disease. They found that the patient's response or lack of response to platinum-based regimens had no effect on postoperative survival.

Because surgery alone is rarely curative, surgical cytoreduction is generally not attempted without a plan for administering postoperative chemotherapy. In the DESKTOP trial[21] women who went on to receive platinum-based chemotherapy regimens after secondary cytoreduction experienced improved survival compared with patients who received other chemotherapy regimens (odds ratio 1.84; 95% confidence interval 1.13–3.01).

Most patients chosen for secondary cytoreduction have by definition platinum-sensitive disease and are candidates for retreatment with platinum-based regimens after surgery. It is difficult to conclude from the published literature whether patients who are not candidates for further platinum treatment will benefit from secondary cytoreduction. We recommend that patients considered for cytoreduction have further chemotherapy options for microscopic tumor control and eradication after surgery.

Other Factors

Additional factors including patient age, performance status, CA-125 levels, histology, tumor grade, and others have also been evaluated in an attempt to predict which patients will benefit from surgery. None of these factors has been shown to significantly influence the results of secondary cytoreduction independently of the other more robust factors previously mentioned.

It is notable that DESKTOP investigators found that both performance status and residual disease after primary surgery were associated with the probability of achieving complete resection during secondary cytoreduction. However, neither factor was associated with survival.

Preoperative Evaluation and Imaging

Predicting preoperatively which patients can be optimally cytoreduced may be challenging. Limited data exist addressing the efficacy of computed tomographic (CT) scanning to predict optimal resectability, and no solitary feature has been consistently associated with unresectability.

Funt and associates[37] attempted to correlate CT findings with surgical outcome in patients undergoing secondary cytoreduction. Two radiologists unaware of surgical outcomes retrospectively reviewed CT images and tried to assess for resectability. Peritoneal carcinomatosis, ascites, nodal disease, perihepatic metastasis, and involvement of bladder, rectum, sigmoid, or vagina were not indicators of tumor resectability. Pelvic sidewall invasion and hydronephrosis were significant independent predictors of suboptimal cytoreduction. It is not entirely clear why pelvic sidewall invasion would be unresectable in the recurrent setting because it is often not found to be unresectable in the primary setting. However, this may be explained by the hypothesis that tumor cells become fibrin-entrapped on previously traumatized peritoneal surfaces.[38] This was a small study of only 36 cases; therefore, the true significance and accuracy of these findings need further evaluation. Currently, there are no reliable CT findings that predict suboptimal cytoreduction, since even extensive hepatic tumors have been demonstrated to be resectable in this setting in experienced centers.[39]

Another imaging modality frequently used in preoperative evaluation is integrated [18]fluorodeoxyglucose-positron emission tomography/CT (FDG-PET/CT). This modality has been shown to be a sensitive post-therapy surveillance modality for the detection of recurrent ovarian cancer and can be useful for the detection of tumor recurrence when conventional imaging is inconclusive or negative.[40,41]

Lenhard and colleagues[42] assessed the predictive value of PET/CT imaging compared with AGO-scoring in patients planned for cytoreductive surgery with recurrent ovarian cancer. The investigators concluded that PET/CT and the AGO score offer good tools for determining candidates for full resectability in recurrent ovarian cancer. PET/CT was found to have a higher negative predictive value and the AGO score a higher positive predictive value; the combination of both improved the diagnostic accuracy.

Bristow and associates[43] used integrated PET/CT to evaluate patients with clinically occult recurrent ovarian cancer before secondary cytoreduction. The overall accuracy of PET/CT for discriminating recurrent disease larger than 1 cm was 81.8%. PET/CT demonstrated high sensitivity (83.3%) as well as a positive predictive value (PPV; 93.8%) for surgically documented recurrent ovarian cancer measuring more than 1 cm. Despite negative or equivocal findings on conventional CT imaging, localized nonphysiologic uptake of FDG on combined PET/CT was a strong predictor of suboptimal-volume recurrent tumor. In addition, lesion-based analysis showed a high PPV (96.1%) for surgically documented macroscopic recurrent tumor. However, PET/CT had only modest lesion-based sensitivity (60.5%), owing primarily to the inability to detect small-volume (less than 7 mm) disease.

This observation raises concerns regarding the clinical impact of PET imaging techniques for patients with suspected recurrent ovarian cancer. As previously discussed, carcinomatosis, usually defined as multiple small lesions, is an important factor in determining prognosis after secondary cytoreduction. A reliable preoperative diagnosis of carcinomatosis would thus be of tremendous importance. If carcinomatosis will not be detected by PET/CT, this modality may not assist in patient selection. Understanding these limitations, currently PET/CT is the most reliable, noninvasive method of identifying larger lesions, which are often not identified on conventional imaging, and can therefore serve as a useful adjunct in the preoperative evaluation and operative planning in patients being considered for secondary cytoreduction.

Procedures, Complications, and Outcome of Secondary Cytoreductive Surgery

The benefit of secondary cytoreduction appears to be seen only when optimal cytoreduction is achieved. In the primary setting, optimal cytoreduction is commonly defined as the maximal size of residual tumor measuring 1 cm. Many authors, however, suggest that the greatest benefit is seen if *all* grossly visible recurrent tumor is resected.[14,16,18,19,21,22] The exact size of residual disease that should be considered optimal is still debatable, but we seek to achieve a complete gross resection in the secondary or tertiary setting. If this is not possible, cytoreduction for tumors up to 5 mm may also be of benefit.[20] Aggressive surgical attempts that leave residual tumor over 5 mm are not warranted except in the palliative setting.

Repeat laparotomy after extensive primary oncologic surgery and chemotherapy is often challenging. When contemplating surgery, two questions regarding the procedure should be answered in assessing the overall benefits versus risks of secondary cytoreduction:

1. What is the rate of optimal cytoreduction or complete gross resection achieved in most series?
2. What are the complications reported and the morbidity described during and after surgical secondary cytoreduction?

In different publications, the rates of achieving optimal secondary cytoreduction, defined as between no residual and less than 2 cm residual tumor, vary widely. Most series report optimal debulking rates of 40% to 60%.[11,12,20,31,33,34] Two series reported optimal rates higher than 80%.[23,27] Complete macroscopic tumor resection rates also vary. A few studies reported rates of approximately 40%,[19,25,32] whereas others reported no residual macroscopic disease in 80% of patients undergoing secondary cytoreduction.[14,15,20] Because of the nonrandomized nature of all series published on this topic, a main confounding factor is patient selection.

Almost all patients with recurrent ovarian cancer have already had their uterus and adnexa removed. To achieve optimal resection or no gross residual disease, often many nongynecologic surgical procedures are required. Several authors have reported the procedures required to achieve optimal residual or no residual disease. These procedures include small and large bowel resections, lymph node dissections, diaphragm stripping/resection, liver resections, and splenectomies.

Morbidity and mortality rates after secondary cytoreduction have been reported to range from 4% to 30% and 0% to 6%, respectively (Table 10-1). In these series, the average blood loss per case was approximately 700 mL with a range of 50 to 3500 mL. Operating time averaged 2.5 to 3.5 hours. Hospital stay was reported to average 9 days, but ranged from 2 days to over 3 months.

Tebes and colleagues[23] reported enterotomy as the most frequently occurring intraoperative complication (8.3%). Other complications such as cystotomy, diaphragm injury, and vascular injury were rare in their experience (1%).

Postoperatively, ileus or bowel obstruction was a relatively common complication. Its incidence varies from 2% to 30% and is somewhat dependent on whether a bowel resection was performed.[31] Wound infection, fistula formation, renal failure, anastomotic leak, pneumonia, and acute respiratory distress syndrome have also been reported.

Table 10-1. Median Overall Survival in Months After Secondary Cytoreduction

Series	N	Number of Patients with No Gross Residual*	Optimal* (months)	Suboptimal* (months)
Segna et al[12]	100	—	27	9
Lichtenegger et al[13]	63	24	n/a	17
Eisenkop et al[14]	106	44	—	19
Zang et al[18]	117	61%†	21%†	4.5%†
Ayhan et al[19]	64	39	19	18
Chi et al[20]	153	—	56	27
Harter et al[21]	267	45	20	20
Salani et al[22‡]	55	50	—	7.2
Tebes et al[23]	85	—	30	17

*In series in which survival was assessed based on no gross residual tumor, the optimal category includes only optimal but gross residual disease.
†5-year overall survival.
‡Median overall survival in the suboptimal category is for any gross residual disease regardless of size.

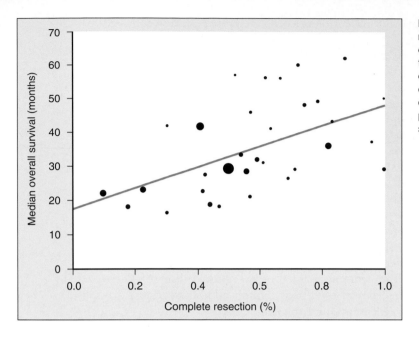

Figure 10-5. Simple linear regression analysis. Median cohort survival time plotted against the proportion of patients in each cohort undergoing complete cytoreductive surgery for recurrent ovarian cancer. Circle size is proportional to the number of subjects in each study.

Survival after Secondary Cytoreduction

Many published retrospective and some prospective nonrandomized series have reported an association between improved survival and optimal secondary surgical cytoreduction (see Table 10-1). Survival ranges from 7 to 27 months for patients without an optimal cytoreduction, 19 to 56 months for patients with optimal cyto-reduction, and 24 to 50 months for patients with no residual disease after secondary cytoreduction. There is obviously a great overlap of reported survival rates among the various series. When taken separately, complete resection is clearly superior, but comparisons across publications demonstrate that the difference between optimal disease and no macroscopic residual is less clear.

Bristow and colleagues[44] recently performed a meta-analysis of studies on cytore-ductive surgery for recurrent ovarian cancer. The purpose of the study was to determine the relative effect of multiple prognostic variables on overall postrecurrence survival time among cohorts of patients with recurrent ovarian cancer undergoing cytoreductive surgery. They analyzed 40 cohorts of patients including over 2000 cases. The only statistically significant clinical variable independently associated with postrecurrence survival time was the percentage of patients undergoing complete cytoreductive surgery. After controlling for all other variables, each 10% increase in the proportion of patients undergoing complete cytoreductive surgery was associated with a 3-month increase in median cohort survival time (Fig. 10-5).

Hyperthermic Intraperitoneal Chemotherapy

An interesting treatment modality being investigated in the setting of recurrent ovarian carcinoma limited to the peritoneal cavity is hyperthermic intraperitoneal chemotherapy (IPHC or HIPEC).[45,46] Hyperthermia has been shown to increase the response to cytotoxic agents in human cell lines and animal models.[47,48] Small series in optimally cytoreduced recurrent ovarian carcinoma have shown some promise.[44,45] However, the infusion must be done over 90 minutes, and therefore the procedure increases operating room times. A mean operating room time of nearly 10 hours was reported by Helm and colleagues.[45] The preliminary reported median survivals do not appear to be strikingly better than those seen in Table 10-1. Although this is an

Box 10-4. Factors Predicting Successful Cytoreduction

The probability of achieving no gross residual disease after secondary cytoreduction is higher when the following criteria are met:

- Good performance status
- Complete resection at first operation
- Initial FIGO stage I/II
- No ascites
- No carcinomatosis
- Long treatment-free interval
- Complete response after first-line therapy
- No extra-abdominal metastasis

Box 10-5. Factors Taken into Account in Management of Recurrent Disease

- Extent of recurrence
- Time from previous treatment
- Recurrence number
- Further chemotherapy options
- Patient performance status

Table 10-2. Selection Criteria for Secondary Cytoreduction (SC)

DFI (months)	One Site	Multiple Sites No Carcinomatosis	Carcinomatosis
6–12	Offer SC	Consider SC	No SC
12–30	Offer SC	Offer SC	Consider SC
>30	Offer SC	Offer SC	Offer SC

DFI, disease-free interval.

interesting concept, supported in part by preclinical data, the clinical application of this more morbid procedure cannot yet be endorsed without more rigorous investigation in a clinical trial setting.

Conclusions and Guidelines

The surgical management of recurrent ovarian cancer is a challenging but integral part of treatment in selected patients. The available data have demonstrated superior survival in the subset of patients who can achieve optimal cytoreduction compared with the subset in whom optimal cytoreduction cannot be achieved. Additional attempts at tumor cytoreduction should be considered and offered in the management of patients with recurrent epithelial ovarian carcinoma who are medically able to undergo surgery and willing to accept additional postoperative chemotherapy. Several factors predict successful cytoreduction and should be evaluated before surgery (Box 10-4).

There is no published randomized trial in the setting of recurrent ovarian cancer addressing the role of surgery. However, this issue is being evaluated in a recently activated GOG trial. While awaiting the results of this trial, the clinician managing patients needs to make critical decisions regarding the potential benefits and risks of further surgical intervention. Box 10-5 summarizes the factors that need to be taken into consideration and Table 10-2 offers suggested selection criteria for secondary cytoreduction for patients with recurrent ovarian cancer.

References

1. Meigs JV: Tumors of the female pelvic organs. New York: Macmillan, 1934.
2. Griffiths CT: Surgical resection of tumor bulk in the primary treatment of ovarian carcinoma. Natl Cancer Inst Monogr 42: 101–104, 1975.
3. Hoskins WJ, Bundy BN, Thigpen JT, Omura GA: The influence of cytoreductive surgery on recurrence-free interval and survival in small-volume stage III epithelial ovarian cancer: a Gynecologic Oncology Group study. Gynecol Oncol 47:159–166, 1992.
4. Hoskins WJ, McGuire WP, Brady MF, et al: The effect of diameter of largest residual disease on survival after primary cytoreductive surgery in patients with suboptimal residual epithelial ovarian carcinoma. Am J Obstet Gynecol 170:974–979, 1994.
5. Norton L: Theoretical concepts and the emerging role of taxanes in adjuvant therapy. The Oncologist 6(Suppl 3):30–35, 2001.
6. Goldie JH, Coldman JA: A mathematical model for relating the drug sensitivity of tumors to their spontaneous mutation rate. Cancer Treat Rep 63:1727–1733, 1979.
7. Chi DS, Liao JB, Leon LF, et al: Identification of prognostic factors in advanced epithelial ovarian carcinoma. Gynecol Oncol 82:532–537, 2001.
8. Bristow RE, Tomacruz RS, Armstrong DK, et al: Survival effect of maximal cytoreductive surgery for advanced ovarian carcinoma during the platinum era: a meta-analysis. J Clin Oncol 20:1248–1259, 2002.
9. Berek JS, Hacker NF, Lagasse LD, et al: Survival of patients following secondary cytoreductive surgery in ovarian cancer. Obstet Gynecol 61:189–193, 1983.
10. Bristow RE, Lagasse LD, Karlan BY: Secondary surgical cytoreduction for advanced epithelial ovarian cancer: patient selection and review of the literature. Cancer 78:2049–2062, 1996.
11. Berek JS, Bertelsen K, du Bois A, et al: Advanced epithelial ovarian cancer: 1998 consensus statements. Ann Oncol 1999; 10(Suppl 1):S87–S92.
12. Segna R, Dottino PR, Mandeli JPP, et al: Secondary cytoreduction for ovarian cancer following cisplatin therapy. J Clin Oncol 11:434–439, 1993.
13. Lichtenegger W, Sehouli J, Buchmann E, et al: Operative results after primary and secondary debulking operations in advanced ovarian cancer (AOC). J Obstet Gynaecol Res 24(6):447–451, 1998.
14. Eisenkop SM, Friedman RL, Spirtos NM: The role of secondary cytoreductive surgery in the treatment of patients with recurrent epithelial ovarian carcinoma. Cancer 88:144–153, 2000.
15. Zang RY, Zhang ZY, Li ZT, et al: Effect of cytoreductive surgery on survival of patients with recurrent epithelial ovarian cancer. J Surg Oncol 75:24–30, 2000.
16. Scarabelli C, Gallo A, Carbone A: Secondary cytoreductive surgery for patients with recurrent epithelial ovarian carcinoma. Gynecol Oncol 83:504–512, 2001.
17. Zang Ry, Li ZT, Zhang ZY, et al: Surgery and salvage chemotherapy for Chinese women with recurrent advanced epithelial ovarian carcinoma: a retrospective case-control study. Int J Gynecol Cancer 13:419–427, 2003.
18. Zang Ry, Li ZT, Tang J, et al: Secondary cytoreductive surgery for patients with relapsed epithelial ovarian carcinoma: who benefits? Cancer 100:1152–1161, 2004.
19. Ayhan A, Gultekin M, Taskiran C, et al: The role of secondary cytoreduction in the treatment of ovarian cancer: Hacettepe University experience. Am J Obstet Gynecol 194:49–56, 2006.
20. Chi DS, McCaughty K, Diaz JP, et al: Guidelines and selection criteria for secondary cytoreductive surgery in patients with recurrent, platinum-sensitive epithelial ovarian carcinoma. Cancer 106:1933–1939, 2006.
21. Harter P, du Bois A, Hahmann M, et al: Surgery in recurrent ovarian cancer: the Arbeitsgemeinschaft Gynaekologische Onkologie (AGO) DESKTOP OVAR trial. Ann Surg Oncol 13:1702–1710, 2006.
22. Salani R, Santillan A, Zahurak ML, et al: Secondary cytoreductive surgery for localized, recurrent epithelial ovarian cancer: analysis of prognostic factors and survival outcome. Cancer 109:685–691, 2007.
23. Tebes SJ, Sayer RA, Palmer JM, et al: Cytoreductive surgery for patients with recurrent epithelial ovarian carcinoma. Gynecol Oncol 106:482–487, 2007.
24. Morris M, Gershenson DM, Wharton JT: Secondary cytoreductive surgery in epithelial ovarian cancer: nonresponders to first-line therapy. Gynecol Oncol 33(1):1–5, 1989.
25. Tay EH, Grant PT, Gebski V, Hacker NF: Secondary cytoreductive surgery for recurrent epithelial ovarian cancer. Obstet Gynecol 99:1008–1013, 2002.
26. Leitao MM, Kardos S, Barakat RR, Chi DS: Tertiary cytoreduction in patients with recurrent ovarian cancer. Gynecol Oncol 95:181–185, 2004.
27. Onda T, Yoshikawa H, Yasugi T, et al: Secondary cytoreductive surgery for recurrent epithelial ovarian carcinoma: proposal for patient selection. Br J Cancer 92:1026–1032, 2005.
28. Munkarah A, Levenback C, Wolf JK, et al: Secondary cytoreductive surgery for localized intra-abdominal recurrences in epithelial ovarian cancer. Gynecol Oncol 81:237–241, 2001.
29. Cormio G, di Vagno G, Cazzolla A, et al: Surgical treatment of recurrent ovarian cancer: report of 21 cases and a review of the literature. Eur J Obstet Gynecol Reprod Biology 86:185–188, 1999.
30. Vaccarello L, Rubin SC, Vlamis V, et al: Cytoreductive surgery in ovarian carcinoma patients with a documented previously complete surgical response. Gynecol Oncol 57:61–65, 1995.
31. Janicke F, Holscher M, Kuhn W, et al: Radical surgery procedure improves survival time in patients with recurrent ovarian cancer. Cancer 70:2129–2136, 1992.
32. Gronlund B, Lundvall L, Christensen IJ, et al: Surgical cytoreduction in recurrent ovarian carcinoma in patients with complete response to paclitaxel-platinum. Eur J Surg Oncol 31:67–73, 2005.
33. Gadducci A, Iacconi P, Cosio S, et al: Complete salvage surgical cytoreduction improves further survival of patients with late recurrent ovarian cancer. Gynecol Oncol 79:344–349, 2000.
34. Gungor M, Ortac F, Arvas M, et al: The role of secondary cytoreductive surgery for recurrent ovarian cancer. Gynecol Oncol 97:74–79, 2005.
35. Harter P, du Bois A: The role of surgery in ovarian cancer with special emphasis on cytoreductive surgery for recurrence. Curr Opin Oncol 17:505–514, 2005.
36. Uzan C, Morice P, Rey A, et al: Outcomes after combined therapy including surgical resection in patients with epithelial ovarian cancer recurrence (s) exclusively in lymph nodes. Ann Surg Oncol 11:658–664, 2004.
37. Funt SA, Hricak H, Abu-Rustum N, et al: Role of CT in the management of recurrent ovarian cancer. AJR Am J Roentgenol 182:393–398, 2004.
38. Sugarbaker PH: Management of peritoneal surface malignancy: appendix cancer and pseudomyxoma peritonei, colon cancer, gastric cancer, abdominopelvic sarcoma, and primary peritoneal malignancy. In Bland KI, Daly JM, Karakousis CP (eds): Surgical Oncology: Contemporary Principles and Practice. New York: McGraw-Hill, 2001, pp 1149–1176.
39. Yoon SS, Jarnagin WR, DeMatteo RP, et al: Resection of recurrent ovarian or fallopian tube carcinoma involving the liver. Gynecol Oncol 91(2):383–388, 2003.
40. Chung HH, Kang WJ, Kim JW, et al: Role of [18F]FDG PET/CT in the assessment of suspected recurrent ovarian cancer: correlation with clinical or histological findings. Eur J Nucl Med Mol Imaging 34(4):480–486, 2007.
41. Torizuka T, Nobezawa S, Kanno T, et al: Ovarian cancer recurrence: role of whole-body positron emission tomography using 2-[fluorine-18]-fluoro-2-deoxy-D-glucose. Eur J Nucl Med Mol Imaging 29(6):797–803, 2002.
42. Lenhard SM, Burges A, Johnson TR, et al: Predictive value of PET-CT imaging versus AGO-scoring in patients planned for cytoreductive surgery in recurrent ovarian cancer. Eur J Obstet Gynecol Reprod Biol 140:263–268, 2008.
43. Bristow RE, del Carmen MG, Pannu HK, et al: Clinically occult recurrent ovarian cancer: patient selection for secondary cytoreductive surgery using combined PET/CT. Gynecol Oncol 90(3):519–528, 2003.
44. Bristow RE, Puri I, Chi DS: Cytoreductive surgery for recurrent ovarian cancer: a meta-analysis. Gynecol Oncol 112:265–274. Epub 2008 Oct 19.
45. Helm CW, Randall-Whitis L, Martin III RS, et al: Hyperthermic intraperitoneal chemotherapy in conjunction with surgery for the treatment of recurrent ovarian carcinoma. Gynecol Oncol 105:90–96, 2007.

46. Cotte E, Glehen O, Mohamed F, et al: Cytoreductive surgery and intraperitoneal chemo-hyperthermia for chemo-resistant and recurrent advanced epithelial ovarian cancer: prospective study of 81 patients. World J Surg 31(9):1813–1820, 2007.

47. Meyn RE, Corry PM, Fletcher SE, et al: Thermal enhancement of DNA damage in mammalian cells treated with cis-diamminechloroplatinum(II). Cancer Res 40:1136–1139, 1980.

48. Alberts DS, Peng YM, Chen HS, et al: Therapeutic synergism of hyperthermia-cis-platinum in a mouse tumor model. J Natl Cancer Inst 65:455–461, 1980.

11 Borderline Epithelial Ovarian Tumors, Sex Cord-Stromal Tumors, and Germ Cell Tumors

J. Stuart Ferriss, Erin R. King, and Susan C. Modesitt

KEY POINTS

- Most borderline tumors are stage I/II, with survival rate approaching 100%.
- Borderline tumors can recur locally even after an extended disease-free interval.
- Microinvasion, advanced stage, and micropapillary histology are associated with increased ovarian cancer recurrence rates.
- Even with advanced disease, adjuvant therapy has not been shown to improve survival in borderline tumors.
- Sex cord-stromal tumors are hormonally active tumors and may manifest as symptoms of either estrogen or androgen excess.
- Primary treatment for sex cord-stromal tumors is surgical and may include postoperative adjuvant chemotherapy (either combination bleomycin/etoposide/cisplatin [BEP] or taxane/platinum) for high-risk or advanced stages of disease.
- Granulosa cell tumors account for 70% to 80% of sex cord-stromal tumors.
- Most sex cord-stromal tumors are diagnosed at an early stage and have a favorable prognosis.
- Dysgerminomas are the most common type of germ cell tumor, followed by immature teratomas and endodermal sinus tumors.
- Peak incidence of ovarian germ cell tumors is from 15 to 19 years of age, and dysgerminomas are frequently diagnosed during pregnancy. Diagnosis requires a comprehensive workup, including tumor markers: α-fetoprotein, β-human chorionic gonadotropin, and lactate dehydrogenase.
- Initial management of germ cell tumors is surgical, with fertility-sparing surgery being preferred except in the case of dysgenetic gonads.
- Adjuvant chemotherapy for germ cell tumors is BEP. Rates of cure approach 95%, and long-term outcomes with regard to ovarian function are favorable.

Borderline Ovarian Tumors

Borderline ovarian tumors (also termed ovarian tumors of low malignant potential) were first officially defined by the World Health Organization (WHO) in 1970 and affect approximately 3000 women yearly in the United States.[1] These tumors represent 15% of all epithelial ovarian cancers, although a recent report from Sweden found that the proportion of borderline tumors increased from 8% of all ovarian neoplasms in 1960 to 1964 to 24% in 2000 to 2005.[1,2] In general, borderline ovarian tumors occur in younger women, are found in earlier stages, and have a more favorable prognosis than epithelial ovarian cancer. They are associated with a 5-year survival rate approaching 100% in early stage.[3] For example, the Swedish population study found that the average age for those with borderline tumors was 55 years compared with 62 years for those with invasive ovarian cancers and that a third of all primary ovarian malignancies in women under 40 years of age were borderline tumors.[2] Overall, these tumors have excellent prognosis with a 93% to 99% 5-year survival rate and an 80% to 90% 15-year survival rate.[3–6]

Histology

Borderline ovarian tumors typically exhibit the following histologic features: architectural complexity of glandular structures, epithelial papillae, cellular stratification, and nuclear atypia, and the requirement for diagnosis is two of these three elements.[6] The key to differentiating between an invasive ovarian cancer and a borderline neoplasm is the lack of stromal invasion. Since these tumors may be large, careful and thorough sectioning is required. Borderline tumors are most frequently serous followed by mucinous, but they can also occur less often as endometrioid, clear, transitional, or mixed types (Table 11-1).

In addition to the histology, other important factors such as extraovarian disease, microinvasion, and micropapillary pattern may be present, and the prognostic significance of each continues to be investigated (Table 11-2). All these features have been linked to increased recurrence rates.

Borderline tumors can have foci of extraovarian disease (often termed implants rather than metastases), and stage remains the most important prognostic factor in this disease. Noninvasive implants can be differentiated from invasive implants by the sharp delineation from normal tissue, a fibrotic or inflammatory stroma, and continued gland formation. In contrast, the invasive implants tend to have infiltration of normal tissue with edematous or myxoid stroma and form nests surrounded by a cleft. To add to the complexity, any given patient may have a mix of implant types,[7-12] although the majority of extraovarian disease remains noninvasive.[11,12] In a review of seven published papers comparing invasive with noninvasive implants, Lu and Bell[3] found that the relapse rate and death due to tumor were significantly increased in the invasive implants (44% versus 19%, and 32% versus 7%, respectively).

Table 11-1. Borderline Ovarian Tumor Histology[3]

Histologic Types	Percentage
Serous	43–75
Mucinous	23–40
Endometrioid	2–10
Clear cell	0–8
Brenner	<1
Mixed	5–10

Data are taken from references 3, 6, 13, 17, and 21.

Table 11-2. Prognostic Features in Borderline Tumors

Clinicopathologic Feature	Significance
Micropapillary histology	Increased rates of extraovarian disease Increased recurrence rates and death due to disease
Stage	The most important factor in predicting recurrence Increased recurrence rates and death due to disease
Microinvasion	Increased rates of recurrence Potential increased rates of recurrence with invasive cancer Increased mortality rates Decreased disease-free and overall survival

Microinvasion has also elicited some controversy as to whether tumors exhibiting this feature represent a subset of borderline tumors or may represent early serous papillary carcinoma. Buttin and colleagues[13] evaluated the impact of microinvasion (defined as invasive foci less than 3 mm in diameter with a total area less than 5% of the tumor) and found that recurrence rates were significantly higher in women with microinvasion compared with rates in women without microinvasion (23% versus 3.5%, $P = .023$). Hogg and colleagues[14] compared serous grade 1 carcinomas with borderline tumors and concluded that borderline tumors with microinvasion represent early carcinomas. This conclusion was based on qualitative histologic similarities between borderline tumors with microinvasion and grade 1 carcinomas and the frequent coexistence of the two entities. Additional support for this supposition may be the fact that borderline tumors may often recur with low-grade serous carcinoma rather than borderline tumors.[15] Finally, Longacre and associates,[16] in an analysis of 276 patients, and Ren and associates,[17] in an analysis of 234 patients, both found that microinvasion was a significant risk factor for decreased survival on multivariate analysis.

Micropapillary architecture within borderline tumors was first described in the 1990s and was added as a subgroup of borderline tumors by the WHO, although debate continues as to whether these tumors should be an entity separate from both borderline and epithelial ovarian carcinoma. These tumors are distinct from the garden variety of borderline tumors in that they have increased cytologic atypia and a papillary proliferation with a hierarchical branching pattern of epithelium. By convention, the micropapillary component must be at least 5 mm.[18,19] There continues to be extensive debate among pathologists as to whether tumors with micropapillary architecture should be classified as a separate entity or as a subset of borderline tumors. Regardless of classification, tumors with micropapillary architecture are more often bilateral, have extraovarian disease, and, in turn, more unfavorable outcomes compared with typical borderline tumors.[3,7,20] In comparing the typical borderline pattern with the micropapillary pattern in seven published studies, Lu and Bell[3] found that both the relapse rate and death due to tumor were significantly increased in the micropapillary type (32% versus 15% and 15% versus 8%, respectively). Since these micropapillary types more often have invasive implants, it is difficult to discern the isolated impact of the micropapillary feature on survival.

Clinical Characteristics

Women with borderline ovarian tumors typically present with pelvic pain and/or a mass that is found incidentally on examination or while imaging for another cause. One study found that pelvic pain was the most common presenting symptom in 39% of patients followed by abdominal distention in 25%; ovarian torsion or hemorrhage may also occur.[21] The typical size of a borderline tumor ranges from 7 to 9 cm[13,22-24] (Fig. 11-1A). Imaging with ultrasound most often identifies an ovarian cyst, which may include other abnormalities including septations or solid components. Gotleib and associates[23] combined their institution's experience with borderline tumors with 11 other studies and found that ultrasound revealed simple cysts in about 9% of patients (17 of 174 patients reported) and septa, solid components, or papillations in 88% (153 of 174). There is no diagnostic imaging modality that is definitive for borderline tumors.

Serum CA-125 measurements are often elevated in borderline tumors and are more commonly increased in serous than in mucinous tumors. Many studies have evaluated the percentage of patients with borderline tumors with elevated CA-125 and found ranges between 24% and 75%.[17,22-26] Other tumor markers such as CEA and CA-19-9 have also been evaluated with conflicting results, but these markers

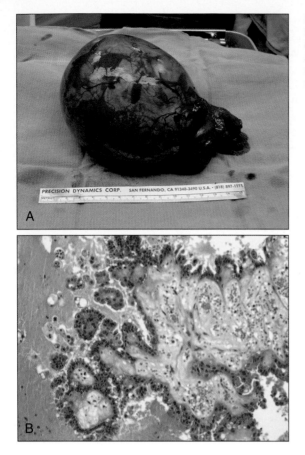

Figure 11-1. A, Gross picture of borderline ovarian tumor. **B,** Micrograph of serous borderline tumor (hematoxylin & eosin, ×400). (B, Courtesy of Dr. Kristen Atkins, Department of Pathology, University of Virginia Health System.)

may be more useful for mucinous borderline tumors.[17,25–26] If elevated, these markers can be used for surveillance.

Diagnosis

Most women with borderline tumors undergo surgical evaluation and treatment that may range from minimal surgery as an ovarian cystectomy to a total salpingo-oophorectomy, hysterectomy, and full staging (omentectomy, washings, peritoneal biopsies, and lymph node dissection), depending on the clinical scenario.

Surgical Management

In general, as in malignant ovarian cancer, there should be a maximal surgical effort to remove as much tumor as possible from women with extraovarian tumors and to assess the extent and need for further staging procedures based on patient characteristics in women whose disease appears confined to the ovary.

Intraoperative Frozen Section

Most often the diagnosis of an ovarian borderline tumor is not known preoperatively, and a frozen section is obtained to establish a definitive diagnosis to guide the nature and extent of surgery required. In general, the pathologic analysis of frozen section to differentiate invasive and noninvasive ovarian tumors demonstrates a sensitivity between 65% and 97% and a specificity of 97% to 100%, as shown on a recent meta-analysis.[27] In borderline tumors, especially large mucinous tumors, that same differentiation may be more difficult. Tempfer and colleagues[28] found that none of their patients was overdiagnosed (defined as a frozen section with borderline or malignant pathology and a subsequent final benign pathology). In contrast, they also found underdiagnosis in almost one third of patients. This was defined as frozen read as normal and final pathology with borderline, or as a frozen diagnosis of borderline and a final malignant pathology. Of note, nearly all the missed underdiagnoses were borderline tumors and not invasive cancers. Increasing tumor size was also a factor in missing the correct diagnosis. In summation, frozen section may lend important information but must be interpreted with caution, especially in centers without gynecologic pathologists.

Extent of Surgery

Women with borderline tumors tend to be younger and often do not have a known diagnosis preoperatively. For women who do not desire future pregnancy, most experts would recommend a bilateral salpingo-oophorectomy, hysterectomy, and staging if indicated (see text that follows). For women who desire reproductive capability, several studies indicate the safety of fertility-sparing surgery with a unilateral oophorectomy or even simple cystectomy if the other ovary and remainder of the surgical exploration are normal.[3,28–32] The performance of fertility sparing surgery does not seem to adversely impact overall survival but does consistently increase recurrence rates in multiple retrospective reviews.[17,29–32] A French study compared cystectomy versus unilateral salpingo-oophorectomy versus bilateral salpingo-oophorectomy and recurrence rates in 313 women with borderline tumors; found were significantly increased recurrence rates with the more limited excisions (30% versus 11% versus 1.7%, respectively; $P < .001$).[32] Morris and associates[29] reviewed 43 patients with borderline tumors treated with fertility-sparing surgery and found that 50% of the women attempting pregnancy conceived (12 of 24 patients for a total of 25 pregnancies) and that the recurrence rate for the entire population was 32%. The recurrence rate of borderline tumors was higher in women treated with cystectomy compared with those treated with oophorectomy (58% versus 23%; $P < .04$). Similarly, Suh-Burgmann[30] found a recurrence rate of 11% in 193 patients treated with conservative surgery with a mean time to recurrence of 4.7 years. Women initially treated with cystectomy were three times more likely to have a recurrence of borderline tumors than women undergoing oophorectomy.[30] In summation, women can safely elect to maintain fertility but must understand the potential increased risk of recurrence and need for additional surgery.

Staging

The role of complete surgical staging for borderline tumors remains controversial. Complete staging would include bilateral salpingo-oophorectomy, hysterectomy, washings, omentectomy, peritoneal biopsies, and lymph node dissection. Proponents of full staging argue that frozen section is unreliable and that if a cancer is found, definitive staging enables a rational adjuvant treatment decision. Furthermore, they contend that full staging will upstage up to 50% of apparent stage I borderline tumors. Opponents of full staging for all patients argue that there is no survival advantage in accurately assessing stage of borderline tumors owing to the lack of evidence for effective adjuvant therapy and that staging may add surgical morbidity (especially if it requires a second surgery to accomplish). Winter and colleagues[33] analyzed 93 consecutive patients with borderline tumors and found that full surgical staging upstaged patients 17% of the time but that retroperitoneal involvement was found only 6% of the time. Furthermore, the overall survival and recurrence rates did not differ between staged and unstaged patients.

Similarly, Longacre and associates[16] found that one third of women undergoing nodal dissection for borderline tumors had positive nodes, but they did not find any significant difference in survival based on nodal status. Finally, a French multicenter study evaluated 360 women with borderline tumors and assessed the impact of surgical restaging of 54 women.[34] The researchers found no impact on survival, but they did find a 14.8% rate of upstaging. This was more common in serous tumors and in women undergoing cystectomy at the initial surgery.[34] In summation, surgical decisions must be made for individual patients and must take into account future fertility wishes, impact on future treatment decisions, and potential surgical morbidity.

Adjuvant Treatment

Stage I Tumors

Since survival rate in stage I patients approaches 100%, few experts suggest any further therapy after surgical excision and simply advocate for long-term surveillance.[35]

Stage II-IV Tumors

Even with advanced-stage borderline tumors, long-term survival rate may be as high as 70%.[3] As previously discussed, these tumors are often associated with adverse prognostic factors including extraovarian disease, microinvasion, and/or micropapillary patterns. Several groups have analyzed whether postoperative adjuvant chemotherapy administration improves survival, but there is limited support for chemotherapy, since most studies have not shown definitive benefit.[1,12,36,37] For example, Barakat and colleagues[36] evaluated postoperative platinum-based chemotherapy in 21 patients (only 40% with macroscopic residual tumor) and found a 62.5% complete response rate at second-look laparotomy; the remainder had stable disease (12.5%), partial response (6%), or progression (19%). In addition, the M.D. Andersen group also failed to demonstrate a survival benefit.[1,12] Finally, an analysis of platinum (cisplatin/cyclophosphamide ± adriamycin) chemotherapy in borderline tumors through the Gynecologic Oncology Group (GOG) found that 9 of 32 patients had persistent disease at second-look laparotomy and that all but one patient was still alive at a median of 32 months (one had died of other causes).[37]

The jury remains out as to whether adjuvant chemotherapy is beneficial, and a randomized trial is not likely forthcoming because of the indolent nature of the disease and the relative rarity of advanced cases. Our current approach is to reserve offering adjuvant chemotherapy to women with macroscopic residual disease and invasive implants, but with full disclosure to the patient about the unknown benefit of this potential therapy as a survival advantage has not been documented.

Surveillance

Most women are followed up with a combination of physical examination, serum tumor markers, and radiologic evaluation if indicated. The frequency of visits depends on the stage and the clinical scenario.

Outcomes

Recurrence

The median time to recurrence is 5 to 7 years for borderline tumors, but late recurrences decades later are also reported. Recurrence can be either a borderline or an invasive epithelial cancer; it is not surprising that invasive recurrences are more likely to result in death.[6,15,16,38] Traditional management of recurrent tumors is secondary cytoreduction with or without postoperative chemotherapy. One of the largest studies on recurrent ovarian borderline tumors was reported by Crispens and associates[15] from the M.D. Anderson experience and showed a 5.6-year median time to recurrence and a further 7.7-year median survival after recurrence. In this study, most women underwent secondary surgery, and optimal cytoreduction was a significant predictor of survival. For all nonsurgical interventions (chemotherapy, hormonal therapy, and radiation therapy), the response rate was only 26%, and 50% of those responses occurred after platinum-based chemotherapy. Similarly, 50% of the patients had stable disease to the nonsurgical options, and again, in order of decreasing efficacy, the therapies were platinum-based chemotherapy (11 of 21 patients), hormonal therapy (8 of 21), other chemotherapy (6 of 21) and radiation therapy (3 of 21). The median duration of stable disease was 12 months.

In summation, women with recurrent borderline tumor should initially be managed surgically (if feasible), and adjuvant treatment may be offered including platinum-based chemotherapy or hormonal treatment.

Sex Cord-Stromal Tumors

Sex cord-stromal tumors consist of a pathologically diverse group of ovarian tumors originating from the sex cords and stroma of the ovary. Their exact histogenesis remains unclear. Collectively, they account for 5% to 8% of all ovarian tumors and can occur in women of any age group, but they are most commonly diagnosed in women in the fifth decade of life. Sex cord-stromal tumors are classified into granulosa cell tumors (GCTs), Sertoli-Leydig tumors, sex cord-stromal tumors with annular tubules, and gynandroblastomas[39] (Table 11-3).

Sex cord-stromal tumors display intermediate malignant behavior in that they can vary from benign to malignant, depending on cell type and level of differentiation. Fortunately, most are diagnosed at an early stage owing to their hormonal activity, which is responsible for the unique presenting symptoms of these tumors. GCTs produce estrogen, whereas Sertoli-Leydig tumors secrete testosterone. Other

Table 11-3. World Health Organization Classification of Sex Cord-Stromal Tumors

Sex Cord-Stromal Tumor Types	Percentage
2.1 Granulosa-stromal cell tumors: Granulosa cell tumors thecoma-fibroma	70
2.2 Sertoli-stromal cell tumors, androblastomas: Well-differentiated, Sertoli-Leydig cell tumor of intermediate differentiation, Sertoli-Leydig cell tumor poorly differentiated (sarcomatoid), retiform	<0.2
2.3 Sex cord tumor with annular tubules	
2.4 Gynandroblastoma	<1
2.5 Unclassified	<1
2.6 Steroid (lipid) cell tumors: Stromal luteoma, Leydig cell tumor, unclassified	<1

From WHO Histological Typing of Ovarian Tumours. Copyright 1999.

sex cord-stromal tumors may also secrete a combination of hormones. In estrogen-secreting tumors, breast enlargement and vaginal bleeding are the most common symptoms. Women of reproductive age may present with menstrual irregularities. The postmenopausal female typically presents with postmenopausal bleeding and breast tenderness. In androgen-secreting tumors, hirsutism, deepening of the voice, male-pattern baldness, breast shrinkage, clitoromegaly, and acne may occur.

Additional nonspecific complaints result from tumor mass, including increased abdominal girth, bloating, and palpable mass on physical examination. Urinary complaints and constipation accompany tumor compression of the bladder and/or rectum.

Overall prognosis is good for these tumors, since most sex cord-stromal tumors are diagnosed at an early stage, have indolent growth, and recur later than their epithelial counterparts. Although some sex cord-stromal tumors are purely benign (e.g., fibromas and thecomas), others have the potential to behave more aggressively. Fortunately, over 90% of sex cord-stromal tumors are diagnosed at stage I. Unequivocally, surgery is the initial step in management for both diagnosis and treatment.

Treatment for sex cord-stromal tumors is controversial because these tumors are relatively rare. The general consensus for postmenopausal women includes total abdominal hysterectomy and bilateral salpingo-oophorectomy with complete surgical staging. Staging should include pelvic washings, peritoneal biopsies, omentectomy, and pelvic and para-aortic lymph node sampling. In a woman who desires future fertility, it is acceptable to leave the remaining ovary and uterus as long as (1) the tumor is confined to one ovary, (2) the contralateral ovary appears normal, and (3) a thorough inspection of the abdomen and pelvis reveals no extraovarian disease.

Unfortunately, for women diagnosed in advanced stages, there are no available randomized controlled trials to guide management, and prospective trials are limited as a consequence of their relative rarity. Most of the available literature is derived from retrospective institutional experiences. In general, for patients with advanced disease, recurrence, or poorly differentiated tumors, adjuvant chemotherapy with bleomycin/etoposide/cisplatin (BEP) or a platinum/taxane regimen is recommended.

Although there is no consensus regarding surveillance of women with sex cord-stromal tumors, given the potential for late recurrence these women require lifetime surveillance. In our current practice, we see these women every 3 to 4 months for the first 2 years, every 6 months in years 3 to 5, and annually thereafter. At each visit, a pelvic examination is performed, and tumor-specific markers are obtained. Some providers obtain periodic CT scans; others acquire only images if there is concern for recurrence.

Because sex cord-stromal tumors are so diverse, each is discussed separately with regard to epidemiology, histology, diagnosis, and treatment recommendations.

Granulosa-Stromal Cell Tumors

Granulosa-stromal cell tumors account for 70% of tumors in the sex cord-stromal group, and 2% to 5% of all ovarian tumors.[40] They encompass GCTs, thecomas, and fibromas. Although GCTs are considered malignant, they grow slowly and do not behave as aggressively as their epithelial counterparts. However, if not detected at an early stage they do have the potential to metastasize and recur. Unlike epithelial-type ovarian tumors, there is no racial or ethnic predilection of GCTs. There is also no identified heritable risk, particularly in the case of *BRCA1* or *BRCA2*, which confer increased risk of epithelial ovarian carcinoma.

Granulosa Cell Tumors

The mean age of diagnosis for the adult subtype of GCT is age 50 to 54,[41] which accounts for 95% of GCTs. However, the juvenile variant manifests at a young age and is responsible for 5% of granulosa-theca cell tumors. Young and associates[42] studied 125 cases of juvenile GCTs and found nearly half in girls under age 10, and less than 3% in women over 30. Although the juvenile subtype falls into the classification of GCTs, histologically this tumor differs from the adult variant.

The cause of GCTs is unclear. Controversy exists as to whether granulosa cells originate from developing gonadal sex cords or from the mesenchyme of the genital ridge. Since granulosa cells proliferate in response to follicle-stimulating hormone (FSH), some have hypothesized that the elevated follicle-stimulating hormone levels observed during menopause may initiate proliferation of granulosa cells and abnormal growth. This would explain the higher incidence of GCTs in postmenopausal women, but does not account for younger women and prepubertal females who develop these tumors. Recent developments have suggested that a potential progenitor granulosa stem cell exists,[43] but the subject warrants more research.

Presentation. With the exception of fibromas, GCTs tend to produce hormones and consequently are diagnosed at an early stage secondary to estrogenic effects. Women with these tumors most commonly present with menstrual cycle disruptions or postmenopausal bleeding, and over 90% of tumors are diagnosed as stage I tumors. In the prepubertal female, 70% to 80% of GCTs cause isosexual precocious puberty.[42] Because of the hemorrhagic nature of GCTs, these tumors may rupture and cause hemoperitoneum; thus, patients may present with acute abdominal pain and peritonitis.

Diagnosis. Symptoms resulting from hyperestrogenism often provoke prompt investigation and early diagnosis. On physical examination, a clinician may detect the presence of an adnexal mass since the average tumor size is 12 cm. Ultrasonography usually reveals a cystic, heterogeneous mass—a nondiagnostic finding. Definitive diagnosis is made at the time of excision and rarely before then.

Histology and Pathology. Grossly, GCTs tend to be gray-to-yellow on the surface, which varies based on the lipid content of the tumor. They often appear hemorrhagic with areas of cystic necrosis (Fig. 11-2A). Most are unilateral; only 2% of GCTs are bilateral. Histologically, Call-Exner bodies are the hallmark of GCTs, occurring in 30% to 60% of GCTs,[40,44,45] and appear as rosettes of granulosa cells surrounded by eosinophilic material (Fig. 11-2B). Other classic findings include the pale coffee-bean grooved nuclei. Since not all GCTs harbor Call-Exner bodies or coffee-bean nuclei, pathologic diagnosis should not rest on these characteristics alone. Some tumors possess only granulosa cells, but most contain theca cells, and some have fibroblasts. These tumors typically have a low mitotic rate, with scant nuclear atypia.

Several pattern subtypes exist: microfollicular (characterized by Call-Exner bodies), macrofollicular (more commonly found in the juvenile subtype), trabecular, and insular. The latter patterns lend themselves to well-differentiated types, whereas poorly differentiated tumors often contain a watered-silk pattern. Immunohistologic staining with inhibin proves useful for the identification of GCTs. Although other immunohistologic markers exist, inhibin remains the most sensitive of the currently available staining reagents.[46]

Grossly, the juvenile subtype appears similar to the adult variant. Histologically, Call-Exner bodies and coffee-bean nuclei are usually absent. In contrast to the adult variant, they are more mitotically active and favor a macrofollicular pattern.

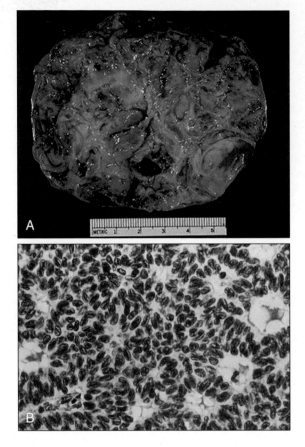

Figure 11-2. A, Gross picture of granulosa cell tumor. **B,** Micrograph of granulosa cell tumor (H&E, ×400). (Courtesy of Dr. Kristen Atkins, Department of Pathology, University of Virginia Health System.)

Treatment. Treatment for GCTs consists of surgery with staging, including total abdominal hysterectomy and bilateral salpingo-oophorectomy. In women who desire fertility, unilateral salpingo-oophorectomy offers a cure rate comparable to complete surgical staging, hysterectomy and bilateral salpingo-oophorectomy,[47,48] provided it is confined to the ovary. See Figure 11-3 for proposed management guidelines. If not performed before surgery, dilation and curettage are recommended to rule out a potential synchronous endometrial cancer. Although concurrent vaginal bleeding may elicit endometrial biopsy on initial intake, if the uterus is not excised in conjunction with the ovaries, endometrial evaluation is essential. This is especially important in the case of abnormal bleeding, or a thickened endometrial stripe larger than 4 mm in a postmenopausal woman. Approximately 30% to 55% of women with GCTs are likely to have endometrial hyperplasia on endometrial biopsy; 5% to 10% will have synchronous endometrial adenocarcinoma.[40,41,44,49]

Adjuvant Therapy. Stage remains the only reproducible factor determining prognosis[50] (Table 11-4; Fig. 11-4). Other factors including age, tumor rupture, and mitotic index may influence prognosis, but these findings are inconsistent from study to study. Between 78% and 91% of GCTs are stage I at the time of initial presentation.[40,45,51-53] and overall prognosis is good: Stage I 5-year survival rates range from 86% to 96%; overall 5-year survival rate for all stages is 75% to 90%. In more advanced-stage tumors, prognosis is less favorable: Stage II tumors have a 5-year survival rate of 55% to 75%; stage III/IV 22% to 50%. In the juvenile subtype, virtually all tumors are detected at an early stage, with a 5-year survival rate of 92%.[42] As

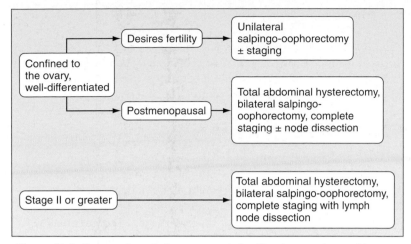

Figure 11-3. Proposed surgical management algorithm for granulosa cell tumors.

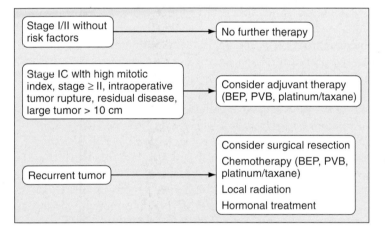

Figure 11-4. Proposed adjuvant treatment algorithm for granulosa cell tumors. BEP, bleomycin/etoposide/cisplatin; PVB, cisplatin, vinblastine, bleomycin.

Table 11-4. Survival Rates in Sex Cord-Stromal Tumors		
Tumor Type		**5-Year Survival Rate**
Granulosa cell tumor	All stages	75–90%
	Stage I	86–96%
	Stage II	55–75%
	Stage III/IV	22–50%
	Juvenile subtype	92%
Fibroma		>90%
Thecoma		>90%
Sertoli-Leydig tumor	Stage I	70–90%
	Advanced stages or poorly differentiated	<20%

in the adult subtype, these juvenile tumors may metastasize, and prognosis declines in advanced stages.

Because advanced-stage GCTs are relatively rare, there is little consensus about adjuvant therapy in the form of chemotherapy or radiation. Generally, there is agreement that if the tumor is at an early stage and excised in its entirety, there is no role for adjuvant therapy. For women with more advanced tumors (i.e., beyond stage II), intraoperative tumor rupture, large tumor (larger than 10 cm), high mitotic rate, increased cellular atypia, or residual disease, adjuvant therapy is often administered. However, the additional benefit remains unclear, since the rarity of advanced-stage disease precludes prospective randomized controlled trials. Retrospective reviews have demonstrated an improvement in progression-free interval, but no improvement in survival.[54-56] Yet in the face of a known high probability of recurrence, some experts recommend adjuvant chemotherapy for these patients.

In the juvenile subtype, chemotherapy is reserved for those with stage II or greater disease, Stage IC with a high mitotic rate (more than 20 per 10 HPFs), or recurrent disease. Evidence is even more sparse in this group than the adult subtype, but chemotherapy may result in longer remission.[42,57]

Surveillance. Women with GCTs require lifetime surveillance owing to the potential for late recurrence of GCTs. At each patient visit we obtain a serum inhibin level and perform a pelvic examination. Granulosa cells produce inhibin, a substance normally secreted by granulosa cells in response to follicle-stimulating hormone during the luteal phase of the menstrual cycle. Inhibin is a heterodimeric polypeptide composed of alpha and beta subunits. The alpha and beta subunits are dimers; the alpha subunit dimers are identical, whereas the beta subunit dimers differ and are termed beta A and beta B. Inhibin is normally absent or undetectable in postmenopausal women, and after surgical excision of a GCT, inhibin levels become undetectable within 1 week. Inhibin remains a useful tool in surveillance for persistence or recurrence.[58-60] Assays exist for both inhibin A and B; however, inhibin B appears to be more sensitive.[58,61] Mucinous ovarian tumors may also produce inhibin. Thus, the molecule is not entirely specific to GCTs.

Other markers that potentially can be used include müllerian-inhibiting substance (MIS), estradiol, and CA-125. Granulosa cells secrete MIS in developing ovarian follicles, and MIS may be superior to inhibin in sensitivity.[62,63] However, MIS has not yet become routinely available in laboratory assays and has not been studied extensively. Since many GCTs secrete estradiol, this could be used as a marker if elevated preoperatively, but not all GCTs produce estradiol. CA-125 is a nonspecific marker that can be elevated in certain GCTs.

Recurrent Disease. Though classified as malignant, GCTs behave indolently and tend to recur later than other ovarian malignancies, thus requiring lifetime surveillance. Most recurrences occur within 4 to 6 years after surgery, but may recur even later. Hines and colleagues[64] documented the latest recorded recurrence at 37 years after surgery. The pelvis and abdomen are the most common sites of recurrence, and surgical resection is appropriate for localized recurrence. In recurrent tumors not amenable to surgical resection as further treatment, chemotherapy offers the best chance for remission. Unfortunately, most patients treated with chemotherapy do not experience long-lasting remission.[65,66] The BEP regimen has shown moderate success but also considerable toxicity. Gershenson and associates[66] documented an 83% response rate with a median survival time of 28 months in a study of nine patients. The GOG[65] also conducted research on the use of BEP in 56 patients with stage II-IV and recurrent sex cord-stromal tumors (48 of which were GCTs) and found a 37% rate of negative findings at the time of second-look laparotomy. Of the patients with advanced stage-disease, 69% were progression-free over 3 years, and 51% of patients with recurrence were progression-free. However, this regimen was associated with significant toxicity (two deaths attributed to bleomycin) and severe granulocytopenia.

Recently, taxanes, in combination with platinum-based agent, have gained attention as potential therapeutic options. Preliminary studies show that they have an efficacy comparable to that with BEP as well as a more favorable toxicity profile.[67–69] The GOG is currently conducting a phase II study of paclitaxel in recurrent ovarian stromal tumors. Less active but reasonable second-line agents include PVB[70] (cisplatin, vinblastine, bleomycin), CAP (cyclophosphamide, doxorubicin, and cisplatin),[71,72] doxorubicin alone,[73] and carboplatin plus etoposide.[74]

Hormonal therapy represents a new option for recurrent GCTs. Hormonal manipulation may play a role in gonadotropin and/or direct tumor suppression. Case reports have documented a prolonged response to tamoxifen and progesterone,[75] gonadotropin-releasing hormone antagonists,[76] and aromatase inhibitors.[77] Hormonal therapy may provide additional longevity in patients who have failed chemotherapy with a favorable side-effect profile.

Though not typically used in the setting of adjuvant therapy, radiation therapy has proved useful in treating recurrent GCTs. Wolf and associates[78] reviewed 14 patients with recurrent GCTs who received external-beam radiation therapy. Of the 14, 6 patients demonstrated a complete response, with 3 patients still living at 10 to 21 years after radiation therapy. Similarly, Savage and colleagues[79] found no improvement in outcomes with adjuvant radiation but found sustained remissions with recurrent disease.

Thecomas

Thecomas also originate from the ovarian stroma and occur primarily in postmenopausal women. They are benign solid masses that are consistently unilateral. Theca cells produce androstenedione, which undergoes conversion to estradiol, and is responsible for the hyperestrogenism. A tumor comprising solely theca cells would correspondingly produce a considerable amount of excess estrogen. Subsequently, most women present with postmenopausal bleeding from endometrial stimulation. Accordingly, the rate of synchronous endometrial adenocarcinoma is 25%.[59]

Thecomas may appear yellowish because of their lipid content. They consist mostly of theca cells, but may contain a few granulosa cells. Since thecomas are benign, treatment involves surgical excision only. In the case of premenopausal women, unilateral salpingo-oophorectomy is acceptable in the documented absence of endometrial hyperplasia or carcinoma. In postmenopausal women, total abdominal hysterectomy and bilateral salpingo-oophorectomy are recommended.

Fibromas

Similar to thecomas, fibromas are usually unilateral and benign and occur in post-menopausal women. Cellular-type fibromas may contain mild atypia and mitotic activity, but should not be confused with fibrosarcomas. Though not hormonally active, fibromas are interesting entities in their own right, since 10% to 15% of those affected present with ascites or Meigs syndrome, and 1% present with hydrothorax. Although the mechanism is not well understood, there is some evidence that vascular epithelial growth factor secreted by fibromas increases capillary permeability, thus contributing to fluid accumulation[80] and the resultant Meigs phenomenon. Pseudo-Meigs syndrome refers to the presence of ascites from a non–fibroma-type ovarian tumor. Treatment includes unilateral salpingo-oophorectomy, which is curative for both the fibroma and the associated Meigs syndrome.

Gorlin's syndrome, an autosomal dominant syndrome also known as nevoid basal cell carcinoma, has also been associated with fibromas. The syndrome results in medulloblastomas, mesenteric cysts, and odontogenic keratocysts. Approximately 75% of affected women develop fibromas, but this predisposition is not well understood.

Sertoli-Leydig Cell Tumors (Androblastomas)

Sertoli-Leydig cell tumors (SLCTs) are rare, accounting for 0.2% of all ovarian tumors. Unlike granulosa-stromal cell tumors, they occur principally in women in the reproductive years with 75% occurring before age 40 and occurring less commonly during menopause or childhood. Similar to theca cells, SLCTs are usually hormonally active and secrete testosterone, thus resulting in androgen excess and potential virilization.

Etiology

The cause of SLCTs remains largely unknown because they originate from the ovarian stromal sex cords but resemble the Sertoli and Leydig cells found in testes. Some hypothesize that they originate from residual undifferentiated sex cord tissue, from mesenchymal, coelomic, or mesonephric cells. More recently, developments point to lack of estrogen, which induces transformation of ovarian follicles into structures resembling seminiferous tubules and Sertoli cells found in the testis.[81] These, in turn, produce MIS and secrete testosterone.

Presentation

The testosterone production associated with SLCTs may cause menstrual disruption, most notably amenorrhea, as well as hirsutism and virilization. Aside from secretion of testosterone, pure Sertoli cell tumors may secrete estrogen or renin. Thus, some patients present with dysfunctional uterine bleeding or hypertension and hypokalemia. Pure Leydig cell tumors secrete only testosterone. However, most tumors are combination SLCTs, and 70% to 85% manifest as virilizing symptoms such as clitoromegaly secondary to androgen secretion (Fig. 11-5).

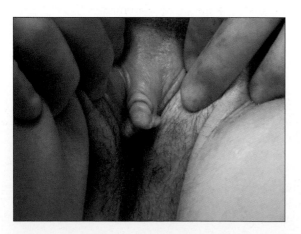

Figure 11-5. Clitoromegaly.

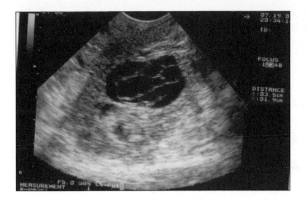

Figure 11-6. Vaginal ultrasound of Sertoli-Leydig tumor.

Diagnosis

In any women presenting with virilization, it is necessary to consider other etiologies including Cushing's syndrome, adrenal tumors, pituitary dysfunction, adrenal hyperplasia, or drug-induced hyperandrogenism. On physical examination, an adnexal mass may be detectable, in conjunction with symptoms associated with androgen excess. As in other ovarian tumors, ultrasound is used for diagnosis. Imaging typically reveals a well-circumscribed unilateral solid mass, or it may reveal a heterogeneously enlarged multicystic ovary (Fig. 11-6). Diagnosis relies on a combination of imaging and laboratory values, but it ultimately rests on surgery.

Pathology

Grossly, over 95% of SLCTs are unilateral and mostly solid, but some have cystic components (Fig. 11-7). They are tan, gray, or white, and their size correlates with the degree of differentiation and prognosis. Thus, larger tumors tend to be poorly differentiated and more aggressive. Well-differentiated tumors are usually 3 to 4 cm and contain retiform (arranged like a net) tissue lending a spongy texture. Poorly differentiated tumors are more likely to contain areas of hemorrhagic necrosis. The hallmark of these tumors is a tubular pattern surrounded by fibrous tissue.

Histologically, SLCTs are classified into five different types: well-differentiated, intermediate differentiation, poorly differentiated, retiform, and mixed with heterologous elements. Heterologous elements include other types of tissue, for example gastrointestinal or cartilaginous. Retiform components may contain hepatocytic differentiation, which results in AFP production. Histology generally determines prognosis.

Surgical Treatment

Definitive treatment for SLCTs is surgery with complete surgical staging. Over 90% of tumors are discovered in stage I, which lends itself to a good prognosis. Five-year survival rate is favorable, and ranges from 70% to 90%. In advanced stages, prognosis is poor and mortality rate approaches 100%. Young and Scully[82] reviewed 207 cases of Sertoli-Leydig tumors and found that none of the well-differentiated tumors, 11% of intermediately differentiated tumors, 59% of poorly differentiated tumors, and 19% of the tumors with heterologous elements behaved malignantly. Thus, differentiation plays a large part in prognosis.

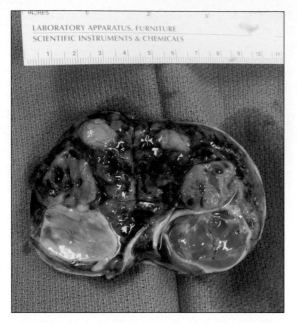

Figure 11-7. Sertoli-Leydig tumor.

Adjuvant Treatment

In the case of advanced disease or poorly differentiated SLCTs, adjuvant chemotherapy may provide benefit. BEP and PVB regimens have shown some response.[66] About 33% of these tumors recur, and accordingly, poorly differentiated tumors are more likely to do so.[83] Unlike GCTs, SLCTs tend to recur early—within 5 years—and sites of recurrence include the abdomen and pelvis.

Surveillance

Postoperatively, testosterone levels decline rapidly and may serve as a useful tumor marker. However, virilization in those with SLCTs may never resolve completely. As in GCTs, patients with SLCTs require lifetime surveillance. Imaging is generally utilized only when there is concern for recurrence by testosterone levels, patient symptoms, or physical examination findings.

Sex Cord Tumor with Annular Tubules

Sex cord tumors with annular tubules (SCTATs) were initially grouped with SLCTs, and some have proposed grouping them with GCTs. Correspondingly, these tumors possess characteristics of both, but they are recognized as a unique entity. Distinctive features include an association with Peutz-Jeghers syndrome in one third of cases, the potential to produce progesterone, and a higher penchant for lymph node metastasis than other sex cord-stromal tumors.[84]

Presentation

The presentation of SCTATs differs based on their association with Peutz-Jeghers syndrome (PJS). In those with Peutz-Jeghers syndrome, tumors are small, bilateral, calcified, and asymptomatic. Given their small size, they are typically not palpable on examination. In contrast, in non–Peutz-Jeghers-associated cases, the population is younger (20s), and tumors are larger, unilateral, and symptomatic.[85] They are hormonally active, often secreting estrogen and/or progesterone, which in a younger target population often presents as menstrual cycle disruptions or dysfunctional uterine bleeding.

Histology

SCTATs are thought of as a combination of granulosa cell and Sertoli-Leydig tumors. The annular (circular) tubules correspond to Sertoli cells, but contain false lumens. They also contain histologic elements consistent with GCTs, and they secrete estradiol. As in GCTs, estradiol is not a useful tumor marker, but inhibin may be useful for surveillance purposes. Progesterone levels also prove useful in the case of progesterone-producing tumors.

Treatment

The recommended treatment for SCTATs is surgical resection. In patients with Peutz-Jeghers syndrome, these tumors are uniformly benign; therefore, treatment consists of unilateral oophorectomy. An interesting association exists between Peutz-Jeghers-associated tumors and malignant adenoma of the cervix, which has been reported in up to 15% of cases.[85] Therefore, these patients require close surveillance with a low threshold for excisional biopsy, since cytology and colposcopy are often nondiagnostic. In non–Peutz-Jeghers–associated cases, tumors behave more aggressively. The risk of extraovarian spread and metastasis is roughly 20% at the time of initial surgery.[85,86] In a study of six patients with SCTATs, lymph node metastases occurred in two patients 7.5 and 10 years after surgery, but all patients were alive at a mean of 7.8 years.[87] Another review examined four patients, one of whom had metastasis to a supraclavicular lymph node, the liver, and the retroperitoneum.[88] Treatment still consists of surgery with complete staging. Adjuvant chemotherapy may offer some additional survival benefit. Typical regimens include BEP or a platinum/taxane combination, but experience is limited.

Gynandroblastomas

Gynandroblastomas are exceedingly rare. They are usually small and benign and occur at an average age of 30, but they may manifest at any age. They are considered a mix of granulosa cell and Sertoli-Leydig tumors, since histologically they consist of both. Average age of presentation is 30, and since gynandroblastomas are part GCT, they secrete estrogen. However, their remaining components may secrete other hormonally active agents, occasionally causing virilization.

Histology

Histologic criteria for diagnosis of gynandroblastomas include at least a 10% GCT component, and some component of well-differentiated or intermediate differentiated Sertoli-Leydig tumor. The remaining elements consist of ovarian tissue and/or heterologous tissue.

Treatment

Gynandroblastomas are consistently benign, and almost all are diagnosed at an early stage. Treatment consists of surgery, and unilateral salpingo-oophorectomy is sufficient. One case of a recurrence was recently reported.[89] These tumors occur so rarely that current available literature supports only conservative surgical management.

Germ Cell Tumors

Malignant ovarian germ cell tumors are a rare, heterogeneous group that account for approximately 1% to 2% of the 21,000 new cases of ovarian cancer each year.[90] Germ cell tumors (benign and malignant) account for 20% to 25% of all ovarian neoplasms and 58% of tumors in women under age 20. As the name implies, these tumors arise from the primordial germ cells of the ovary and thus share characteristics with malignant germ cell tumors of the testis. In fact, given that ovarian germ cell tumors occur at about one tenth the rate of testicular tumors, many of the advances in therapy, particularly in chemotherapy regimens, were first studied in male patients, and then extrapolated to women.[91] Another characteristic of germ cell tumors is the possibility of primary extragonadal tumors whose location (e.g., retroperitoneal or mediastinal) corresponds to the track taken by germ cells during embryonic development.[92]

Histology

Ovarian germ cell tumors comprise a number of different histologic types (Table 11-5). In terms of incidence, dysgerminomas are the most common malignant ovarian germ cell tumors (Fig. 11-8), followed by immature teratomas (Fig. 11-9) and endodermal sinus tumors (Fig. 11-10), although mixed varieties containing disparate tumor components also exist. Other histologic types such as embryonal carcinomas, nongestational choriocarcinomas, struma ovarii, and so on, are more rare. Surveillance, Epidemiology and End Results (SEER) Program data from 1973 to 2002 identified 1262 cases of ovarian germ cell tumors: 414 (32.8%) dysgerminomas, 449 (35.6%) immature teratomas, and 362 (28.7%) mixed histologies.[93] For simplicity, these tumors may be divided into two broad categories: dysgerminomas (the counterpart to the male seminoma) and nondysgerminomas.[94]

Table 11-5. Histologic Classification Scheme of Ovarian Germ Cell Tumors

I. Primitive germ cell tumors
   A. Dysgerminoma
   B. Endodermal sinus tumor (yolk sac tumor)
   C. Embryonal carcinoma
   D. Polyembryoma
   E. Nongestational choriocarcinomas
   F. Mixed germ cell tumor

II. Biphasic or triphasic teratoma
   A. Immature teratoma
   B. Mature teratoma
      1. Solid
      2. Cystic
         a. Dermoid cyst
         b. Fetiform teratoma (homunculus)

III. Monodermal teratoma and somatic-type tumors associated with group II (above)
   A. Thyroid (struma ovarii)
   B. Carcinoid
   C. Neuroectodermal
   D. Carcinoma
   E. Melanocytic
   F. Sarcoma
   G. Sebaceous
   H. Pituitary type
   I. Others

Adapted from World Health Organization classification of tumors.

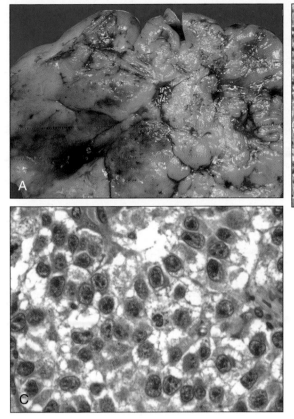

Figure 11-8. A, Gross picture of dysgerminoma. **B,** Micrograph of dysgerminoma. **C,** High-power micrograph of dysgerminoma. (Courtesy of Dr. Kristen Atkins, Department of Pathology, University of Virginia Health System.)

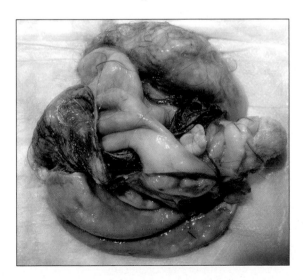

Figure 11-9. Gross picture of cystic teratoma. (Courtesy of Dr. Kristen Atkins, Department of Pathology, University of Virginia Health System.)

Grossly, dysgerminomas are fleshy, solid tumors that have a gray-white appearance. At histologic examination, they are composed of sheets of vesicular cells separated by fibrous stroma.[95] Immature teratomas are generally bulky tumors with a smooth surface. Microscopically, they are characterized by areas of necrosis and hemorrhage. As in their benign counterparts, bone, cartilage, hair and sebaceous

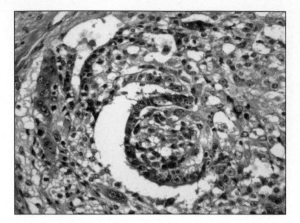

Figure 11-10. Endodermal sinus tumor demonstrating characteristic Schiller-Duval body. Present in nearly 50% of endodermal sinus tumors, Schiller-Duval bodies are pathognomonic for this tumor and are said to resemble a glomerulus (H&E, ×400). (Courtesy of Dr. Kristen Atkins, Department of Pathology, University of Virginia Health System.)

Table 11-6. Differential Expression of Tumor Markers in Malignant Ovarian Germ Cell Tumors

	Tumor Marker		
Tumor	**AFP**	**β-hCG**	**LDH**
Dysgerminoma	Usually normal	Usually normal	**Elevated**
Immature teratoma	Usually normal	Usually normal	—
Endodermal sinus tumor	**Elevated**	Normal	—
Embryonal carcinoma	**Elevated**	**Elevated**	—
Nongestational choriocarcinoma	Normal	**Elevated**	—

material may be present. The immature components are typically glandular, bone, muscle or nervous tissue.[95] Endodermal sinus tumors (yolk sac tumors) have pathognomonic structures that resemble a renal glomerulus, the Schiller-Duval body (see Fig. 11-10).

Based on the underlying histologic makeup of the germ cell tumor, specific blood proteins (tumor markers) may be elevated (Table 11-6). Classically, dysgerminomas and pure immature teratomas have no specific tumor markers, but dysgerminomas may have an elevated lactate dehydrogenase. Endodermal sinus tumors usually have an elevated AFP, which may correlate with disease burden, but a normal β-human chorionic gonadotropin (β-hCG). Choriorcarcinomas have the opposite picture with an elevated β-hCG and a normal AFP. Embryonal carcinomas usually have elevations in both AFP and β-hCG. Tumors of mixed histology may have elevations in some or all of these tumor markers, depending on the cell types present.

Clinical Characteristics

The peak incidence of ovarian germ cell tumors is between ages 15 and 19 years, and one third of these tumors are malignant.[90] Ovarian germ cell tumors are generally rapid-growing and thus nearly 85% of patients present with abdominal and pelvic pain/pressure and a palpable mass.[94,96] Rupture, hemorrhage, and torsion are often seen and can mimic the picture of acute appendicitis. A few patients may present with signs of precocious puberty as a result of the production of hormones such as β-hCG and estrogen.[93,94] Given that the peak incidence of ovarian germ cell tumors is in the reproductive years, they are often seen in the setting of pregnancy. In one study including over 9000 adnexal masses found during pregnancy, 44% of the 81 cancers were germ cell tumors; of these, dysgerminoma (41%) was the most common histology.[97]

Seventy percent of patients present with International Federation of Gynecology and Obstetrics (FIGO) stage I-II disease, with the bulk of the remaining 30% representing stage III tumors.[98] Most tumors are unilateral with the notable exception of dysgerminomas, which are reported to be bilateral in 10% to 15% of cases. Nevertheless, one series of 26 cases over 15 years noted a 23% rate of bilateral involvement.[98] Despite this, bilaterality does not necessarily equate with malignancy, since benign cystic teratomas of the contralateral ovary are also seen in 5% to 10% of cases.[94]

Diagnosis

The diagnostic workup of ovarian germ cell tumors begins with a comprehensive history and physical examination. Particular attention should be paid to the presence or absence of menstruation and secondary sex characteristics, since malignant germ cell tumors can arise in the setting of dysgenetic gonads. Thus, a preoperative karyotype is especially important and indicated for premenarchal girls.[92] Additional baseline evaluation for all patients should include: blood studies, liver function testing, serum tumor markers (see Table 11-6), and appropriate imaging such as a pelvic ultrasound. Dysgerminomas are classically solid tumors with areas of hemorrhage, and they thus appear as solid masses on ultrasound. Teratomas and endodermal sinus tumors are more complex in appearance with cystic and solid components. For these tumors, a chest x-ray is needed during the diagnostic evaluation, since they often metastasize to the lungs and/or mediastinum. Computed tomography or magnetic resonance imaging constitutes an acceptable alternative.

Prognosis

Prognostic indicators in ovarian germ cell tumors have yet to be formalized into a scoring system such as that used in testicular tumors.[99] However, several studies have demonstrated that FIGO stage, elevated tumor markers, nondysgerminoma or immature teratoma histology, sarcomatous elements, and lymph node involvement all are associated with poor outcomes.[100–103]

In a review of 113 patients with ovarian germ cell tumors, Murugaesu and associates[101] found that when both AFP and β-hCG are elevated, there is a dramatic decrease in overall survival: One-year survival for patients with normal tumor markers was 89.6% compared with 50.4% for those who had elevations of both. Despite accruing 113 patients, the authors noted that this study was not sufficiently powered to establish threshold values for either AFP or β-hCG. Lai and associates,[103] in a review of 93 patients, demonstrated that patients with dysgerminoma or immature teratoma histology had a 100% 5-year survival rate compared with 83.3% for those with other histologies. This confirms prior observations that patients with endodermal sinus or choriocarcinomas have a worse prognosis. Malagon and associates[100] reviewed 46 cases of germ cell tumors in which sarcomatous elements were found (e.g., embryonal rhabdomyosarcoma, angiosarcoma, and leiomyosarcoma) and compared them with historical controls matched for age and stage of disease who lacked these elements. They found that patients who lack sarcomatous components were more likely to show no evidence of disease after therapy than those with these elements.

More recently, Kumar and colleagues,[102] in a review of SEER data, found that lymph node metastasis was associated with an almost threefold risk of death (HR 2.87, 95% CI 1.44–5.73), regardless of age, stage, grade, and histology. In addition, the data demonstrate a possible survival benefit of lymphadenectomy, since patients who received a lymph node dissection had a 5-year survival rate of 94% compared with 89% in those who had no lymph nodes removed. Of note, increasing grade of the tumor was associated with lymph node metastasis, but this was not statistically significant. However, O'Connor and colleagues[104] demonstrated that tumor grade is the most important prognostic indicator of overall survival in the setting of immature teratomas. Finally, whereas age has not been shown to be an independent predictor of outcome in ovarian germ cell tumors, a Pediatric Intergroup Study of 109 girls with primary extragonadal germ cell tumors demonstrated a significant decrease in overall survival for girls 12 years old or older at diagnosis.[105]

Surgical Management

The initial management of ovarian germ cell tumors is surgical, with fertility-sparing surgery being preferred, given the young age of the majority who present with these tumors. One contraindication to a fertility-sparing procedure would be the case of dysgenetic gonads, further emphasizing the importance of a comprehensive preoperative evaluation. In the absence of dysgenetic gonads, the outcomes of patients who received fertility-sparing surgery are comparable to those who received complete removal of both ovaries, regardless of stage or disease burden.[97,106]

The principles of cytoreductive surgery in epithelial ovarian cancer have been applied to the initial treatment of ovarian germ cell tumors. This is based on the findings of GOG protocols that have demonstrated at least some benefit to surgical debulking.[107,108] Thus, the current management schema includes peritoneal washings, removal of the affected ovary, bilateral pelvic and para-aortic lymphadenectomy, omentectomy, and careful inspection of all peritoneal surfaces with excision of any suspicious lesions or systematic peritoneal biopsies in the absence of visible lesions[94] (Fig. 11-11). Even so, given the high sensitivity of ovarian germ cell tumors to chemotherapy, significant tumor debulking is advised only if it can be accomplished without increasing morbidity or delaying the initiation of chemotherapy.[91] These recommendations hold regardless of histology, although some authors have suggested that lymphadenectomy is not necessary in the setting of immature teratomas, given their propensity for peritoneal spread (rather than nodal spread), or in the setting of

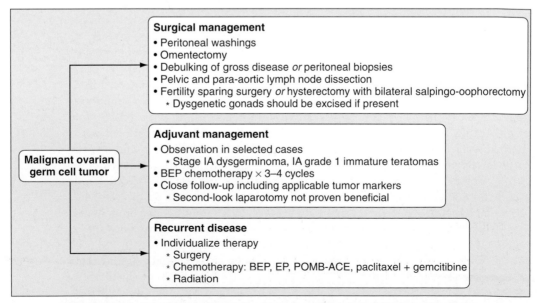

Figure 11-11. Proposed management schema for malignant ovarian germ cell tumors.

endodermal sinus tumors for which chemotherapy is recommended regardless of nodal status.[92]

Adjuvant Treatment

Adjuvant therapy decisions are based on stage, histology, and grade of the tumor. For example, stage IA dysgerminomas and stage IA, grade 1 immature teratomas can be observed without the need for further therapy.[47] Currently, it is recommended that those with all other stages and grades (regardless of histology) should receive adjuvant chemotherapy.

For dysgerminomas, adjuvant therapy has consisted of radiation therapy or chemotherapy. Before the advent of platinum-based chemotherapy, dysgerminomas were successfully managed with external-beam radiation therapy, with the major side effect being nearly universal ovarian failure, despite attempts at surgically displacing the ovaries.[94] Given the success of platinum-based chemotherapy, and the observation that most patients demonstrate normal ovarian function after treatment, chemotherapy has essentially replaced radiation in the setting of adjuvant treatment for dysgerminomas.[93]

Modern chemotherapy for malignant germ cell tumors of the ovary incorporates BEP. In the 1970s, initial chemotherapy experience in ovarian germ cell tumors came from the GOG, which demonstrated the value of combination chemotherapy with vincristine, dactinomycin and cyclophosphamide (VAC),[107] followed later by cisplatin, vinblastine and bleomycin (PVB), which proved superior.[109] BEP had been shown to be superior in testicular tumors, and its activity in ovarian germ cell tumors was evaluated in GOG 90, which demonstrated that BEP was superior to PVB in this setting.[110] The importance of bleomycin as a component of BEP was proved later in an Eastern Cooperative Oncology Group (ECOG) trial, in which patients treated with BEP had an overall survival rate of 95% compared with 86% for patients treated with etoposide and cisplatin alone.[111]

Reflecting on data collected in testicular cancer trials, the optimal number of cycles of chemotherapy with BEP is not predetermined but can be altered by the clinical picture of the patient. One trial, which compared three cycles with four cycles of BEP in patients with low-risk testicular cancer, found that the outcomes were generally similar.[112] The advantage of one less cycle of chemotherapy is a reduction of early and late side effects of therapy, not the least of which are the pulmonary toxicity associated with bleomycin and the potential late onset of treatment-related leukemias. Studies looking at treatment of favorable (i.e., surgically staged, little to no residual disease) ovarian germ cell tumors have also reported good outcomes with three cycles of BEP.[113] However, patients with bulky residual disease should receive four cycles of chemotherapy because no other regimen to date has proved superior.[91]

Increasingly, surgery has been advocated as the sole primary therapy for selected cases of germ cell tumors. In a prospective, single-institution study, Bonazzi and associates[114] followed up 32 patients with pure ovarian immature teratomas, all stages I-II, grades 1-2. In this series, 22 were treated with surgery alone. There were two recurrences, both salvaged with chemotherapy. Marina and colleagues[115] reviewed 50 patients with pure immature teratomas, 23 of whom had malignant foci (grades 1-3) and were treated with surgical excision alone. There were four recurrences in this group, and all were salvaged by chemotherapy. Dark and associates[116] recently updated their experience with surgery followed by close observation, with chemotherapy reserved for recurrent disease. Briefly, the original study examined a surveillance policy that followed surgical excision in 24 patients with malignant ovarian germ cell tumors stage IA, including nine dysgerminomas, nine immature teratomas, and six endodermal sinus tumors. Seven of eight recurrences were salvaged with chemotherapy, and the only death was due to pulmonary embolism while undergoing treatment. In the updated dataset, the relapse rate was 22% for dysgerminomas and 36% for nondysgerminomas. Ten of 11 recurrences were successfully salvaged; one death was due to chemoresistant disease. All recurrences were noted within 13 months of initial surgery, and the overall disease-specific survival rate was 94%.[117] Results such as these from single-institution studies have prompted the Children's Oncology Group to study surgical excision alone in stage I tumors. The data are forthcoming.

Surveillance

Once therapy is completed, the method of surveillance is based on the clinical and histologic characteristics of the primary tumor. For example, dysgerminomas and pure immature teratomas often have low or normal tumor markers at diagnosis and thus can be followed up only with a combination of interval history, physical examination, and imaging as clinically indicated. In contrast, endodermal sinus tumors (with their characteristically elevated AFP) have a sensitive, reproducible marker of persistent or recurrent disease. In the setting of mixed tumors, surveillance can be individualized when one or more tumor markers were elevated before therapy and have responded as expected to definitive management.

In general, follow-up should be at regular intervals for at least 2 years, since 75% of recurrences occur within the first year after completion of therapy.[92] Although no recommendations for contraception have been formalized, it is reasonable to delay pregnancy (if possible) during the first year of follow-up if tumor markers are being used for disease surveillance.

Second-look laparotomy has not been shown to improve outcomes for patients with dysgerminomas or early-stage immature teratomas.[98,108] However, some have suggested that in the setting of advanced-stage immature teratomas, second-look laparotomy may be of benefit since these tumors have no reliable tumor markers.[92] There have been no studies comparing post-therapy imaging as a replacement for second-look surgery in this setting.

Outcomes

Because most tumors are early stage at diagnosis—and even advanced tumors are exquisitely sensitive to chemotherapy—those with malignant ovarian germ cell tumors generally have an excellent prognosis.[98,118] Several retrospective studies have demonstrated that with current platinum-based chemotherapy, 5-year survival rates are 95% to 97%, keeping in mind that the majority of patients are stage I at diagnosis.[108,119] Even in disseminated cancer, Lai and associates[103] noted an 88% 5-year survival rate for stage III-IV disease.

Recurrent disease may be managed with chemotherapy, radiation therapy, surgery, or some combination of therapeutic modalities. If the patient was only under surveillance after surgery, chemotherapy with BEP is indicated. In the setting of persistence or recurrence after chemotherapy with BEP, options include radiation therapy, high-dose chemotherapy with etoposide, cisplatin, and bone marrow transplantation, or the POMB-ACE regimen (cisplatin, vincristine, methotrexate, bleomycin, dactinomycin, cyclophosphamide, and etoposide).[92] Recently, a phase II study of paclitaxel and gemcitabine as salvage therapy in the setting of heavily pretreated, recurrent germ cell tumors demonstrated a 31% objective response (12.5% durable complete response).[120]

The focus of long-term follow-up in addition to surveillance for disease recurrence has been concerned with the late effects of chemotherapy: infertility and risk of secondary malignancy. Many published retrospective reviews have demonstrated a favorable outcome with regard to return of ovarian function (i.e., return of menstruation and ability to conceive) following combination chemotherapy.[121-125] In one study, 61.7% of women who were menarchal before cheomotherapy developed amenorrhea while receiving treatment.[122] Return of menses after therapy has been estimated to be between 91.5% and 100%.[121,122,125]

Fertility outcomes after chemotherapy are not as clearly estimated, since it is not always known how many women have actually attempted conception after therapy. One study that collected this information noted that of 38 women who attempted conception, 29 (76%) were successful.[123] In addition, a more recent study noted a similar success rate (75%) among women attempting pregnancy.[124] The long-term cancer risk of combination chemotherapy seems to be related to the use of alkylating agents such as etoposide and is dose-related. One study of 616 children who received alkylating agents for treatment of germ cell tumors found that the 10-year incidence of treatment-related acute leukemias was 1% for children who received chemotherapy alone and 4.2% for those who received combination chemotherapy and radiation therapy.[126] The apparent threshold dose of etoposide is 2000 mg/m^2, with patients who received more than this amount having a risk of leukemia approaching that seen in patients with both chemotherapy and radiation.[92]

References

1. Gershenson DM: Clinical management of potential tumors of low malignancy. Best Pract Res Clin Obstet Gynaecol 16:513–527, 2002.
2. Skirnisdottir I, Garmo H, Wilander E, et al: Borderline ovarian tumors in Sweden 1960–2005: trends in incidence and age at diagnosis. Int J Cancer 15:123(8):1897–1901, 2008.
3. Lu KH, Bell DA: Borderline ovarian tumors. In Gershenson DM, McGuire WP, Gore M, et al (eds): Gynecologic Cancer: Controversies in Management. Philadelphia: Elsevier, 2004, pp 519–526.
4. Harlow BL, Weiss NS, Lofton S: Epidemiology of borderline ovarian tumors. J Natl Cancer Inst 78:71–74, 1987.
5. Silverberg SG, Bell DA, Kurman RJ, et al: Borderline ovarian tumors: key points and workshop summary. Hum Pathol 35:910–917, 2004.
6. Jones MB: Borderline ovarian tumors: current concepts for prognostic factors and clinical management. Clin Obstet Gynecol 49:517–525, 2006.
7. Gershenson DM: Is micropapillary serous carcinoma for real? Cancer 95:677–680, 2002.
8. Bell DA, Weinstock MA, Scully RE: Peritoneal implants of ovarian serous borderline tumors: histologic features and prognosis. Cancer 62:2212–2222, 1988.
9. Russell P: Borderline epithelial tumours of the ovary: a conceptual dilemma. Clin Obstet Gynecol 11:259–277, 1984.
10. Michael H, Roth LM: Invasive and noninvasive implants in ovarian serous tumors of low malignant potential. Cancer 57:1240–1247, 1986.
11. Gershenson DM, Silva EG, Tortolero-Luna G, et al: Ovarian serous borderline tumors with noninvasive peritoneal implants. Cancer 83:2157–2163, 1998.
12. Gershenson DM, Silva EG, Levy L, et al: Ovarian serous borderline tumors with invasive peritoneal implants. Cancer 82:1096–1103, 1998.
13. Buttin BM, Herzog TJ, Powell MA, et al: Epithelial ovarian tumors of low malignant potential: the role of microinvasion. Obstet Gynecol 99:11–17, 2002.
14. Hogg R, Scurry J, Kim SN, et al: Microinvasion links serous borderline tumor and grade 1 invasive carcinoma. Gynecol Oncol 106:44–51, 2007.
15. Crispens MA, Bodurka D, Deavers M, et al: Response and survival in patients with progressive or recurrent serous ovarian tumors of low malignant potential. Obstet Gynecol 99:3–10, 2002.
16. Longacre TA, McKenney JK, Tazelaar HD, et al: Ovarian serous tumors of low malignant potential (borderline tumors): outcome-based study of 276 patients with long-term (− 5 years) follow-up. Am J Surg Pathol 29:707–723, 2005.
17. Ren J, Peng Z, Yang B: A clinicopathologic multivariate analysis affecting recurrence of borderline ovarian tumors. Gynecol Oncol 110:162–167, 2008.
18. Seidman JD, Kurman RJ: Treatment of micropapillary serous ovarian carcinoma (the aggressive variant of serous borderline tumors). Cancer 95:675–676, 2002.
19. Bristow RE, Gossett DR, Shook DR, et al: Micropapillary serous ovarian carcinoma: surgical management and clinical outcome. Gynecol Oncol 86:163–170, 2002.
20. Eichhorn JH, Bell DA, Young RH, et al: Ovarian serous borderline tumors with micropapillary and cribiform patterns: a study of 40 cases and comparison with 44 cases without these patterns. Am J Surg Pathol 23:397–409, 1999.
21. Boran N, Cil AP, Tulunay G, et al: Fertility and recurrence results of conservative surgery for borderline ovarian tumors. Gynecol Oncol 97:845–851, 2005.
22. But I: Serum Ca-125 level as a reflection of proliferative activity of serous borderline ovarian tumor. Int J Gynecol Obstet 71:289–291, 2000.
23. Gotleib WH, Soriano D, Achiron R, et al: Ca-125 measurement and ultrasonography in borderline tumors of the ovary. Am J Obstet Gynecol 183:541–546, 2000.
24. Rice LW, Lage JM, Berkowitz RS, et al: Preoperative Ca-125 levels in borderline tumors of the ovary. Gynecol Oncol 46(2):226–229, 1992.
25. Engelen MJA, de Bruijn HWA, Hollema H, et al: Serum CA-125, cardinoembryonic antigen, and CA19-9 as tumor markers in borderline ovarian tumors. Gynecol Oncol 78:16–20, 2000.
26. Tamakoshi K, Kikkawa F, Shibata K, et al: Clinical value of Ca-125, Ca-19-9, CEA, CaA 72-4 and TPA in borderline ovarian tumor. Gynecol Oncol 62:67–72, 1996.

27. Geomini P, Bremer G, Kruitwagen R, et al: Diagnostic accuracy of frozen section diagnosis of the adnexal mass: a metaanalysis. Gynecol Oncol 96:1–9, 2005.

28. Tempfer CB, Polterauer S. Bentz EK, et al: Accuracy of intra-operative frozen section analysis in borderline tumors of the ovary: a retrospective analysis of 96 cases and review of the literature. Gynecol Oncol 107:248–252, 2007.

29. Morris RT, Gershenson DM, Silva EG, et al: Outcome and reproductive function after conservative surgery for borderline ovarian tumors. Obstet Gynecol 95:541–547, 2000.

30. Suh-Burgmann E: Long-term outcomes following conservative surgery for borderline tumor of the ovary: a large population based study. Gynecol Oncol 103:841–847, 2006.

31. Boran N, Cil AP, Tulunay G, et al: Fertility and recurrence rates of conservative surgery for borderline ovarian tumors. Gynecol Oncol 97:845–851, 2005.

32. Poncelet C, Fauvet R, Boccara J, et al: Recurrence after cystectomy for borderline ovarian tumors: results of a French multicenter study. Ann Surg Oncol 13:565–571, 2006.

33. Winter WE, III, Kucera PR, Rodgers W, et al: Surgical staging in patients with ovarian tumors of low malignant potential. Obstet Gynecol 100:671–676, 2002.

34. Fauvet R, Boccara J, Dufournet C, et al: Restaging surgery for women with borderline ovarian tumors: results of a French multicenter study. Cancer 100:1145, 2004.

35. Barnhill DR, Kurman RJ, Brady MD, et al: Preliminary analysis of the behavior of stage I ovarian tumors of low malignant potential: a Gynecologic Oncology Group Study. J Clin Oncol 13:2752–2756, 1995.

36. Barakat RR, Benjamin I, Lewis JL, Jr, et al: Platinum-based chemotherapy for advanced-stage serous ovarian carcinoma of low malignant potential. Gynecol Oncol 59:390–393, 1995.

37. Sutton GP, Bundy BN, Omura GA, et al: Stage III ovarian tumors of low malignant potential treated with cisplatin combination therapy (a Gynecologic Oncology Group Study). Gynecol Oncol 41:230–233, 1991.

38. Bristow RE, Gossett DR, Shook DR, et al: Recurrent micropapillary serous ovarian carcinoma: the role of secondary cytoreductive surgery. Cancer 95:791–800, 2002.

39. Scully R, Sobin, L: Histological Typing of Ovarian Tumours, vol. 9. New York: Springer Berlin, 1999. Copyright 1999 World Health Organization.

40. Evans AT, III, Gaffey TA, Malkasian GD, Jr, et al: Clinicopathologic review of 118 granulosa cell and 82 theca cell tumors. Obstet Gynecol 55:231, 1980.

41. Schumer ST, Cannistra SA: Granulosa cell tumor of the ovary. J Clin Oncol 21:1180–1189, 2003.

42. Young RH, Dickerson GR, Scully RE: Juvenile granulosa cell tumor of the ovary: a clinicopathologic analysis of 125 cases. Am J Surg Pathol 8:575–596, 1984.

43. Rodgers RJ, Irving-Rodgers HF, van Wezel IL, et al: Dynamics of the membrane granulosa during expansion of the ovarian follicular antrum. Mol Cell Endocrinol 172:41–48, 2001.

44. Fox H, Agrawal K, Langley FA: A clinicopathologic study of 92 cases of granulosa cell tumor of the ovary with special reference to the factors influencing prognosis. Cancer 35:231–241, 1975.

45. Stenwig JT, Hazekamp JT, Beecham JB: Granulosa cell tumors of the ovary. A clinicopathological study of 118 cases with long-term follow-up. Gynecol Oncol 7:136–152, 1979.

46. McCluggage WG: Recent advances in immunohistochemistry in the diagnosis of ovarian neoplasms. J Clin Pathol 53:327–334, 2000.

47. Gershenson DM: Management of early ovarian cancer: germ cell and sex cord-stromal tumors. Gynecol Oncol 55: S62, 1994.

48. Zhang M, Cheung MK, Shin JY, et al: Prognostic factors responsible for survival in sex cord stromal tumors of the ovary—an analysis of 376 women. Gynecol Oncol 104:396–400, 2007.

49. Gusberg SB, Kardon P: Proliferative endometrial response to theca-granulosa cell tumors. Am J Obstet Gynecol 111:633–643, 1971.

50. Miller BE, Barron BA, Wan JY, et al: Prognostic factors in adult granulosa cell tumor of the ovary. Cancer 79:1951–1955, 1997.

51. Bjorkholm E, Silfversward C: Prognostic factors in granulosa-cell tumors. Gynecol Oncol 11:261–274, 1981.

52. Malmstrom H, Hogberg T, Risberg B, et al: Granulosa cell tumor of the ovary: prognostic factors and outcome. Gynecol Oncol 52:50–55, 1994.

53. Schneider DT, Calaminus G, Wessalowski R, et al: Ovarian sex cord stromal tumors in children and adolescents. J Clin Oncol 21:2357–2363, 2003.

54. Al-Badawi IA, Brashner PM, Ghatage P, et al: Postoperative chemotherapy in advanced ovarian granulosa cell tumors. Int J Gynecol Cancer 12:119–123, 2002.

55. Chan JK, Zhang M, Khaleb V, et al: Prognostic factors responsible for survival in sex cord stromal tumors of the ovary-a multivariate analysis. Gynecol Oncol 96:204–209, 2005.

56. Zanagnolo V, Pasinetti B, Sartori E: Clinical review of 63 cases of sex cord stromal tumors. Eur J Gynaecol Oncol 25:431–438, 2004.

57. Calaminus G, Wessalowski R, Harms D, et al: Juvenile granulosa cell tumors of the ovary in children and adolescents: results from 33 patients registered in a prospective cooperative study. Gynecol Oncol 65:447–452, 1997.

58. Lapphon RE, Burger HG, Bouma J, et al: Inhibin as a marker for granulosa-cell tumors. N Engl J Med 321:790–793, 1989.

59. Jobling T, Mamers P, Healy DL, et al: A prospective study of inhibin in granulosa cell tumors of the ovary. Gynecol Oncol 55:285–289, 1984.

60. Boggess JF, Soules MR, Goff BA, et al: Serum inhibin and disease status in women with ovarian granulosa cell tumors. Gynecol Oncol 64:64–69, 1997.

61. Mom CH, Engelen MJ, Willemse PH, et al: Granulosa cell tumors of the ovary: the clinical value of serum inhibin A and B levels in a large single center cohort. Gynecol Oncol 105:365–372, 2007.

62. Rey RA, Lhomme C, Marcillac I, et al: Antimullerian hormone as a serum marker of granulosa cell tumors of the ovary: comparative study with serum alpha inhibin and estradiol. Am J Obstet Gynecol 174:958–965, 1996.

63. Lane AH, Lee MM, Fuller AF, et al: Diagnostic utility of mullerian inhibiting substance determination in patients with primary and recurrent granulosa cell tumors. Gynecol Oncol 73:51–55, 1999.

64. Hines JF, Khalifa MA, Moore JL, et al: Recurrent granulosa cell tumor of the ovary 37 years after initial diagnosis: a case report and review of the literature. Gynecol Oncol 60:484–488, 1996.

65. Homesley HD, Bundy BN, Hurteau JL, et al: Bleomycin, etoposide, and cisplatin combination therapy of granulosa cell tumors and other stromal cell malignancies: a Gynecologic Oncology Group study. Gynecol Oncol 72:131–137, 1999.

66. Gershenson DM, Morris M, Burke TW, et al: Treatment of poor-prognosis sex cord-stromal tumors of the ovary with the combination of bleomycin, etoposide, and cisplatin. Obstet Gynecol 87:527–531, 1996.

67. Brown J, Shvartsman HS, Deavers MT, et al: The activity of taxanes in the treatment of sex cord-stromal ovarian tumors. J Clin Oncol 22:3517–3523, 2004.

68. Brown J, Shvartsman HS, Deavers MT, et al: The activity of taxanes compared with bleomycin, etoposide, and cisplatin in the treatment of sex cord-stromal ovarian tumors. Gynecol Oncol 97:489–496, 2005.

69. Chiara S, Merlini L, Campora E, et al: Cisplatinum-based chemotherapy in recurrent or high-risk ovarian granulosa cell tumor patients. Europ J Gynaecol Oncol 14:314–317, 1993.

70. Zambetti M, Escobedo A, Pilotti S, et al: Cisplatinum/vinblastine/bleomycin combination chemotherapy in advanced or recurrent granulosa cell tumors of the ovary. Gynecol Oncol 36:317–320, 1990.

71. Gershenson DM, Copeland LJ, Kavanaugh JJ, et al: Treatment of metastatic stromal tumors of the ovary with cisplatin, doxorubicin, and cyclophosphamide. Obstet Gynecol 70:765–769, 1987.

72. Muntz HG, Goff BA, Fuller AF: Recurrent ovarian granulosa cell tumor: role of combination chemotherapy with a report of a long-term response to a cyclophosphamide, doxorubicin, and cisplatin regimen. Eur J Gynaecol Oncol 11:263–268, 1990.

73. Disaia P, Saltz A, Kagan AR, et al: A temporary response of recurrent granulosa cell tumor to adriamycin. Obstet Gynecol 52:355–358, 1978.

74. Powell JL, Otis CN: Management of advanced juvenile granulosa cell tumor of the ovary. Gynecol Oncol 64:282–284, 1997.

75. Hardy R, Bell J, Nicely C, et al: Hormonal treatment of a recurrent granulosa cell tumor of the ovary: case report and review of the literature. Gynecol Oncol 96:865–869, 2005.

76. Fishman AP, Kudelka, Tresukosol D, et al: Leuprolide acetate for treating refractory or persistent ovarian granulosa cell tumor. J Reprod Med 41:393–396, 1996.
77. Freeman S, Modesitt S: Anastrozole therapy in recurrent ovarian adult granulosa cell tumors: a report of 2 cases. Gynecol Oncol 103:755–758, 2006.
78. Wolf JK, Mullen J, Eifel PJ, et al: Radiation treatment of advanced or recurrent granulosa cell tumors of the ovary. Gynecol Oncol 73:35–41, 1999.
79. Savage P, Constenla D, Fisher C, et al: Granulosa cell tumors of the ovary: demographics, survival, and management of advanced disease. J Clin Oncol 10:242–245, 1998.
80. Ishiko O, Yoshida H, Sumi T, et al: Vascular endothelial growth factor levels in pleural and peritoneal fluid in Meigs syndrome. Eur J Obstet Gynecol Reprod Biol 98:129–130, 2001.
81. Britt KL, Findlay JK: Regulation of the phenotype of ovarian somatic cells by estrogen. Mol Cell Endocrinol 202:11–17, 2003.
82. Young RH, Scully RE: Ovarian Sertoli-Leydig cell tumors: a clinicopathologic analysis of 207 cases. Am J Surg Pathol 9:543–569, 1985.
83. Latthe P, Shafi MI, Rollason TP: Recurrence of Sertoli-Leydig cell tumor in contralateral ovary. Case report and review of the literature. Eur J Gynaecol Oncol 21:62–63, 2000.
84. Young RH: Sex cord stromal tumors of the ovaries and testis: their similarities and differences with consideration of selected problems. Mod Pathol 18:S81, 2005.
85. Young RH, Welch RH, Dickerson GR, et al: Ovarian sex cord tumor with annular tubules: review of 74 cases including 27 with Peutz-Jeghers syndrome and four with adenoma malignum. Cancer 50:1384–1402, 1982.
86. Puls LE, Hamous J, Morrow MS, et al: Recurrent ovarian sex cord tumor with annular tubules: tumor marker and chemotherapy experience. Gynecol Oncol 54:396–401, 1994.
87. Hart WR, Kumar N, Crissman JD: Ovarian neoplasms resembling sex cord tumors with annular tubules. Cancer 45:2352–2563, 1980.
88. Ahn GH, Chi JG, Lee SK: Ovarian sex cord tumor with annular tubules. Cancer 57:1066–1073, 1986.
89. Chikvula M, Hunt J, Carter G, et al: Recurrent gynandroblastoma of ovary–a case report: a molecular and immunohistochemical analysis. Int J Gynecol Pathol 26:30–33, 2007.
90. Quirk JT, Natarajan N, Mettlin CJ: Age-specific ovarian cancer incidence rate patterns in the United States. Gynecol Oncol 99(1):248–250, 2005.
91. Williams SD: Malignant ovarian germ cell tumors. In Gershenson DM, McGuire WP, Gore M, et al (eds): Gynecologic Cancer: Controversies in Management. Philadelphia: Churchill Livingstone, 2005, pp 499–502.
92. Berek JS, Hacker NF: Nonepithelial ovarian and fallopian tube cancers. In Berek JS, Hacker NF (eds): Practical Gynecologic Oncology, 4th ed. Philadelphia: Lippincott Williams & Wilkins, 2005, pp 511–542.
93. Pectasides D, Pectasides E, Kassanos D: Germ cell tumors of the ovary. Cancer Treat Rev 34(5):427–441, 2008.
94. Gershenson DM: Management of ovarian germ cell tumors. J Clin Oncol 25(20):2938–2943, 2007.
95. Crum CP: The female genital tract. In Kumar V, Abbas AK, Fausto N (eds): Robbins and Cotran Pathologic Basis of Disease, 7th ed. Philadelphia: Elsevier, 2005.
96. Imai A, Furui T, Tamaya T: Gynecologic tumors and symptoms in childhood and adolescence: 10-years' experience. Int J Gynaecol Obstet 45(3):227–234,1994.
97. Leiserowitz GS, Xing G, Cress R, et al: Adnexal masses in pregnancy: how often are they malignant? Gynecol Oncol 101(2):315–321, 2006.
98. Schwartz PE, Chambers SK, Chambers JT, et al: Ovarian germ cell malignancies: the Yale University experience. Gynecol Oncol 45(1):26–31,1992.
99. International Germ Cell Consensus Classification: A prognostic factor-based staging system for metastatic germ cell cancers: International Germ Cell Cancer Collaborative Group. J Clin Oncol 15(2):594–603, 1997.
100. Malagon HD, Valdez AM, Moran CA, et al: Germ cell tumors with sarcomatous components: a clinicopathologic and immunohistochemical study of 46 cases. Am J Surg Pathol 31(9):1356–1362, 2007.
101. Murugaesu N, Schmid P, Dancey G, et al: Malignant ovarian germ cell tumors: identification of novel prognostic markers and long-term outcome after multimodality treatment. J Clin Oncol 24(30):4862–4866, 2006.
102. Kumar S, Shah JP, Bryant CS, et al: The prevalence and prognostic impact of lymph node metastasis in malignant germ cell tumors of the ovary. Gynecol Oncol 110(2):125–132, 2008.
103. Lai CH, Chang TC, Hsueh S, et al: Outcome and prognostic factors in ovarian germ cell malignancies. Gynecol Oncol 96(3):784–791, 2005.
104. O'Connor DM, Norris HJ: The influence of grade on the outcome of stage I ovarian immature (malignant) teratomas and the reproducibility of grading. Int J Gynecol Pathol 13(4):283–289, 1994.
105. Marina N, London WB, Frazier AL, et al: Prognostic factors in children with extragonadal malignant germ cell tumors: a pediatric intergroup study. J Clin Oncol 24(16):2544–2548, 2006.
106. Peccatori F, Bonazzi C, Chiari S, et al: Surgical management of malignant ovarian germ-cell tumors: 10 years' experience of 129 patients. Obstet Gynecol 86(3):367–372, 1995.
107. Slayton RE, Park RC, Silverberg SG, et al: Vincristine, dactinomycin, and cyclophosphamide in the treatment of malignant germ cell tumors of the ovary. A gynecologic oncology group study (a final report). Cancer 56(2):243–248, 1985.
108. Williams S, Blessing JA, Liao SY, et al: Adjuvant therapy of ovarian germ cell tumors with cisplatin, etoposide, and bleomycin: a trial of the gynecologic oncology group. J Clin Oncol 12(4):701–706, 1994.
109. Williams SD, Blessing JA, Moore DH, et al: Cisplatin, vinblastine, and bleomycin in advanced and recurrent ovarian germ-cell tumors. A trial of the Gynecologic Oncology Group. Ann Intern Med 111(1):22–27, 1989.
110. Williams SD, Blessing JA, Hatch KD, et al: Chemotherapy of advanced dysgerminoma: trials of the Gynecologic Oncology Group. J Clin Oncol 9(11):1950–1955, 1991.
111. Loehrer PJ S, Johnson D, Elson P, et al: Importance of bleomycin in favorable-prognosis disseminated germ cell tumors: an Eastern Cooperative Oncology Group trial. J Clin Oncol 13(2):470–476, 1995.
112. Einhorn LH, Williams SD, Loehrer PJ, et al: Evaluation of optimal duration of chemotherapy in favorable-prognosis disseminated germ cell tumors: a southeastern cancer study group protocol. J Clin Oncol 7(3):387–391, 1989.
113. Williams SD, Blessing JA, DiSaia PJ: Second-look laparotomy in ovarian germ cell tumors: the gynecologic oncology group experience. Gynecol Oncol 52(3):287–291, 1994.
114. Bonazzi C, Peccatori F, Colombo N, et al: Pure ovarian immature teratoma, a unique and curable disease: 10 years' experience of 32 prospectively treated patients. Obstet Gynecol 84(4):598–604, 1994.
115. Marina NM, Cushing B, Giller R, et al: Complete surgical excision is effective treatment for children with immature teratomas with or without malignant elements: a pediatric oncology group/children's cancer group intergroup study. J Clin Oncol 17(7):2137–2143, 1999.
116. Dark GG, Bower M, Newlands ES, et al: Surveillance policy for stage I ovarian germ cell tumors. J Clin Oncol 15(2):620–624, 1997.
117. Patterson DM, Murugaesu N, Holden L, et al: A review of the close surveillance policy for stage I female germ cell tumors of the ovary and other sites. Int J Gynecol Cancer 18(1):43–50, 2008.
118. Bafna UD, Umadevi K, Kumaran C, et al: Germ cell tumors of the ovary: Is there a role for aggressive cytoreductive surgery for nondysgerminomatous tumors? Int J Gynecol Cancer 11(4):300–304, 2001.
119. Billmire D, Vinocur C, Rescorla F, et al: Outcome and staging evaluation in malignant germ cell tumors of the ovary in children and adolescents: an intergroup study. J Pediatr Surg 39(3):424–429; discussion 424–429, 2004.
120. Einhorn LH, Brames MJ, Juliar B, et al: Phase II study of paclitaxel plus gemcitabine salvage chemotherapy for germ cell tumors after progression following high-dose chemotherapy with tandem transplant. J Clin Oncol 25(5):513–516, 2007.
121. Brewer M, Gershenson DM, Herzog CE, et al: Outcome and reproductive function after chemotherapy for ovarian dysgerminoma. J Clin Oncol 17(9):2670–2675, 1999.
122. Low JJ, Perrin LC, Crandon AJ, et al: Conservative surgery to preserve ovarian function in patients with malignant ovarian

germ cell tumors. A review of 74 cases. Cancer 15:89(2):391–398, 2000.

123. Tangir J, Zelterman D, Ma W, et al: Reproductive function after conservative surgery and chemotherapy for malignant germ cell tumors of the ovary. Obstet Gynecol 101(2):251–7, 2003.

124. de La Motte Rouge T, Pautier P, Duvillard P, et al: Survival and reproductive function of 52 women treated with surgery and bleomycin, etoposide, cisplatin (BEP) chemotherapy for ovarian yolk sac tumor. Ann Oncol 19(8):1435–1441, 2008.

125. Kang H, Kim TJ, Kim WY, et al: Outcome and reproductive function after cumulative high-dose combination chemotherapy with bleomycin, etoposide and cisplatin (BEP) for patients with ovarian endodermal sinus tumor. Gynecol Oncol Jul 23, 2008.

126. Schneider DT, Hilgenfeld E, Schwabe D, et al: Acute myelogenous leukemia after treatment for malignant germ cell tumors in children. J Clin Oncol 17(10):3226–3233, 1999.

Conclusion

12

*Robert E. Bristow and
Deborah K. Armstrong*

Ovarian cancer remains the leading cause of gynecologic cancer–related morbidity and mortality in developed countries. This volume contains contributions from many of the leading authorities in the clinical management of ovarian cancer as well as those at the cutting edge of basic research and translational science. Although the epidemiology of ovarian cancer has been relatively well defined, continued advances are being made with respect to understanding the molecular and genetic basis for disease. These advances have led to (1) progress in identifying women who have an increased risk of developing ovarian cancer and to (2) the development of more effective disease prevention strategies. Radiographic imaging is an integral part of ovarian cancer detection, diagnosis, management, and post-treatment surveillance.

A number of imaging modalities are available, and a variety of new techniques, especially molecular imaging approaches, are being developed to facilitate detection of early-stage disease as well as to define the extent of metastatic tumor in women with a more advanced stage of disease. This information is critical to the effective planning of surgical and adjuvant therapy.

As described in this volume, the goal of primary surgery for advanced stage ovarian cancer is to accurately establish a diagnosis and leave little or no residual disease by using a variety of cytoreductive surgical techniques and approaches. Advances in the use of chemotherapy for ovarian cancer have contributed to recent improvements in the expected survival times for women with advanced-stage tumors. Both novel therapeutic agents as well as delivery mechanisms have been integrated into routine clinical practice.

Despite important gains in early detection and primary treatment, a significant proportion of women with ovarian cancer will ultimately experience disease recurrence. Recent evidence indicates that for a select group of patients, a repeat attempt at cytoreductive surgery may be indicated, with successful tumor removal being associated with a clinically meaningful prolongation of survival time. Selection of second-line adjuvant therapy should be evidence-based and done according to guidelines that consider the treatment-free interval, prior therapy received, and prior toxicity. The role of chemoresistance and chemosensitivity testing in the setting of recurrent disease remains to be further defined. A number of encouraging therapeutic agents, including angiogenesis inhibitors, are currently in clinical trials and may ultimately be shown to be effective against ovarian cancer in both the primary and recurrent disease settings.

In the coming years, improvements in the early detection and management of ovarian cancer will depend on incremental, but nevertheless forward-leaning, scientific discoveries as well as more effective and less toxic therapies. Equally important is the seamless integration of a multidisciplinary clinical care team, including the specialties of gynecologic and medical oncology, radiology, critical care, pharmacy, genetic counseling, nursing, social work, and psychiatry to deliver optimum therapy and ultimately make meaningful gains in both survival time and quality of life.

Index

Note: Page numbers followed by f indicate figures; those followed by t indicate tables; and those followed by b indicate boxed material.

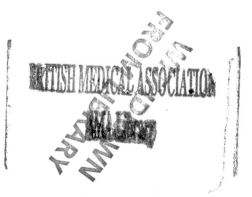